SPECIALTY IMAGING™

PITFALLS AND CLASSIC SIGNS OF THE ABDOMEN AND PELVIS

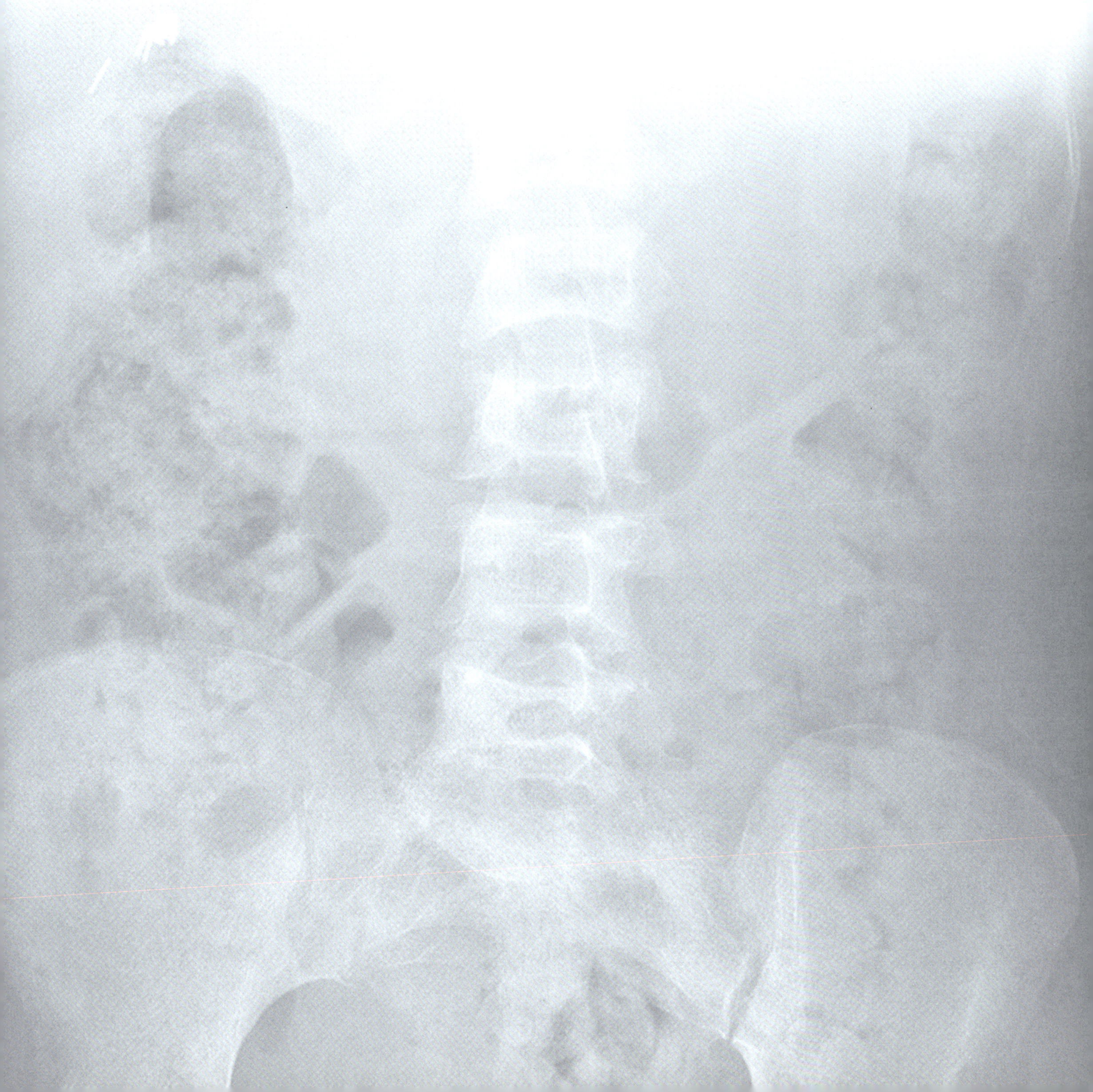

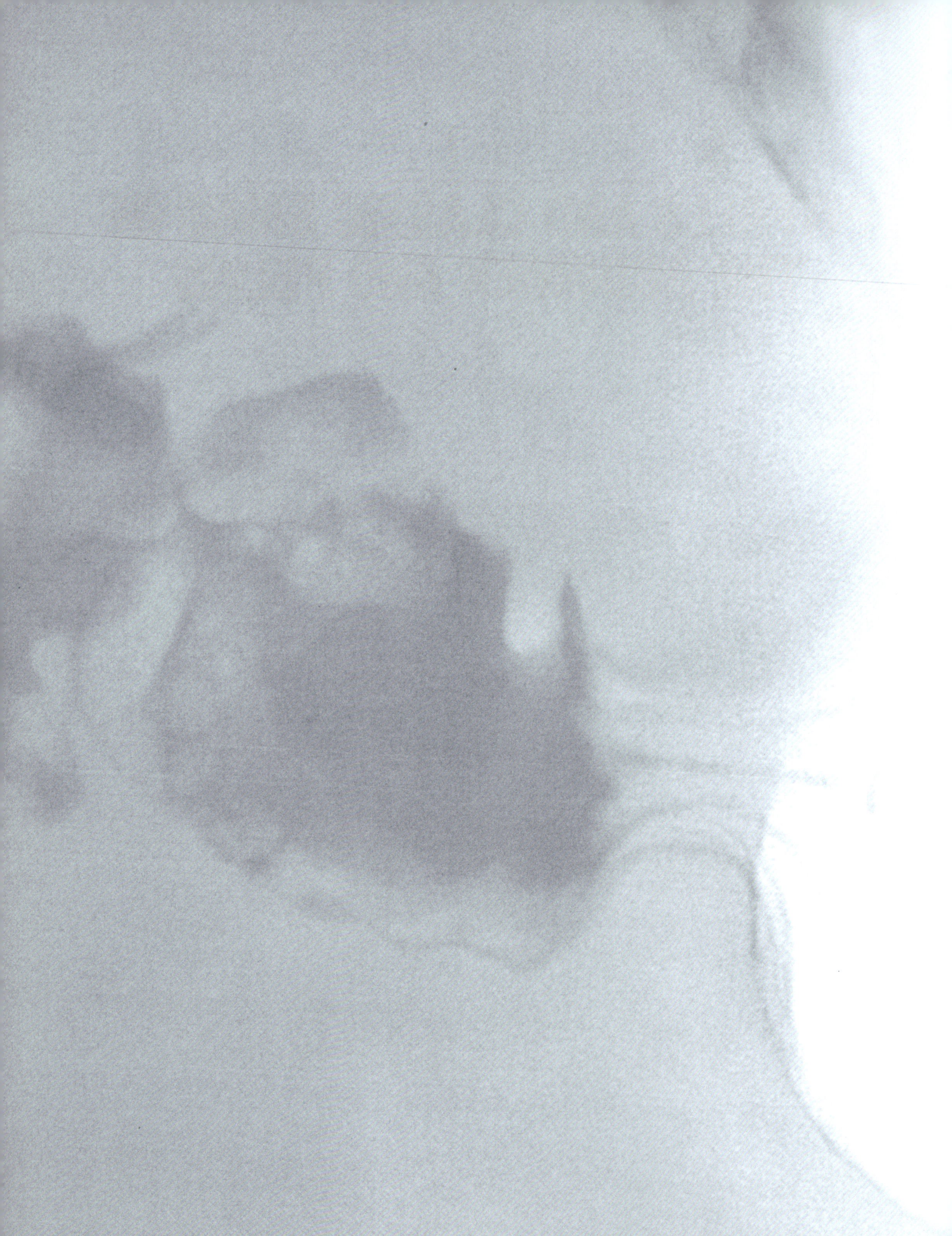

SPECIALTY IMAGING™

PITFALLS AND CLASSIC SIGNS OF THE ABDOMEN AND PELVIS

Khaled M. Elsayes, MD
Associate Professor
Department of Diagnostic Radiology
The University of Texas M.D. Anderson Cancer Center
Houston, Texas

Akram M. Shaaban, MBBCh
Associate Professor (Clinical)
Department of Radiology
University of Utah School of Medicine
Salt Lake City, Utah

Christine O. Menias, MD
Professor of Radiology
Mayo Clinic School of Medicine
Scottsdale, Arizona
Adjunct Professor of Radiology
Washington University School of Medicine
St. Louis, Missouri

ELSEVIER

1600 John F. Kennedy Blvd.
Ste 1800
Philadelphia, PA 19103-2899

SPECIALTY IMAGING: PITFALLS AND CLASSIC SIGNS OF THE ABDOMEN AND PELVIS ISBN: 978-1-937242-18-3

Notices

Knowledge and best practice in this field are constantly changing. As new research and experience broaden our understanding, changes in research methods, professional practices, or medical treatment may become necessary.

Practitioners and researchers must always rely on their own experience and knowledge in evaluating and using any information, methods, compounds, or experiments described herein. In using such information or methods they should be mindful of their own safety and the safety of others, including parties for whom they have a professional responsibility.

With respect to any drug or pharmaceutical products identified, readers are advised to check the most current information provided (i) on procedures featured or (ii) by the manufacturer of each product to be administered, to verify the recommended dose or formula, the method and duration of administration, and contraindications. It is the responsibility of practitioners, relying on their own experience and knowledge of their patients, to make diagnoses, to determine dosages and the best treatment for each individual patient, and to take all appropriate safety precautions.

To the fullest extent of the law, neither the Publisher nor the authors, contributors, or editors, assume any liability for any injury and/or damage to persons or property as a matter of products liability, negligence or otherwise, or from any use or operation of any methods, products, instructions, or ideas contained in the material herein.

Publisher Cataloging-in-Publication Data

Specialty imaging : pitfalls and classic signs of the abdomen and pelvis /
[edited by] Khaled M. Elsayes and Akram M. Shaaban.
pages ; cm
Pitfalls and classic signs of the abdomen and pelvis
Includes bibliographical references and index.
ISBN 978-1-937242-18-3 (hardback)
1. Abdomen--Imaging--Atlases. 2. Pelvis--Imaging--Atlases.
I. Elsayes, Khaled M. II. Shaaban, Akram M. IV. Title: Pitfalls and
classic signs of the abdomen and pelvis.
[DNLM: 1. Radiography, Abdominal--Atlases. 2. Abdomen--abnormalities--Atlases.
3. Pelvis--abnormalities--Atlases. WI 17]
RC944 .S64 2014
617.550754--dc23

International Standard Book Number: 978-1-937242-18-3

Cover Designer: Tom M. Olson, BA
Cover Art: Lane R. Bennion, MS

Printed in Canada by Friesens, Altona, Manitoba, Canada

Last digit is the print number: 9 8 7 6 5 4 3 2 1

First and foremost, I would like to dedicate this time to the Almighty God, who has guided me to gain this knowledge.

To the memory of my parents.

To my wife and children.

I also take this opportunity to extend my appreciation to those individuals who have been instrumental in my career in radiology and those who have inspired me to complete this project.

To my mentors, friends and all colleagues in:

-MD Anderson Cancer Center, especially, Chusilp Charnsangavej, Marshall Hicks, Joel Vikas Kundra, Randy Ernst, and Aliya Qayyum

-University of Michigan, especially, Isaac Francis, Joel Platt, James Ellis, Rich Cohan, and Hero Hussain

- Egypt, especially, Hazem Moharram, Mamdouh Mahfouz, Tarek Eldiasty, Ikram Hamed, Ahmed Samy, Mohamed Moustafa, Moustafa Ismail, Omar Moawyah, Ihab Fathy, and Amr Nasef

- Mallinckrodt Institute of Radiology, especially, Jeffrey J. Brown, Vamsidhar R. Narra, Jay Heiken, and Christine Menias

- Elsewhere, especially, John Leyendecker (Wake Forest), Rich Baron (Chicago), Haitham Elsamalouty (Toledo), and Akram Shaaban (Utah)

To all contributors of this book.

To all of my medical students and residents.

KME

To my parents, who taught me the value of perseverance & hard work.
To my wife Inji, my son Karim, and my daughters May and Jena, the jewels of my life, thanks for your understanding & tremendous support.
To all my residents and fellows, whose challenging questions made me a better radiologist.

AMS

I'd like to dedicate this book to all my former residents, fellows, colleagues, and teachers, who continue to donate to the "Cooky Jar," and continue to teach me. It has truly been a privilege. This work could not have been completed without them.

COM

CONTRIBUTORS

Miral P. Gupta, MD
Diagnostic Radiology Resident
University of Texas-Houston
Houston, Texas

Eslam Y. Wassal, MD, MSc
Research Intern
Department of Diagnostic Radiology
The University of Texas M.D. Anderson Cancer Center
Houston, Texas

Hubert H. Chuang, MD, PhD
Assistant Professor
Department of Nuclear Medicine
Division of Diagnostic Imaging
The University of Texas M.D. Anderson Cancer Center
Houston, Texas

Gregory C. Ravizzini, MD
Assistant Professor
Department of Nuclear Medicine
Division of Diagnostic Imaging
The University of Texas M.D. Anderson Cancer Center
Houston, Texas

Yehia M. ElGuindy, MD
Resident
Department of Radiology
University of Toledo
Toledo, Ohio

Rafael Andrés Vicéns, MD
Abdominal Radiologist
Department of Radiology
Auxilio Mutuo Hospital
San Juan, Puerto Rico

Kamran Ali, MD
Associate Professor of Radiology
Department of Radiology
University of Kansas School of Medicine-Wichita
Wichita, Kansas

Eniola F. Mudasiru-Dawodu, MD
Radiologist
West Houston Radiology Associates
Houston, Texas

Tina E. Sprouse, MD
Women's Imaging Fellow
Georgetown University Hospital
Department of Radiology
Washington, District of Columbia

Ketan Yogesh Shah, MD
PGY3 Radiology Resident
Baylor College of Medicine
Houston, Texas

Richard L. Baron, MD
Professor of Radiology
Department of Radiology
University of Chicago Pritzker School of Medicine
Chicago, Illinois

Ahmad A. Khan, MD
Fellow, Abdominal Imaging
Department of Radiology
The University of Texas M.D. Anderson Cancer Center
Houston, Texas

Ehab H. Youssef, MD, FRCR
Clinical Lecturer of Radiology
Department of Radiology
University of Michigan
Ann Arbor, Michigan

Nicolaus A. Wagner-Bartak, MD
Assistant Professor of Diagnostic Radiology
Section of Abdominal Imaging
Department of Diagnostic Radiology
The University of Texas M.D. Anderson Cancer Center
Houston, Texas

Veral D. Amin, MD
Diagnostic Radiology, PGY3 Resident
Department of Radiology
Baylor College of Medicine
Houston, Texas

Mohammed S. Al-Natour, MD
PGY5 Radiology Resident
Department of Radiology
University of Toledo Medical Center
Toledo, Ohio

Ravinder S. Legha, MD/MS
Assistant Professor of Radiology
Department of Diagnostic Imaging
The University of Texas M.D. Anderson Cancer Center
Houston, Texas

Corey T. Jensen, MD
Assistant Professor of Radiology
Department of Radiology
The University of Texas M.D. Anderson Cancer Center
Houston, Texas

Kareem F. Ahmed, MD
Research Assistant II
Department of Diagnostic Radiology
The University of Texas M.D. Anderson Cancer Center
Houston, Texas

Amit Pandya, MD, RDMS, RVT, RDCS
Assistant Professor of Radiology
Department of Radiology
University of Michigan
Ann Arbor, Michigan

Mohammad K. Eldomery, MD
Postdoctoral Research Fellow of Genetics
Department of Molecular & Human Genetics
Baylor College of Medicine
Houston, Texas

Ahmed Abdelbaki, MD
Surgery Resident
Guthrie Clinic/Robert Packer Hospital
Sayre, Pennsylvania

Ajaykumar C. Morani, MBBS, DNB, MD
Assistant Professor of Radiology
Department of Diagnostic Radiology
The University of Texas M.D. Anderson Cancer Center
Houston, Texas

Priya Bhosale, MD
Associate Professor of Radiology
Department of Abdominal Imaging
The University of Texas M.D. Anderson Cancer Center
Houston, Texas

Ania Z. Kielar, MD, FRCPC
Department of Radiology
Associate Professor, University of Ottawa
Ottawa, Ontario, Canada
Adjunct Professor, University of Toronto
Toronto, Ontario, Canada

Ahmed M. Zaki, MD
Research Assistant in Abdominal Imaging
Department of Diagnostic Radiology
The University of Texas M.D. Anderson Cancer Center
Houston, Texas

Stephen R. Lee, MD
Clinical Fellow in Radiology
Abdominal Imaging and Intervention, Department of Radiology
Massachusetts General Hospital
Boston, Massachusetts

Abdelhameed M. Nienaa
Medical Student
Alexandria University Faculty of Medicine
Alexandria, Egypt

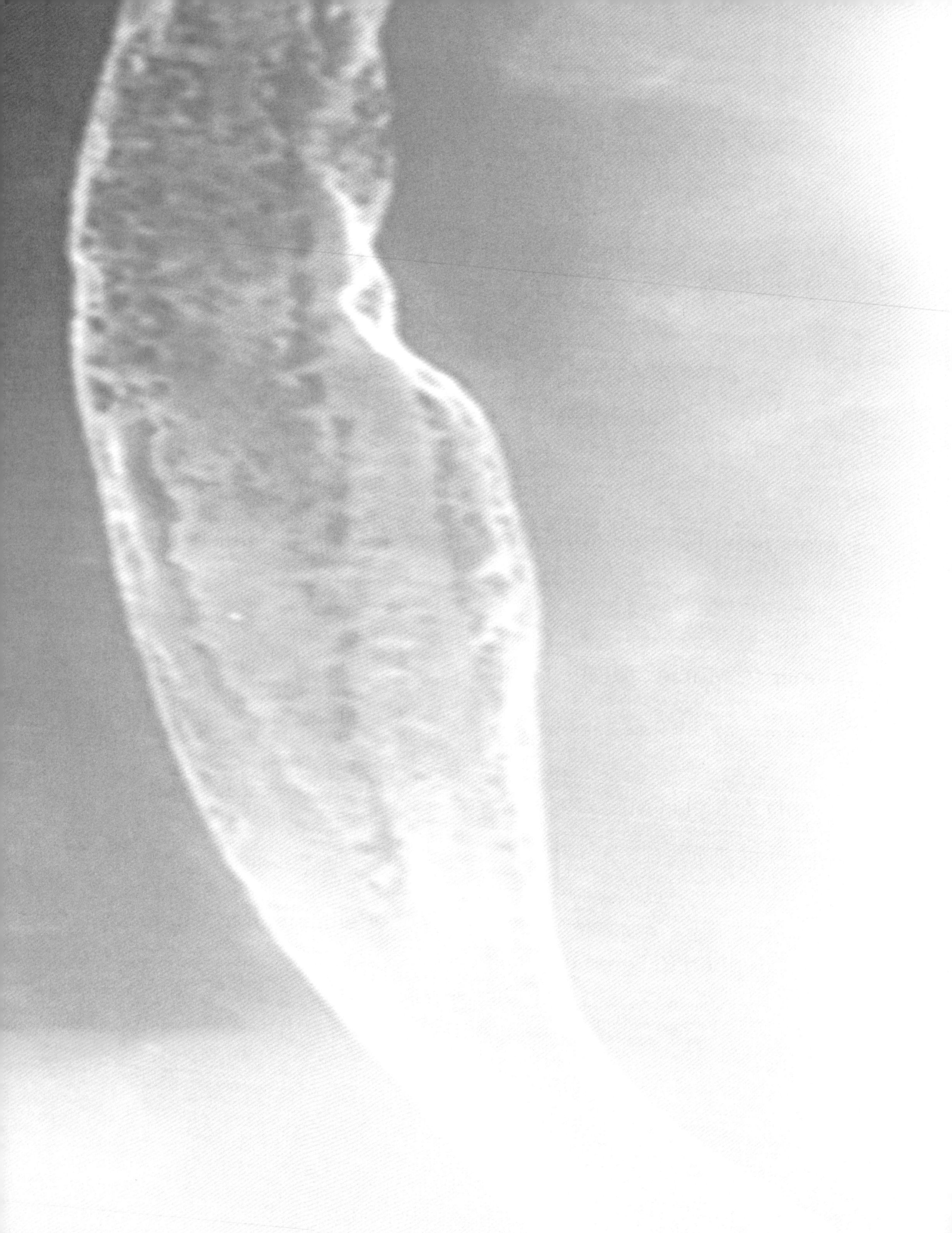

PREFACE

Diagnostic imaging has become widely available and plays an increasing role in clinical diagnosis and therapy. In most practices, there is a wide range of commonly misinterpreted cases in the abdomen and pelvis, mainly because many radiologists are not completely familiar with anatomical, morphological, physiological, hemodynamic, and biological principles as well as a lack of clinical and radiological knowledge. This leads to frequent misinterpretations, which further results in wrong management and potentially negative outcomes.

Addressing these problems starts with understanding the spectrum of basic concepts and principles in a case-based approach. In *Specialty Imaging: Pitfalls and Classic Signs of the Abdomen and Pelvis,* each chapter contains several cases that could be misinterpreted, followed by a thorough discussion of the reason for these misinterpretations, the basic principles, and a systematic approach to help avoid such misinterpretation.

This text provides practicing radiologists and radiology residents with the level of knowledge necessary to avoid misinterpretation and help make precise diagnosis in the presence of certain classic pathognomonic features.

Unlike other texts on the subject, this book treats diagnosis from a practical point of view. The cases walk you through a radiology expert's analysis of imaging pitfalls and classic signs of the abdomen and pelvis. These cases are presented progressively, with the expert's thought process described in detail. The cases highlight clinical presentation, relevant pathology, anatomy, and physiology as well as pertinent imaging features of common disease processes.

As with all Amirsys references, all of the information is distilled into succinct, bulleted text with thousands of images and illustrations. Coupled with a companion eBook, this volume is an irreplaceable textbook for anyone confronted with the challenges of imaging in the abdominal and pelvic areas.

We hope that *Specialty Imaging: Pitfalls and Classic Signs of the Abdomen and Pelvis* will find a handy spot on your library shelf and in your reading room (after the radiology residents have read it in its entirety).

Khaled M. Elsayes, MD
Associate Professor
Department of Diagnostic Radiology
The University of Texas M.D. Anderson Cancer Center
Houston, Texas

Akram M. Shaaban, MBBCh
Associate Professor (Clinical)
Department of Radiology
University of Utah School of Medicine
Salt Lake City, Utah

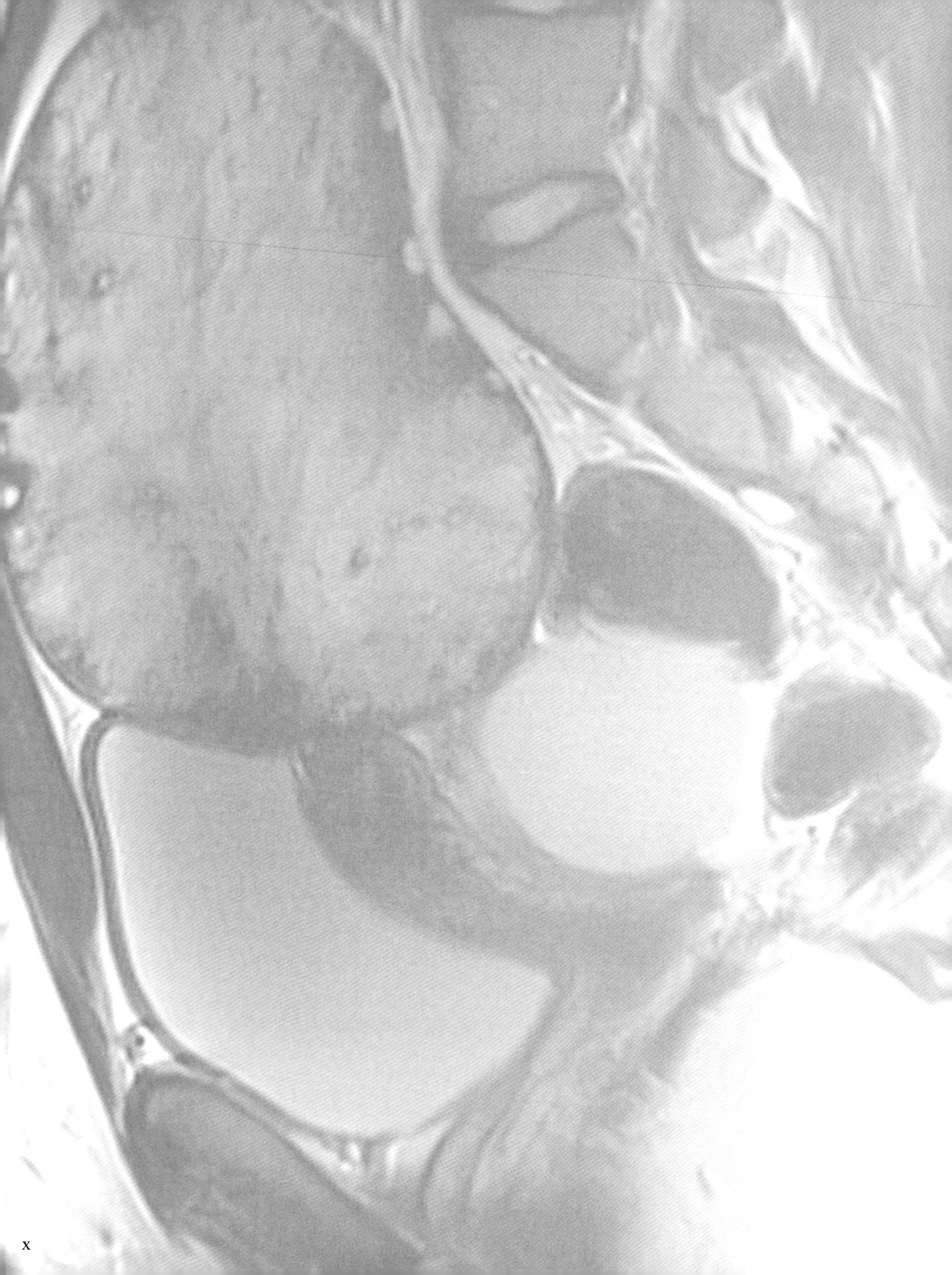

ACKNOWLEDGMENTS

Text Editors

Dave L. Chance, MA, ELS
Arthur G. Gelsinger, MA
Sarah J. Connor, BA
Tricia L. Cannon, BA

Image Editors

Jeffrey J. Marmorstone, BS
Lisa A. M. Steadman, BS

Medical Editors

Behrang Amini, MD, PhD

Illustrations

Laura C. Pliego, MA
Lane R. Bennion, MS
Richard Coombs, MS

Art Direction and Design

Laura C. Pliego, MA
Tom M. Olson, BA

Lead Editor

Angela M. Green Terry, BA

Publishing Leads

Katherine L. Riser, MA
Rebecca L. Hutchinson, BA

AMIRSYS®
Names you know. Content you trust.®

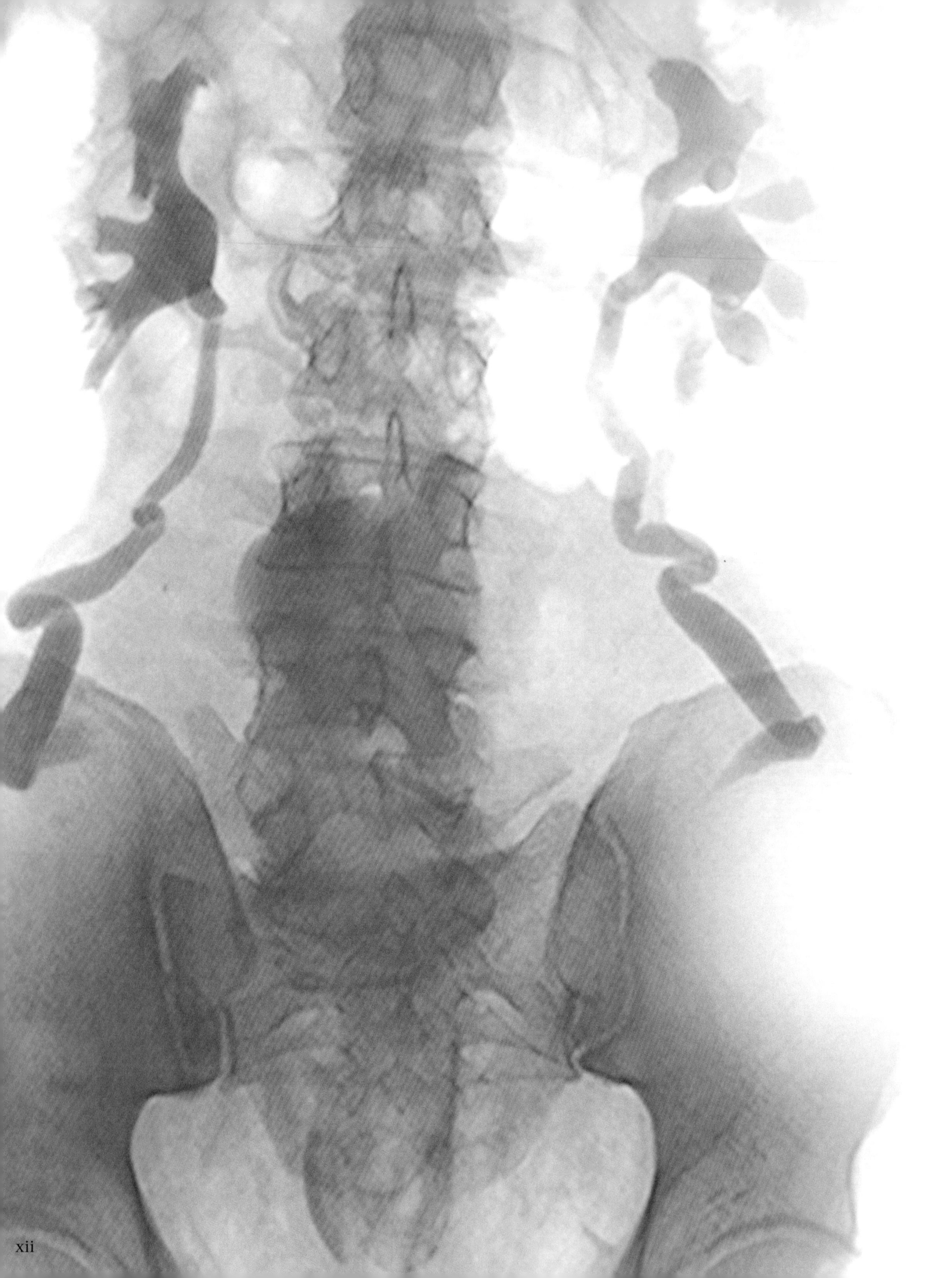

SECTIONS

TABLE OF CONTENTS

SECTION 1
Liver

Technique-Related Pitfalls

Benign Conditions Simulating Malignancy

Malignant Lesions Mimicking Benign Conditions

Treatment-Related Conditions Simulating Diseases

Fat-Related Pitfalls

Vascular-Related Pitfalls

SECTION 4
Spleen

Technique-Related Pitfalls

Benign Conditions Simulating Malignancy

Treatment-Related Conditions Simulating Diseases

Classic Signs and Appearances

SECTION 5
Abdominal Wall, Peritoneum, Retroperitoneum, and Diaphragm

Benign Conditions Simulating Malignancy

Treatment-Related Conditions Simulating Diseases

Classic Signs and Appearances

SECTION 6
Gastrointestinal Tract

Benign Conditions Simulating Malignancy

Malignant Lesions Mimicking Benign Conditions

Classic Signs and Appearances

SECTION 7
Adrenal Gland

Benign Conditions Simulating Malignancy

Pitfalls in Adenoma Evaluation

Malignant Lesions Mimicking Benign Conditions

Classic Signs and Appearances

SECTION 10
Scrotum

Benign Lesions Simulating Malignancy

Malignant Lesions Mimicking Benign Conditions

SECTION 11
Female Pelvis

Technique-Related Pitfalls

Benign Conditions Simulating Malignancy

SECTION 1
Liver

Technique-Related Pitfalls

Benign Conditions Simulating Malignancy

Malignant Lesions Mimicking Benign Conditions

Treatment-Related Conditions Simulating Diseases

Fat-Related Pitfalls

Vascular-Related Pitfalls

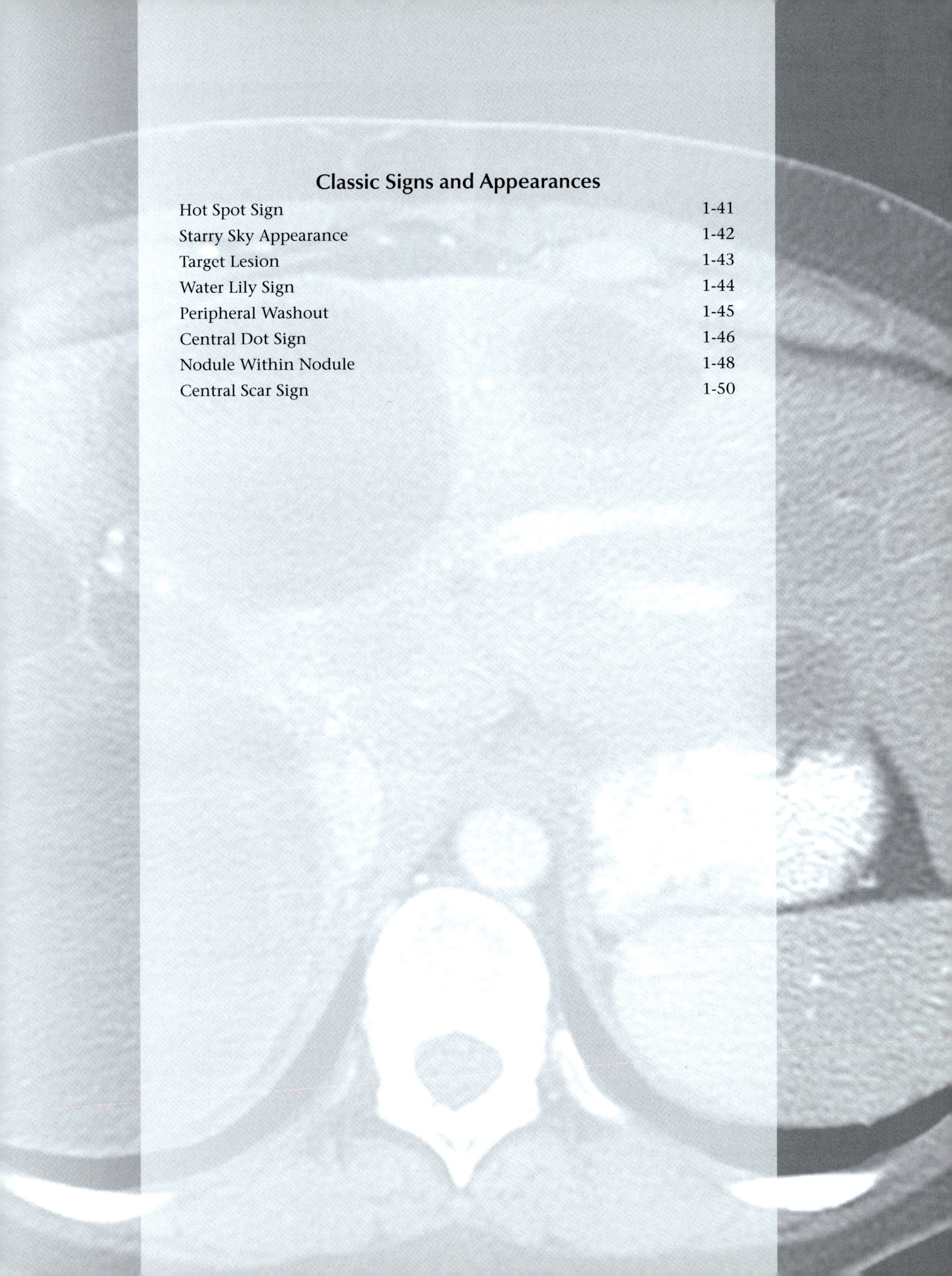

Classic Signs and Appearances

ULTRASOUND MIRROR IMAGE ARTIFACT

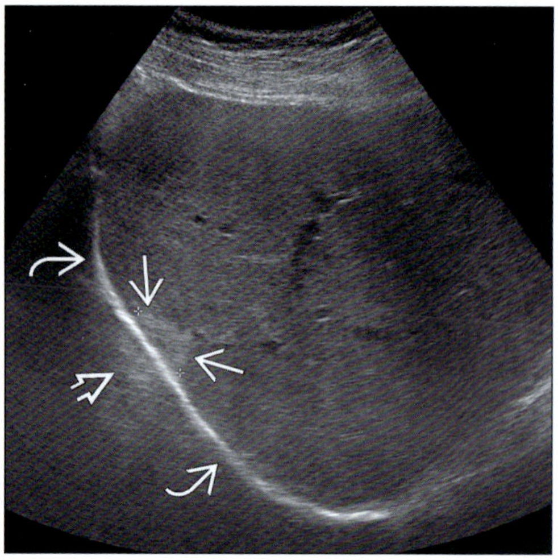

Longitudinal US shows a hepatic right lobe echogenic lesion → and a duplicated echogenic structure → projecting on the other side of the diaphragm → at the expected location of lung parenchyma.

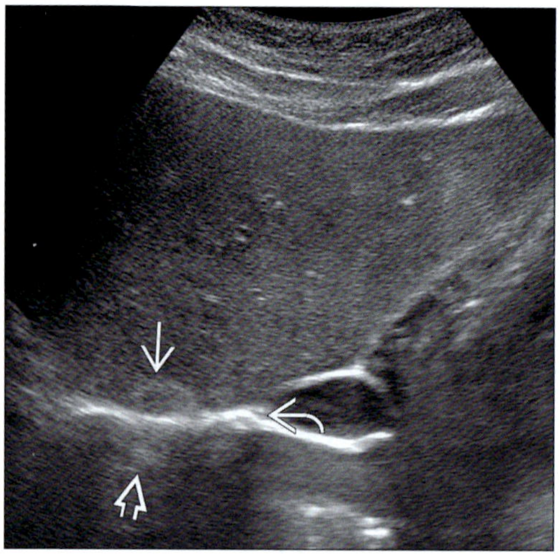

Transverse US shows a hepatic right lobe echogenic lesion → and a duplicated echogenic structure → projecting on the other side of the diaphragm →.

CLINICAL SCENARIO

History

- 45-year-old man with history of colon cancer and known right lobe hepatic hemangioma

IMAGE INTERPRETATION

Pitfalls

- Echogenic subcapsular mass that involves liver and appears to straddle diaphragm to involve the lung base

Actual Diagnosis

- Right lobe hepatic hemangioma
- Apparent involvement of diaphragm and lung is due to known ultrasound mirror image artifact

Clues to Correct Diagnosis

- Mirror image is more hypoechoic and somewhat more blurred and distorted than image of original structure
  - Due to absorption of ultrasound beam when passing through a long pathway
- Changing patient position and transducer angle may result in disappearance of artifact

BACKGROUND

Relevant Physics

- Mirror image artifact results from object located on one side of highly reflective interface distant from transducer head, appearing on other side of reflective surface
  - Both virtual and artificial images have equal distance to reflector from opposite directions
- Occurs when strong reflector causes structures that lie in front of reflector to appear as if they lie behind it, just as something viewed in mirror appears to lie behind it
- Generated by false assumption that echo returns to ultrasound transducer after single reflection
  - Primary beam encounters highly reflective interface (pleural-air interface in this case)
  - Reflected echoes then encounter back side of hepatic hemangioma and are reflected back toward reflective interface before being reflected to transducer for detection
  - Display shows duplicated structure equidistant from but deep to strongly reflective interface
- Reflecting surface should be large and relatively smooth so as to reflect sound as a mirror reflects light
- Same phenomenon is rarely observed at both transabdominal and transvaginal obstetric ultrasound
  - May result in erroneous diagnosis of heterotopic pregnancy (intrauterine and ectopic pregnancy)

IMAGING FEATURES

US

- Structure (mass) within liver has duplicate image on other side of diaphragm

CT and MR

- Ultrasound-related artifact
- No corresponding lesions should be identified on CT or MR

RELATED REFERENCES

1. Miglietta F et al: Mirror-image artifact of early pregnancy on transvaginal sonography. J Ultrasound Med. 31(11):1858-9, 2012
2. Feldman MK et al: US artifacts. Radiographics. 29(4):1179-89, 2009
3. Lim BH et al: The mirror image artifact of early pregnancy. Ultrasound Obstet Gynecol. 21(5):518-20, 2003

DISAPPEARING LIVER LESION ON T2WI

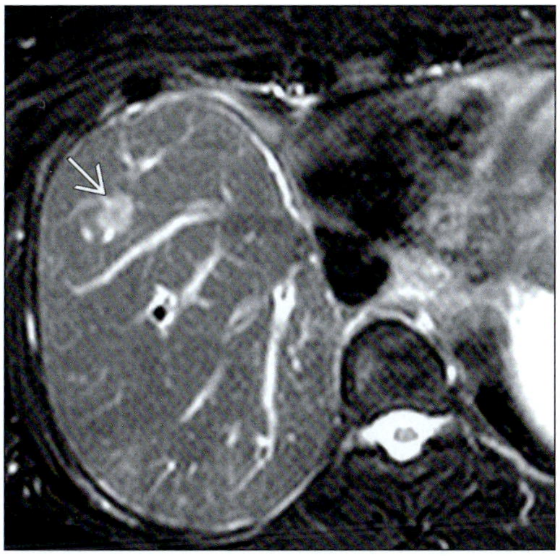

Axial T2WI MR obtained by fast spin-echo (FSE), which is a routine T2WI, demonstrates a focal lesion ➔ exhibiting mildly increased signal intensity within the right hepatic lobe.

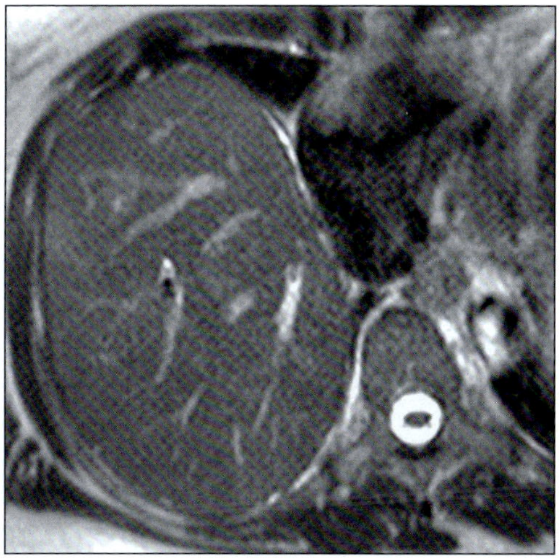

Axial T2WI MR obtained by single-shot fast spin-echo (SSFSE), which is a heavily T2WI, demonstrates no definite evidence of abnormal signal intensity to correlate with right hepatic lobe focal lesion.

CLINICAL SCENARIO

History

- Patient with history of hepatitis B

IMAGE INTERPRETATION

Pitfalls

- Heavily T2WI (e.g., single-shot fast spin-echo [SSFSE]) may not demonstrate malignant solid lesions seen on routine T2WI

Actual Diagnosis

- Small focus of hepatocellular carcinoma (HCC)

Clues to Correct Diagnosis

- Mass is seen on routine T2WI (fast spin-echo [FSE]) as mildly increased signal intensity compared to surrounding liver parenchyma
- Malignant lesions often become isointense to liver parenchyma on heavily T2WI as opposed to benign lesions such as hemangiomas and cysts

IMAGING FEATURES

MR

- Routine and heavily T2WI can be used to differentiate between benign and malignant liver lesions
- On routine T2WI (TE 90 ms)
  - Benign lesions (such as cysts and hemangiomas) demonstrate markedly increased signal intensity
  - Malignant lesions (such as HCC in cirrhotic livers & metastases in presence of primary malignancy) demonstrate mildly increased signal intensity
- On heavily T2WI (TE > 160 ms)
  - Benign lesions demonstrate further increase in signal intensity
  - Malignant lesions demonstrate less signal intensity and can appear isointense to surrounding liver and can be missed

Explanation

- Malignant solid lesions have relaxation times (81 ms) close to spleen (53 ms), which explain mildly increased signal intensity of HCC & metastases on routine T2WI
- Benign lesions such as cysts & hemangiomas appear markedly hyperintense on T2WI (higher than spleen), as they have relaxation times around 165 ms for hemangioma & 550 ms for cysts
- Markedly increased signal intensity of benign lesions persists on heavily T2WI and suppresses for solid malignant lesions

Key Teaching Point

- Malignant solid lesions (including HCC, which typically demonstrates mildly increased signal intensity on routine T2WI) can be missed on heavily T2WI
- In screening patients with chronic liver disease for HCC, changes in T2 signal intensity can be important clue to suspect HCC development
  - Radiologist must not use the heavily T2WI as the only T2 sequence (often obtained because it is fast), as it will fail to detect these early signal changes seen with early HCC development

RELATED REFERENCES

1. Siegelman ES et al: MR characterization of focal liver lesions: pearls and pitfalls. Magn Reson Imaging Clin N Am. 22(3):295-313, 2014
2. Cieszanowski A et al: Discrimination of benign from malignant hepatic lesions based on their T2-relaxation times calculated from moderately T2-weighted turbo SE sequence. Eur Radiol. 12(9):2273-9, 2002
3. Ito K et al: Hepatic lesions: discrimination of nonsolid, benign lesions from solid, malignant lesions with heavily T2-weighted fast spin-echo MR imaging. Radiology. 204(3):729-37, 1997
4. Semelka RC et al: Malignant lesions of the liver identified on T1- but not T2-weighted MR images at 1.5 T. J Magn Reson Imaging. 4(3):315-8, 1994

INFLAMMATORY PSEUDOTUMOR

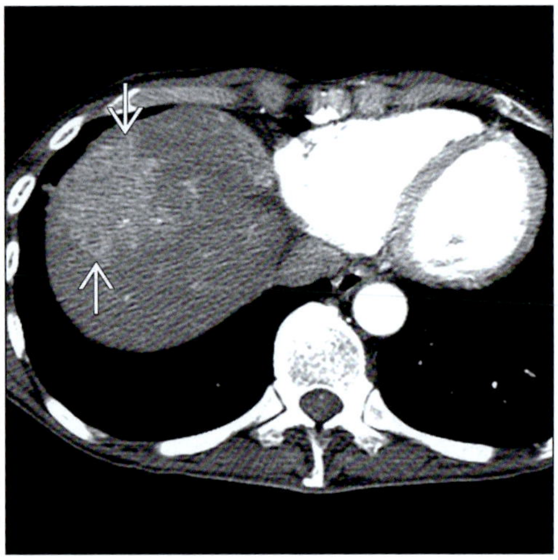

Axial CECT demonstrates an irregular enhancing mass within the right hepatic lobe ➔.

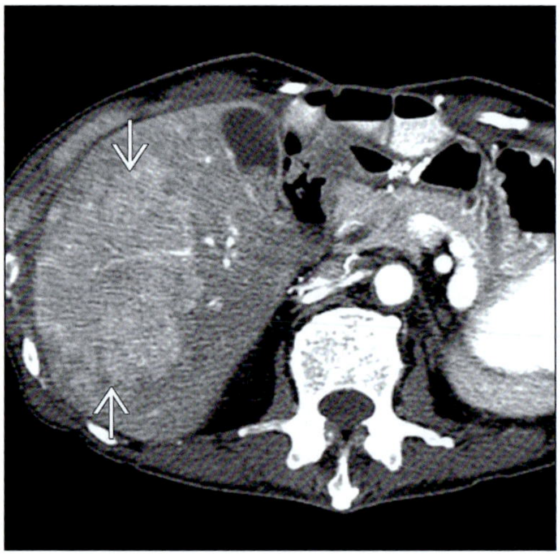

Axial CECT at a lower level demonstrates the large heterogeneously enhancing mass ➔ extending to occupy a large portion of the right hepatic lobe.

CLINICAL SCENARIO

History

- 48-year-old man with abdominal pain and weight loss
- Past history of splenectomy due to Epstein-Barr virus (EBV)

Relevant Laboratory Tests

- ↑ AST, alkaline phosphatase, bilirubin, and ↑ total leukocyte count

IMAGE INTERPRETATION

Pitfalls

- IPT may be misdiagnosed as 1 of following liver lesions, as they share similar enhancement patterns on CT and MR
  - Metastasis
  - Atypical HCC (especially if risk factors like viral hepatitis or cirrhosis)
  - Intrahepatic cholangiocarcinoma
  - Liver abscess with partial liquefaction or granulation

Actual Diagnosis

- Inflammatory pseudotumor of liver

Clues to Correct Diagnosis

- IPT should be considered in patients with solid liver lesions and 1 or more of the following
  - Systemic illness (fever, pain, fatigue, weight loss)
  - Inflammatory blood picture
  - Normal hepatic tumor markers (AFP, CA19)
  - History of IPT

BACKGROUND

Epidemiology

- Rare, most frequently seen in Asia
- M > F, usually in young adults
- IPT can occur in various organs including lung (most commonly affected), liver, spleen, mediastinum, and mesentery

Relevant Pathology

- Exact cause is unknown (various causes include infection [e.g., EBV], vascular, or autoimmune)
- Microscopic: Spindle-shaped cells, myofibroblasts, mixed inflammatory cells (plasma cells, lymphocytes, neutrophils, eosinophils) in addition to fibrous stroma

IMAGING FEATURES

General

- Commonly single lesion (81%), rarely multiple (19%)

US

- Hypoechoic or hyperechoic mass

CT

- NECT: Single or multiple hypoattenuating lesions
- CECT: Usually heterogeneous, peripheral enhancement with central low attenuation & occasional delayed enhancement

MR

- T1WI: Hypointense
- T2WI: Hyperintense
- T1WI C+: Usually peripheral enhancement in arterial phase with occasional delayed enhancement

PET/CT

- May show abnormal metabolic activity with high standardized uptake value

RELATED REFERENCES

1. Kong WT et al: The analysis of enhancement pattern of hepatic inflammatory pseudotumor on contrast-enhanced ultrasound. Abdom Imaging. 39(1):168-74, 2014
2. Park JY et al: Clinical features, image findings, and prognosis of inflammatory pseudotumor of the liver: a multicenter experience of 45 cases. Gut Liver. 8(1):58-63, 2014

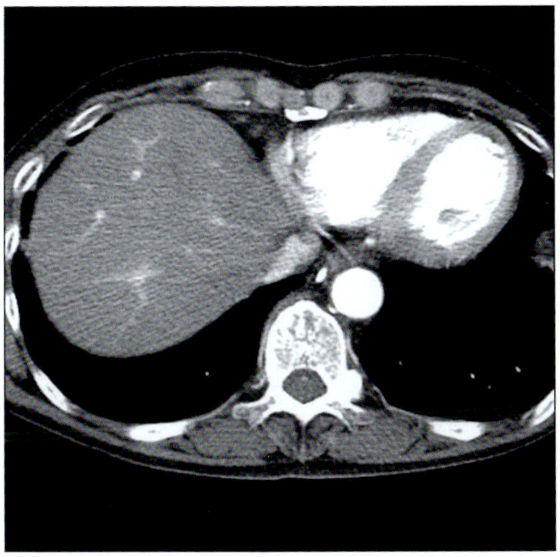

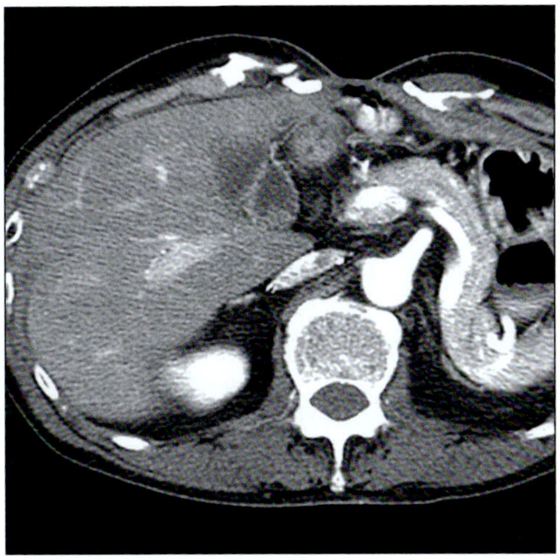

(Left) *Axial CECT at the mass level demonstrates significant resolution of the enhancing mass after intake of of anti-inflammatory medication.* ***(Right)*** *Axial CECT at a lower level in the same patient demonstrates almost near complete clearance of the enhancing mass.*

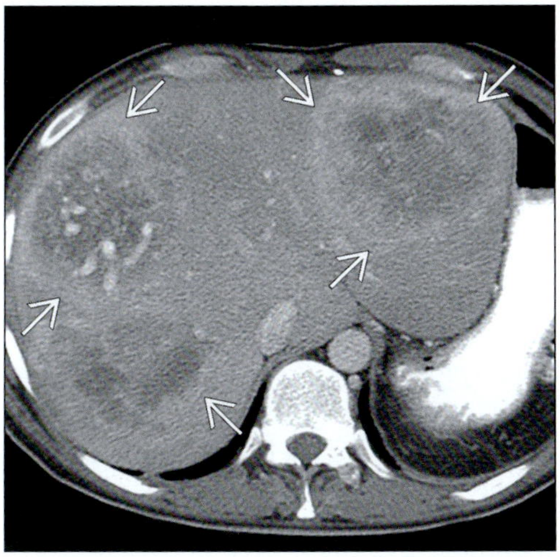

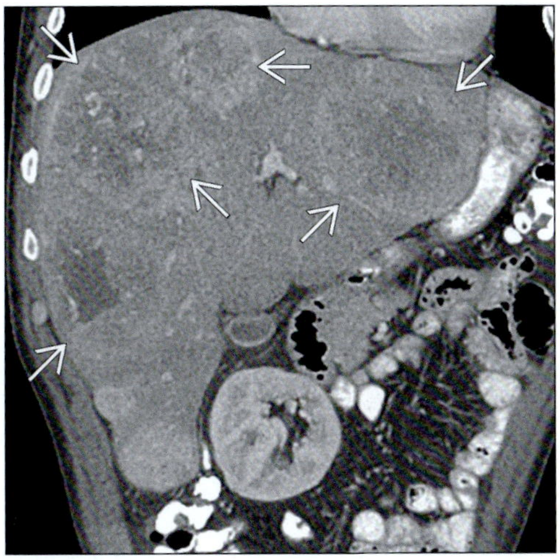

(Left) *Axial CECT In a 48-year-old man with a history of EBV demonstrates multiple bilobar masses ➔ exhibiting peripheral enhancement.* ***(Right)*** *Coronal CECT in early venous phase shows multiple peripherally enhancing masses scattered within both hepatic lobes ➔.*

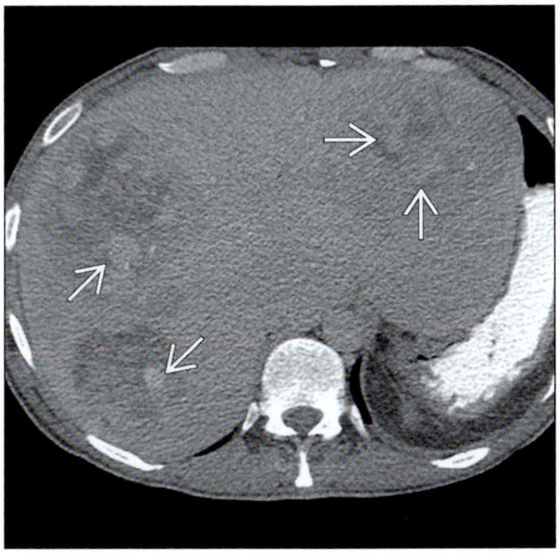

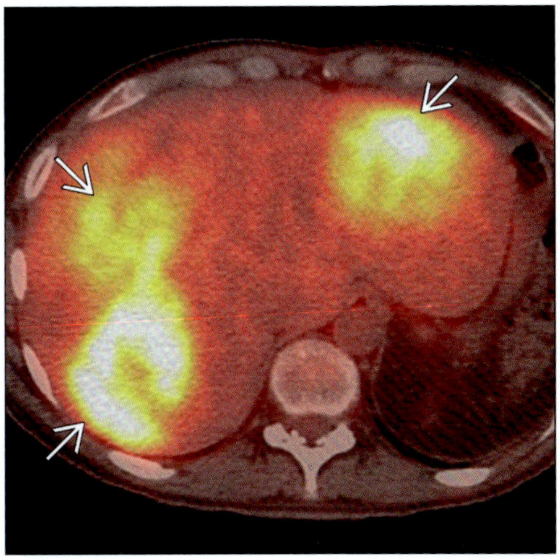

(Left) *Axial CECT in delayed phase shows progressive central enhancement of the masses ➔.* ***(Right)*** *Axial FDG PET scan demonstrates increased FDG uptake of the masses ➔.*

GIANT REGENERATIVE CIRRHOTIC NODULE

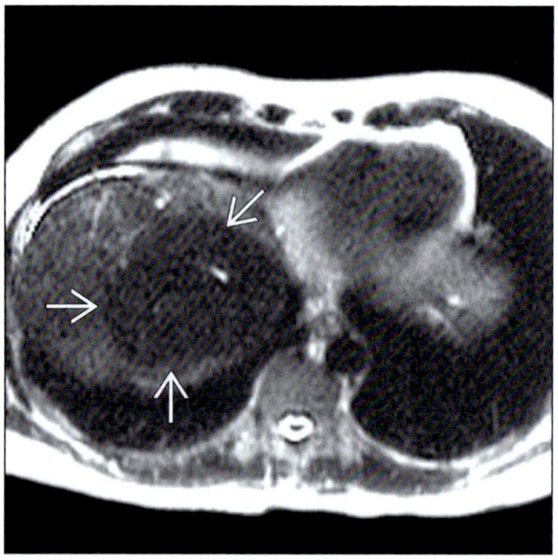

Axial T2WI MR demonstrates a well-circumscribed large ovoid mass ➔ exhibiting relatively low signal intensity compared to the surrounding liver parenchyma.

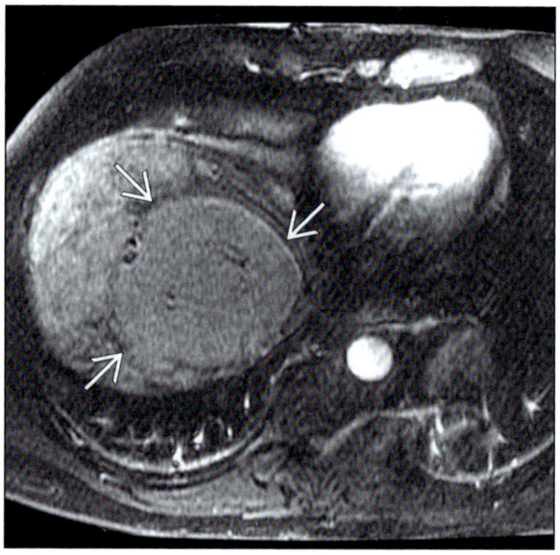

Axial T1WI C+ MR demonstrates isointensity of the mass ➔ compared to the surrounding liver parenchyma, indicating a similar degree of enhancement.

CLINICAL SCENARIO

History

- 64-year-old man with history of primary sclerosing cholangitis and cirrhosis

IMAGE INTERPRETATION

Pitfalls

- Can be misinterpreted as hepatocellular carcinoma (HCC) especially with its large size in the background of cirrhotic liver

Actual Diagnosis

- Giant regenerative cirrhotic nodule

Clues to Correct Diagnosis

- Hypointense signal intensity on T2WI, whereas HCC demonstrates high signal intensity on T2WI
- No arterial enhancement or delayed enhancement washout as opposed to HCC

BACKGROUND

General

- Liver cirrhosis is characterized by irreversible remodeling of hepatic architecture with bridging fibrosis and spectrum of hepatocellular nodules
- Cirrhosis-associated hepatocellular nodules result from localized proliferation of hepatocytes and supporting stroma in response to liver injury
- Regenerative cirrhotic nodules are usually surrounded by fibrous septa
- Regenerative nodules may be monoacinar or multiacinar, depending on whether they contain 1 or more terminal portal tracts
- Regenerative nodules also may be classified according to size as either micronodules (< 3 mm) or macronodules (≥ 3 mm)
  - Though rare, giant regenerative nodules with diameter of 5 cm have been reported
- Hepatic nodules usually develop in previously damaged livers; damage to liver can be caused by several factors
- HCC is believed to develop from cirrhotic liver nodules in a stepwise fashion
  - Regenerative nodule → low-grade dysplastic nodule → high-grade dysplastic nodule → small HCC → large HCC

Pathology

- Regenerative nodules have intact reticulin framework
  - Normal vascular profile
  - Preserved hepatocellular and phagocytic functions
  - Hepatocytes in regenerative nodules resemble those in adjacent liver parenchyma, although subtle nuclear pleomorphism may be observed

IMAGING FEATURES

CT

- Regeneration nodules are usually isoattenuating to surrounding liver parenchyma with no significant post-contrast enhancement
  - Can be hyperattenuating when containing iron (siderotic)

MR

- T1WI: Usually isointense or hypointense (when siderotic) compared to adjacent liver parenchyma
- T2WI: Iso- or hypointense to liver
- T1WI C+: No abnormal enhancement (enhances similar to surrounding liver parenchyma)

RELATED REFERENCES

1. Hanna RF et al: Cirrhosis-associated hepatocellular nodules: correlation of histopathologic and MR imaging features. Radiographics. 28(3):747-69, 2008
2. Hussain SM et al: MR imaging of hepatocellular carcinoma. Magn Reson Imaging Clin N Am. 10(1):31-52, v, 2002

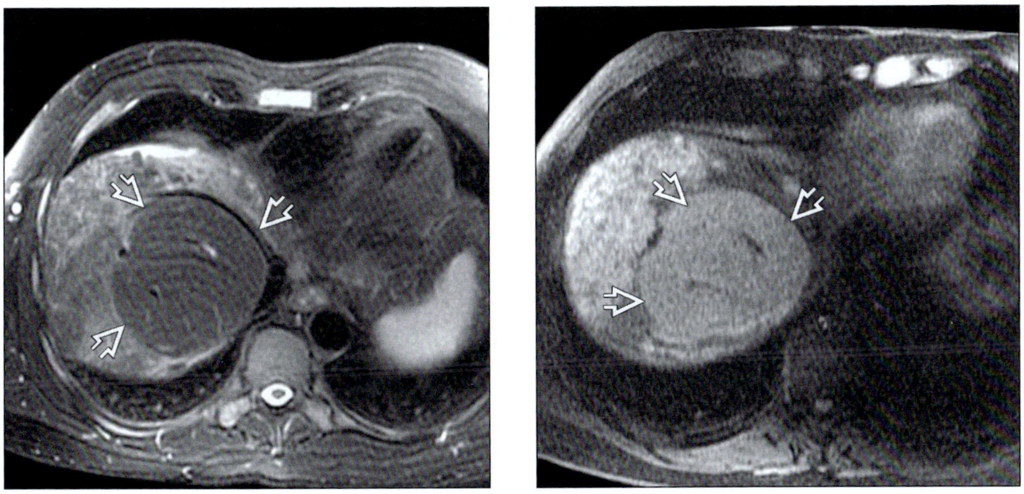

(Left) *Axial T2WI MR confirms the hypointensity of the mass* ➲*.* ***(Right)*** *Axial T1WI MR without intravenous contrast demonstrates isointensity of the mass compared to the surrounding liver parenchyma.*

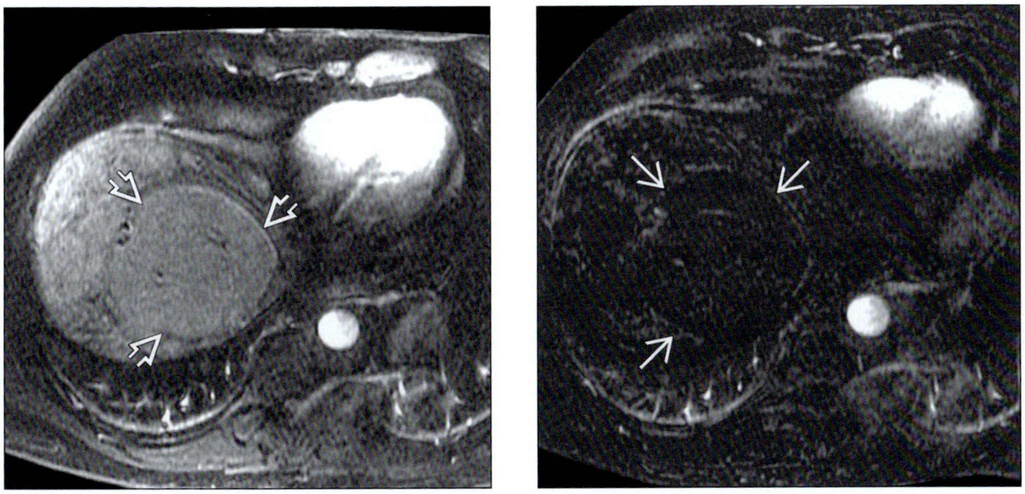

(Left) *Axial T1WI C+ MR in arterial phase demonstrates isointensity of the mass* ➲ *to the surrounding liver parenchyma indicating similar degree of enhancement compared to the surrounding liver parenchyma.* ***(Right)*** *Axial subtraction image demonstrates no significant enhancement of the mass* ➔*.*

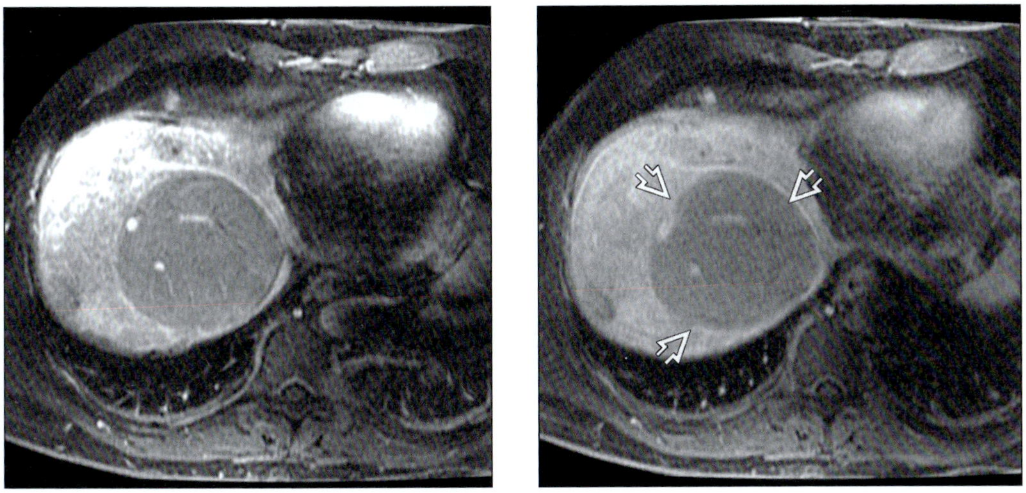

(Left) *Axial T1WI C+ MR in venous phase demonstrates persistent nonenhancement by the mass.* ***(Right)*** *Axial T1WI C+ MR in delayed phase demonstrates persistent nonenhancement by the mass* ➲*.*

FOCAL CONFLUENT FIBROSIS

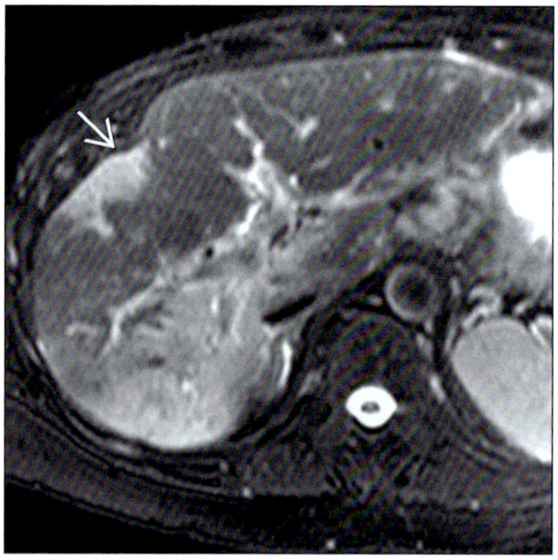

Axial T2WI FS MR demonstrates an ill-defined, wedge-shaped area within the anterior segment of the right hepatic lobe and medial segment of the left hepatic lobe exhibiting high signal intensity ➔.

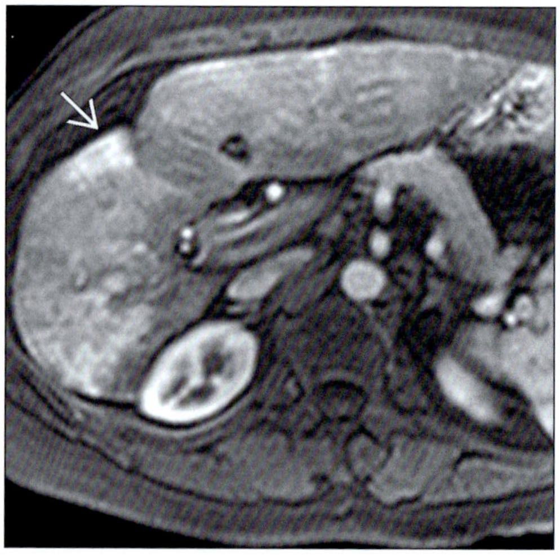

Axial T1WI FS C+ MR demonstrates slight enhancement of an ill-defined, wedge-shaped area ➔, associated with capsular retraction.

CLINICAL SCENARIO

History

- 45-year-old man with history of alcoholic cirrhosis

IMAGE INTERPRETATION

Findings

- Wedge-shaped enhancing area in anterior segment of right hepatic lobe with capsular retraction

Pitfalls

- Can be confused with cholangiocarcinoma (peripheral), treated malignancies, hepatic cavernous hemangioma (especially within cirrhotic liver)

Actual Diagnosis

- Focal confluent fibrosis

Clues to Correct Diagnosis

- Characteristic location (medial segment of left lobe, anterior segment of right lobe, or both)
- Wedge-shaped with capsular retraction
- Review of previous imaging in cirrhotic liver confirms progress of fibrosis and often makes diagnosis

BACKGROUND

General

- Fibrosis is present in most cirrhotic livers (90% of cases)
- Retraction of overlying capsule (90%) with volume loss

Epidemiology

- 14% of patients with advanced cirrhosis
- Most in cirrhosis 2° to primary sclerosing cholangitis (56%); other causes: Viral and alcoholic hepatitis
- Gender: M > F (related to prevalence of cirrhosis)

Relevant Anatomy

- 90% involve medial segment of left lobe &/or anterior segment of right lobe, spare caudate and lateral segments

IMAGING FEATURES

General Features

- Wedge-shaped in typical location with volume loss, delayed enhancement, and capsular retraction
- May radiate from porta hepatis and extend to capsule
- Peripheral foci may be band-shaped or curvilinear, usually total lobar or segmental distribution

CT

- NECT
  - Wedge- or band-like area of low attenuation
  - Retraction of overlying liver capsule (90%)
  - May affect entire segment or lobe with marked volume loss, even absence of affected segment
- CECT
  - Usually same attenuation as liver parenchyma on venous phase (occasionally slightly hypo- or hyperattenuating)
  - Delayed persistent enhancement similar to fibrotic lesions
  - Crowding of blood vessels or bile ducts within collapsed area of liver

MR

- T1WI: Hypointense to adjacent liver parenchyma
- T2WI: Hyperintense due to edema or active fibrosis
- T1WI C+
  - Slightly hypointense to liver on immediate post-gadolinium sequences (80%)
  - In later phase, may become iso-/hyperintense to liver
  - Progressive enhancement on PV and delayed phases
  - May be hyperenhancing in early phase and retain contrast in late phases if active fibrosis

RELATED REFERENCES

1. Brancatelli G et al: Focal confluent fibrosis in cirrhotic liver: natural history studied with serial CT. AJR Am J Roentgenol. 192(5):1341-7, 2009
2. Brancatelli G et al: Cirrhosis: CT and MR imaging evaluation. Eur J Radiol. 61(1):57-69, 2007

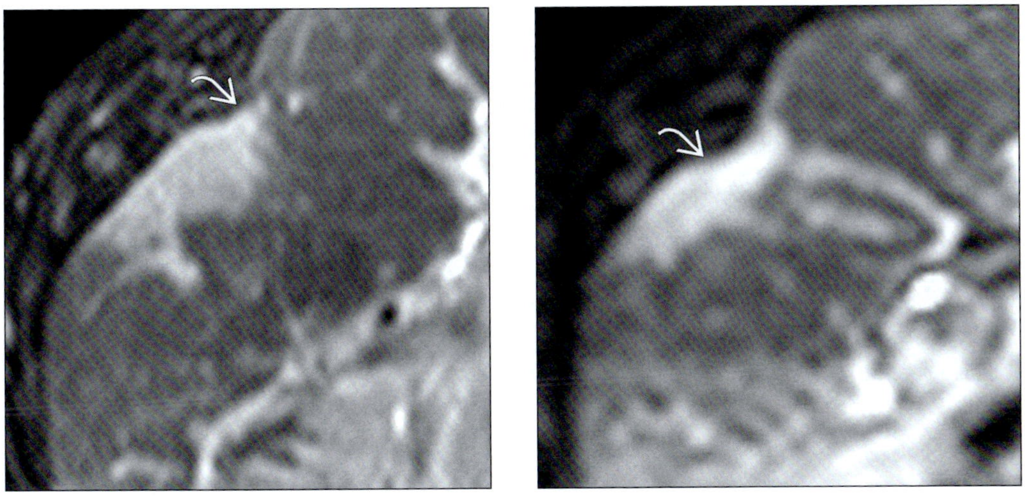

(Left) *Axial T2WI FS MR demonstrates the high signal intensity, ill-defined area within the anterior segment of the right hepatic lobe and the medial segment of the left hepatic lobe with associated capsular retraction ↷.* ***(Right)*** *Axial DWI demonstrates increased signal intensity (with low signal intensity on ADC [not shown]), indicating corresponding restricted diffusion in the subcapsular region ↷.*

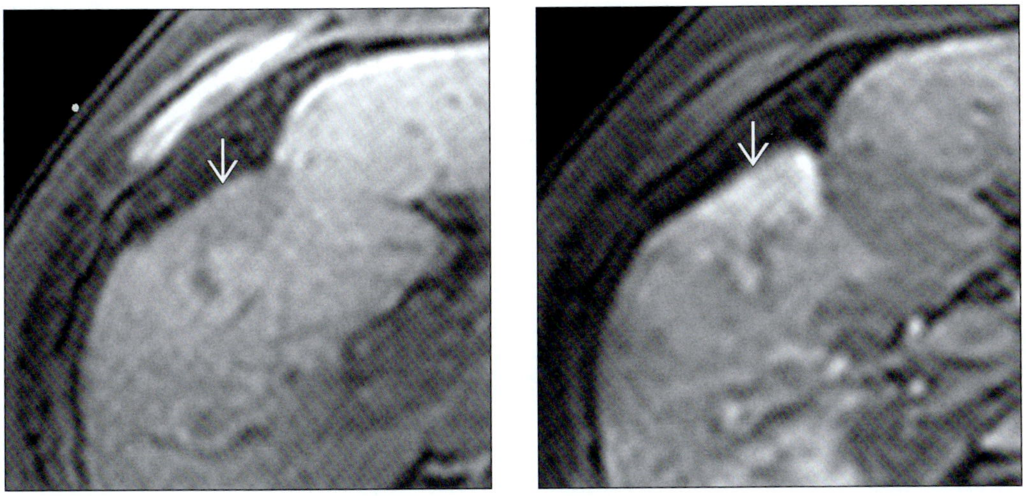

(Left) *Axial T1WI FS MR without contrast demonstrates low signal intensity of the subcapsular region →.* ***(Right)*** *Axial T1WI FS C+ MR in the arterial phase demonstrates patchy slight enhancement in the subcapsular region →.*

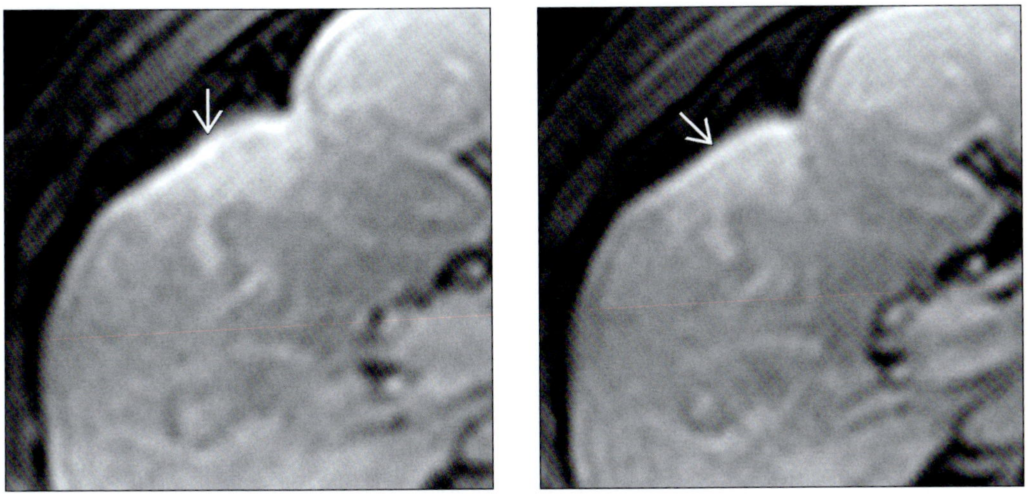

(Left) *Axial T1WI FS C+ MR in the venous phase demonstrates persistent enhancement of the subcapsular region →.* ***(Right)*** *Axial T1WI FS C+ MR in delayed phase demonstrates persistent enhancement →. Associated capsular retraction is noted.*

SCLEROSED HEMANGIOMA

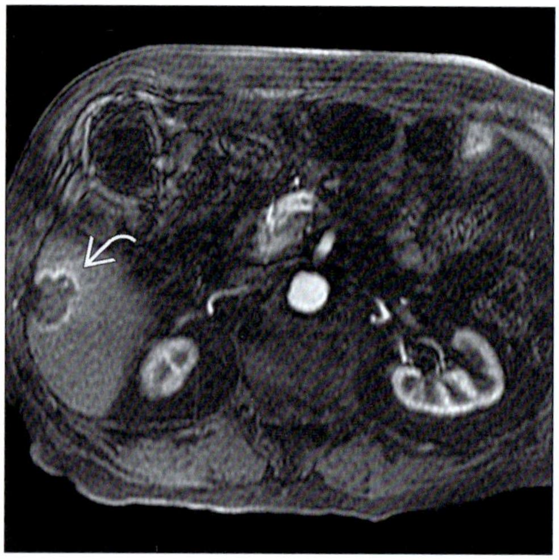

Axial T1WI FS C+ MR during arterial phase reveals a hypointense mass within segment VI of the right lobe of the liver with a continuous rim enhancement ➔.

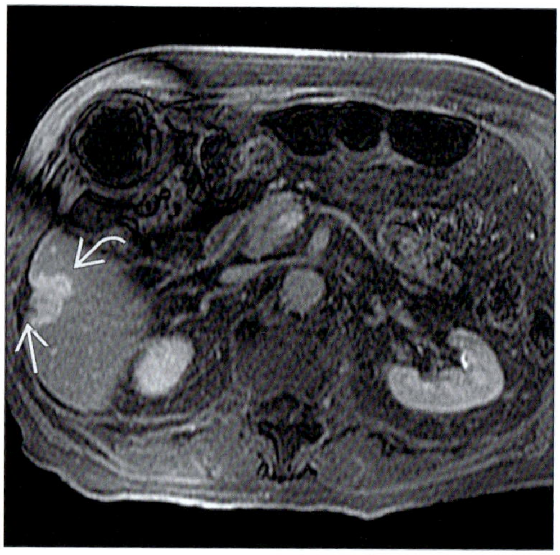

Axial T1WI FS C+ MR reveals a homogeneous central enhancement of the mass within segment VI of the liver on late venous phase ➔. Note associated capsular retraction ➔.

CLINICAL SCENARIO

History

- 87-year-old man with sigmoid adenocarcinoma

IMAGE INTERPRETATION

Pitfalls

- Can be mistaken for metastasis in light of history and peripheral continuous enhancement

Actual Diagnosis

- Sclerosed hemangioma

Clues to Correct Diagnosis

- Features suggestive of sclerosed hemangiomas include
  - Geographic pattern
  - Capsular retraction
  - Decrease in size over time
  - Loss of previously seen regions of enhancement
  - Presence of transient hepatic attenuation difference
  - Rim enhancement during the arterial phase
  - Nodular regions of intense enhancement as seen in typical hemangioma

BACKGROUND

General

- Sclerosed hemangioma is subtype that undergoes fibrosis or hyalinization of its stroma and blood vessel

Relevant Anatomy

- Most occur in periphery in geographic pattern
- Many result in capsular retraction

Relevant Pathology

- Microscopically, multiple dilated blood-filled vessels in a background of fibrocollagenous stroma
- Occasional dystrophic calcifications &/or with hemorrhage, thrombus, and hemosiderin

IMAGING FEATURES

US

- Heterogeneously hyperechoic

CT

- Hypodense ± calcifications on NECT
- Peripheral discontinuous nodular or continuous rim enhancement on arterial phase
- Centripetal enhancing nodules on portal venous phase
- Progressive delayed centripetal enhancement

MR

- T1WI: Hypointense
- T2WI: Isointense or hyperintense
- Same post-contrast enhancement pattern as on CT
- Hepatobiliary agents: No uptake

PET/CT

- Low FDG uptake is slightly higher or similar to liver background (< 2.5 SUV)

KEY TEACHING POINTS

Misinterpretation

- Sclerosed hemangioma is rare entity that can be mistaken for a metastasis
- Diagnosis should be considered with enhancement pattern, peripheral continuous rim enhancement, &/or capsular retraction

RELATED REFERENCES

1. Doyle DJ et al: Imaging features of sclerosed hemangioma. AJR Am J Roentgenol. 189(1):67-72, 2007
2. Makhlouf HR et al: Sclerosed hemangioma and sclerosing cavernous hemangioma of the liver: a comparative clinicopathologic and immunohistochemical study with emphasis on the role of mast cells in their histogenesis. Liver. 22(1):70-8, 2002
3. Vilgrain V et al: Imaging of atypical hemangiomas of the liver with pathologic correlation. Radiographics. 20(2):379-97, 2000

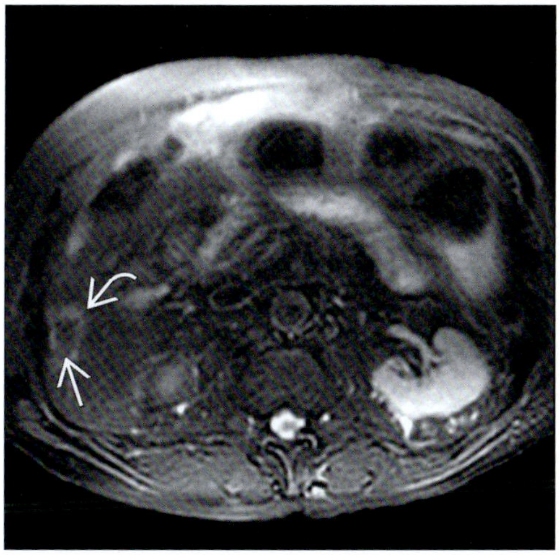

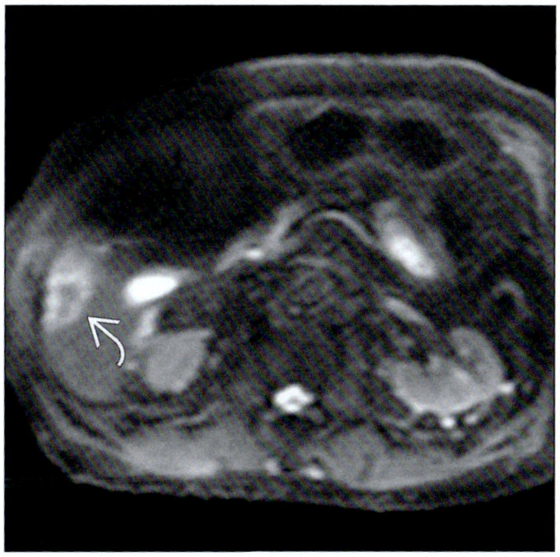

(Left) *Axial T2WI MR shows a right lobe hepatic mass with central hypointense signal and a peripheral high signal intensity rim.* ***(Right)*** *Axial DW MR shows a peripheral high signal intensity, indicating diffusion restriction.*

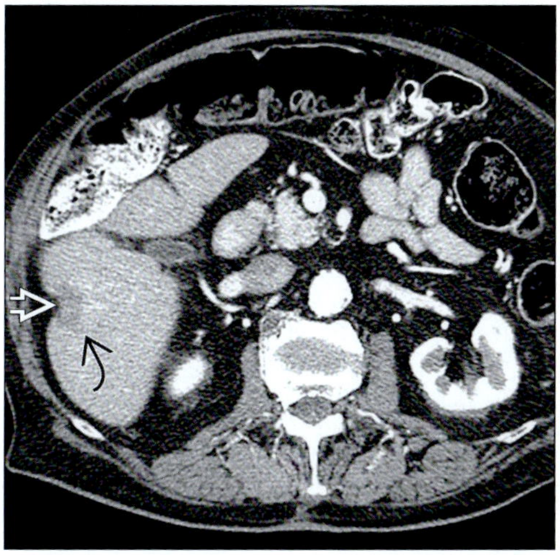

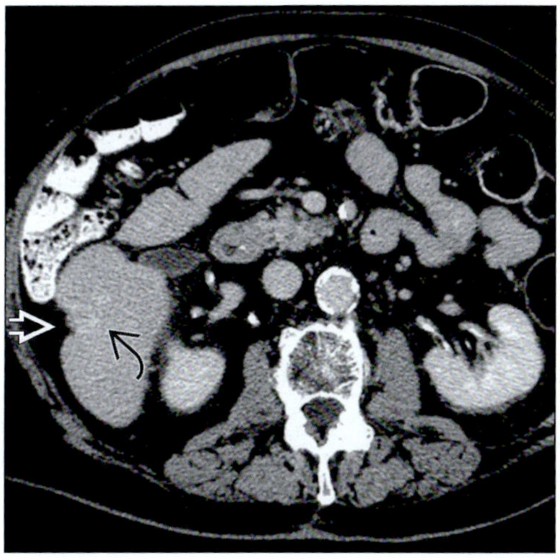

(Left) *Axial CECT during the arterial phase shows a peripheral hypodense mass with ill-defined peripheral enhancement. There is an associated capsular retraction.* ***(Right)*** *Axial CECT during the delayed phase shows a peripheral mass with a centripetal progressive enhancement. There is an associated capsular retraction.*

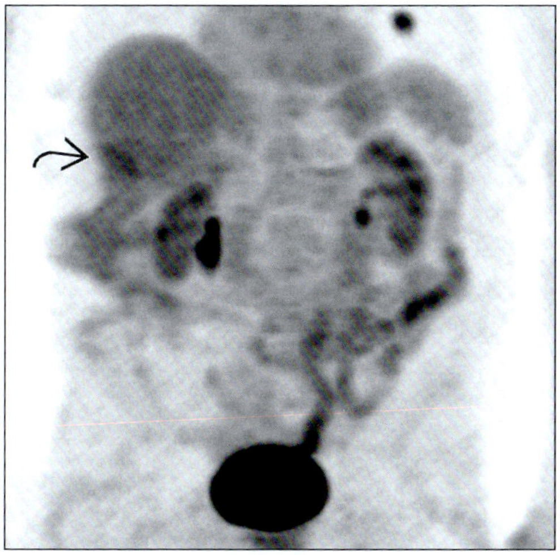

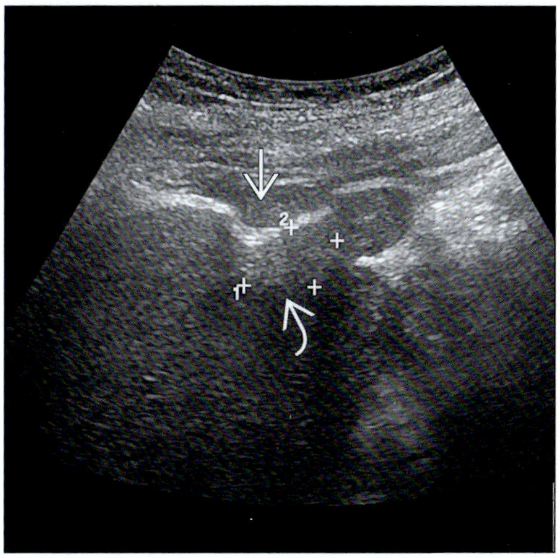

(Left) *Magnified planar PET image shows mild FDG uptake in the right hepatic lobe correlating with the mass.* ***(Right)*** *Prebiopsy grayscale ultrasound shows the mass in the liver as hyperechoic associated with capsular retraction.*

SIDEROTIC NODULE MIMICKING HCC

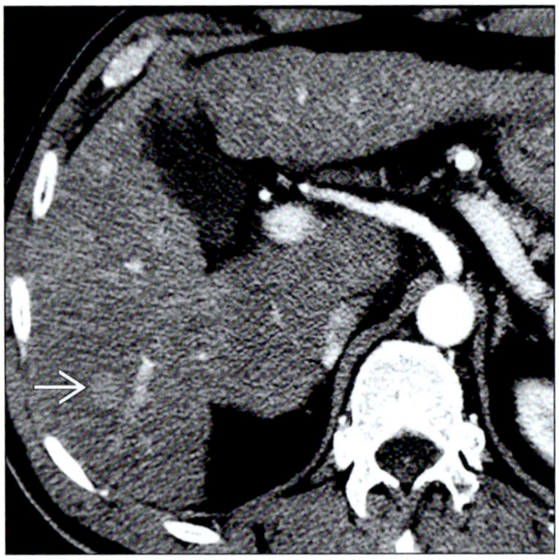

Axial CECT in arterial phase shows a cirrhotic morphology of the liver with a 1.5 cm nodule ➡ within the right hepatic lobe that appears hyperdense relative to surrounding liver parenchyma.

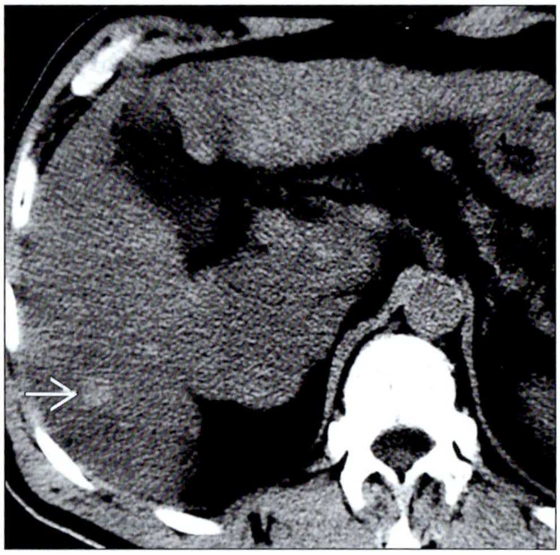

Axial NECT shows that the lesion was originally hyperdense ➡ (not enhancing), indicating siderotic regenerative nodule.

CLINICAL SCENARIO

History

- 67-year-old man with chronic liver disease

IMAGE INTERPRETATION

Pitfalls

- Hyperdense siderotic nodule (SN) may mimic enhancing focal lesion on CECT, hence, can be misinterpreted as hepatocellular carcinoma (HCC), particularly in presence of liver cirrhosis

Actual Diagnosis

- Siderotic regenerative nodule

Clues to Correct Diagnosis

- Siderotic nodule appears hyperattenuating to liver in CECT, thus can simulate enhancing lesions such as HCC
- It is necessary to review NECT for evaluation of enhancement

BACKGROUND

General

- Benign lesions simulating HCC can be encountered in cirrhotic livers
- Cross-sectional imaging (preferably contrast MR) is used to characterize cirrhotic liver nodules

Epidemiology

- HCC represents 5th most common malignancy worldwide and 33rd most common cause of death
- Risk is greatest among patients with hepatitis B or C
- Patients at increased risk undergo routine imaging surveillance

Relevant Pathology

- Cirrhotic liver nodules can be broadly categorized as regenerative (RN), dysplastic (DN) and HCC
- RN represents a region of parenchyma enlarged in response to necrosis, altered circulation, or other stimuli
- When the nodule is surrounded by fibrous septa and banded by septa, it is also called cirrhotic nodule
- When RNs contain iron, they are further categorized as siderotic, or iron containing

IMAGING FEATURES

General

- Presence of iron within SN is characteristic (echogenic on US, hyperdense in CT, and hypointense on MR)

US

- Heterogeneous cirrhotic morphology of liver
- SN can be demonstrated as nonspecific echogenic foci

CT

- NECT: Hyperdense
- CECT: Can also appear hyperdense but with no significant post-contrast enhancement
- Delayed phase: No significant enhancement or washout

MR

- Heterogeneous cirrhotic morphology of liver
- T1WI: Hypointense
- T2WI: Heterogeneous hypointense
- Can demonstrate blooming artifact on in-phase compared to out-of-phase (longer echo time)

RELATED REFERENCES

1. Brancatelli G et al: Helical CT screening for hepatocellular carcinoma in patients with cirrhosis: frequency and causes of false-positive interpretation. AJR Am J Roentgenol. 180(4):1007-14, 2003
2. Baron RL et al: From the RSNA refresher courses: screening the cirrhotic liver for hepatocellular carcinoma with CT and MR imaging: opportunities and pitfalls. Radiographics. 21 Spec No:S117-32, 2001

LARGE REGENERATIVE NODULES, BUDD-CHIARI

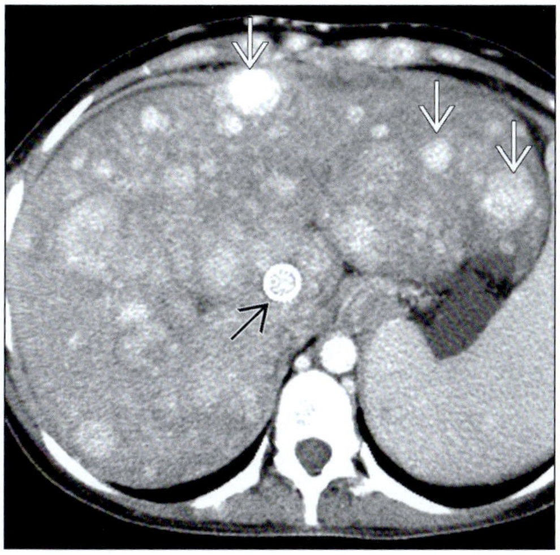

Axial CECT in arterial phase demonstrates multiple enhancing focal lesions ➡ in both hepatic lobes. A stent is noted within the contrast-enhanced IVC ⇨.

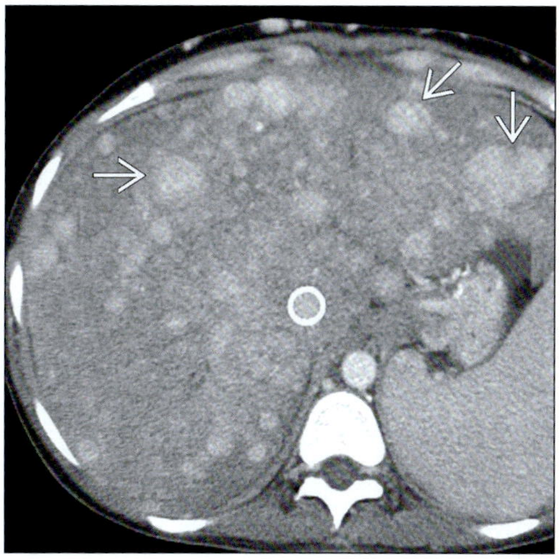

Axial CECT in venous phase demonstrates decreased enhancement of multiple enhancing focal lesions ➡ in both hepatic lobes (but no washout).

CLINICAL SCENARIO

History

- 63-year-old woman with history of Budd-Chiari syndrome secondary to IVC stenosis treated by stenting

IMAGE INTERPRETATION

Pitfalls

- Could be misinterpreted as hepatocellular lesions
  - Multiple adenomas or focal nodular hyperplasia, multifocal hepatocellular carcinoma (HCC), metastases

Actual Diagnosis

- Large regenerative nodules (LRNs) associated with Budd-Chiari syndrome

Clues to Correct Diagnosis

- History of Budd-Chiari syndrome (with IVC stent present)
- LRNs are typically multiple
- Homogeneous and usually intense enhancement during arterial phase
- No washout on delayed phase of contrast enhancement (unlike HCC & metastases)

BACKGROUND

Terminology

- LRNs have long been confused with nodular regenerative hyperplasia (NRH)

Relevant Pathology

- LRN & NRH are different types of hepatocellular nodules
  - LRNs usually occur with Budd-Chiari syndrome
    - Hyperplastic larger lesions (5 mm to 5 cm)
    - Nodules typically enhance after IV contrast administration
  - NRH usually occurs with organ transplantation, myeloproliferative or autoimmune disease
    - Multiple (1 mm), regenerative small lesions without fibrous septa
    - Nodules do not enhance after IV contrast administration

IMAGING FEATURES

US

- Nodules may be inconspicuous
- Heterogeneous echotexture or distortion of normal architecture may be sole finding
- Visible nodules are well circumscribed, homogeneous, and hypoechoic but may be hyperechoic
- Color Doppler: Changes of Budd-Chiari (irregular vessel distribution & high peak systolic velocity)

CT

- NECT: Multiple hypoattenuating lesions
- CECT: Lesions enhance on arterial or venous phase
  - Delayed phase: Isoattenuating (no washout)

MR

- T1WI: Homogeneous and slightly hyperintense (due to presence of copper within nodules)
- T2WI: Isointense or hypointense
- T1WI C+: May enhance in arterial or venous phase, become isointense on delayed phase
  - Central scar & perilesional halo: Occasionally seen

PET/CT

- No abnormal FDG uptake (similar to liver uptake)

RELATED REFERENCES

1. Ames JT et al: Distinguishing clinical and imaging features of nodular regenerative hyperplasia and large regenerative nodules of the liver. Clin Radiol. 64(12):1190-5, 2009
2. Rha SE et al: Nodular regenerative hyperplasia of the liver in Budd-Chiari syndrome: CT and MR features. Abdom Imaging. 25(3):255-8, 2000

HEPATIC PSEUDOANEURYSM

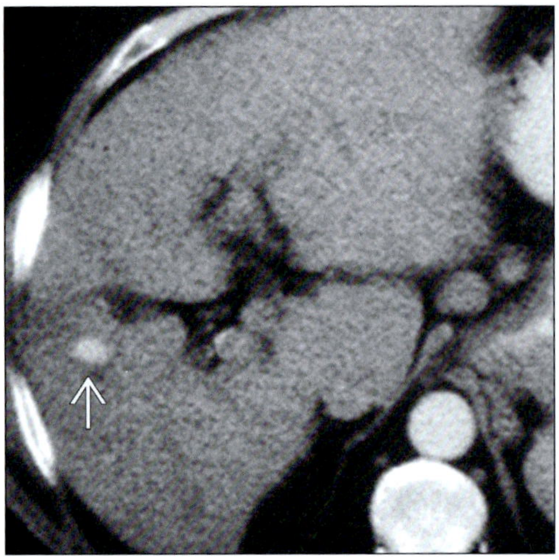

Axial CECT demonstrates a small enhancing nodule ➔ in the background of cirrhotic liver morphology. Patient was scheduled for a liver biopsy under ultrasound guidance.

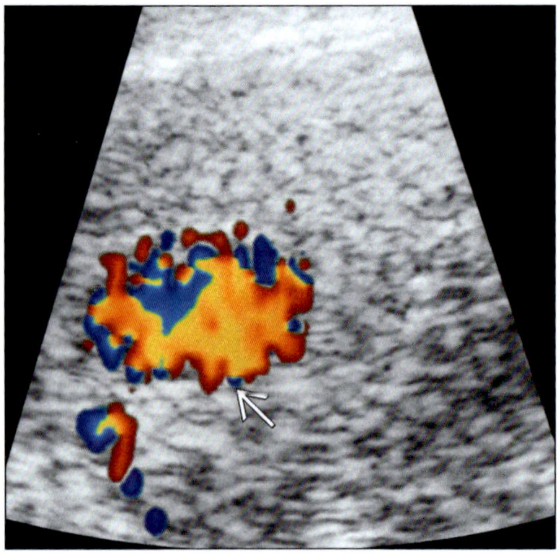

Color Doppler performed prebiopsy showed the classic to-and-fro pattern of swirling blood in the lesion ➔.

CLINICAL SCENARIO

History

- 45-year-old patient with history of chronic liver disease

IMAGE INTERPRETATION

Pitfalls

- May be misinterpreted as arterially enhancing mass (e.g., HCC, especially in background of chronic liver disease)
- Flash-filling hemangioma can have similar appearance on CT

Actual Diagnosis

- Post-biopsy pseudoaneurysm (PSA)

Clues to Correct Diagnosis

- History of liver biopsy
- Similar attenuation to arterial structures
- Signal void on T1WI and T2WI

BACKGROUND

Epidemiology

- Many small lesions can enhance vigorously and homogeneously in liver during arterial phase in patients with chronic liver disease
- Only 10–30% of arterially enhancing nodules in patients with chronic liver disease are HCC
- Post-biopsy PSA and AVM are commonly seen in patients with chronic liver disease who undergo frequent biopsies to evaluate disease progression
- PSAs complicate 0.3-2.1% of liver transplantation and 0.6% of laparoscopic cholecystectomies; also reported after trauma, percutaneous liver biopsy, percutaneous biliary drainage, and TIPS

Relevant Pathology

- a.k.a. false aneurysm, results from leakage of blood from artery into adjacent tissue with a consequent communication between native artery and resultant adjacent cavity
- PSA formation is more likely to occur when only 1 side of arterial wall is injured
- Although commonly asymptomatic, PSAs are at risk of rupture, resulting in life-threatening hemorrhage

IMAGING FEATURES

US

- Anechoic, well-circumscribed rounded structure
- Vascular yin-yang pattern

CT

- Well-circumscribed enhancing rounded structure

MR

- T1WI: Signal void
- T2WI: Signal void
- T1WI C+: High intensity similar to major arterial structures at early phase contrast-enhanced MR without washout on delayed images
- Communicating with an arterial structure
- DWI: No diffusion restriction

PET/CT

- No abnormal FDG uptake

Key Teaching Points

- PSA can complicate hepatic procedures, such as biopsy
- May simulate arterially enhancing lesion such as HCC
- PSAs exhibit high attenuation similar to major arterial structures at early phase contrast-enhanced CT and MR without washout on delayed images

RELATED REFERENCES

1. Own A et al: Bleeding hepatic pseudoaneurysm complicating percutaneous liver biopsy with interventional treatment options. Eur Radiol. 15(1):183-5, 2005

DELAYED ENHANCING METASTASIS

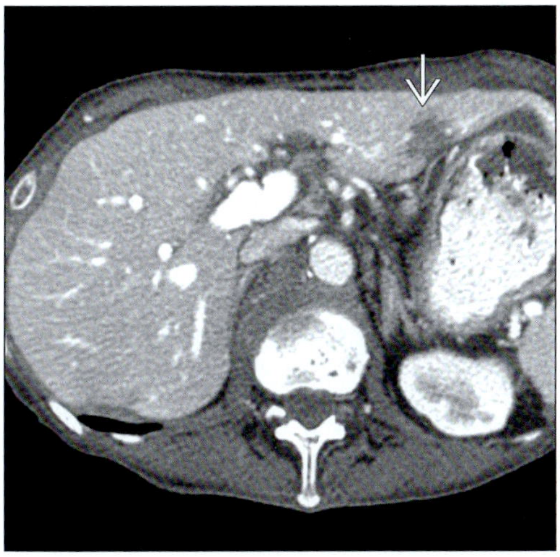

Axial CECT in portal venous phase demonstrates a hypoattenuating lesion ➡ within the lateral segment of the left hepatic lobe.

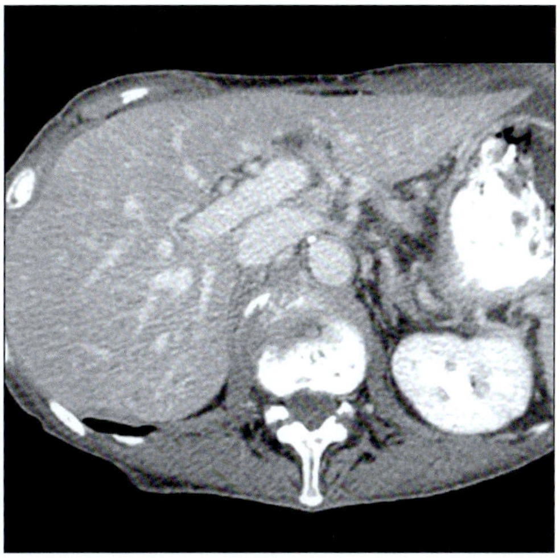

Axial CECT in delayed phase shows enhancement of the left lobe lesion, which becomes isoattenuating to liver on delayed phase (as opposed to hemangioma, which appears isoattenuating to vasculature).

CLINICAL SCENARIO

History

- 88-year-old man with right upper quadrant pain and history of resected colorectal cancer

IMAGE INTERPRETATION

Pitfalls

- Centripetal filling of contrast in delayed phase can be misdiagnosed as hemangioma

Actual Diagnosis

- Metastatic colonic adenocarcinoma

Clues to Correct Diagnosis

- History of primary malignancy
- Peripheral rim enhancement in arterial phase can be continuous and not nodular, discontinuous puddling as in hemangioma
- Similar enhancement to liver parenchyma (CT isoattenuation/MR isointensity) is seen on delayed phase
  - In contrast to hemangioma, which follows blood pool (enhances similar to vasculature)
- Hemorrhage and necrosis point to malignancy

BACKGROUND

General

- Some metastases show delayed enhancement in intratumoral desmoplastic areas during delayed phase due to contrast retention in fibrosed tissue
- In addition, fibrotic metastases may be missed in post-contrast late phase due to delayed enhancement, which is isodense/isointense to liver parenchyma
  - Metastases can be 2° to colorectal (most common), pancreatic or gallbladder adenocarcinoma, and cholangiocarcinoma
- Colon cancer is 3rd most common cancer
  - Metastasis is most common hepatic malignancy
  - Right liver lobe is more commonly affected
- 50,000 colorectal cancer patients develop hepatic metastasis annually

IMAGING FEATURES

CT

- Single or multiple hypoattenuating nodules of variable sizes and shapes
- Peripheral continuous rim enhancement is frequently seen in arterial phase
- Can demonstrate filling on delayed post-contrast phase, thus appears isoattenuating to liver parenchyma
- Central necrosis may occur
- Capsular retraction in subcapsular lesions may occur due to desmoplastic reaction
- Intralesional calcification may occur in metastatic mucinous adenocarcinoma and also after chemotherapy treatment

MR

- T1WI: Hypointense to liver
- T2WI: Hyperintense to liver
- T1WI C+: Less enhancement compared to surrounding liver parenchyma
  - Peripheral rim enhancement in arterial phase is frequently encountered
  - Centripetal extension of contrast on delayed phase (becomes isodense to liver parenchyma)

PET/CT

- Increased FDG uptake

RELATED REFERENCES

1. Kanematsu M et al: Imaging liver metastases: review and update. Eur J Radiol. 58(2):217-28, 2006
2. Sica GT et al: CT and MR imaging of hepatic metastases. AJR Am J Roentgenol. 174(3):691-8, 2000
3. Gabata T et al: Delayed MR imaging of the liver: correlation of delayed enhancement of hepatic tumors and pathologic appearance. Abdom Imaging. 23(3):309-13, 1998

CYSTIC LIVER METASTASIS

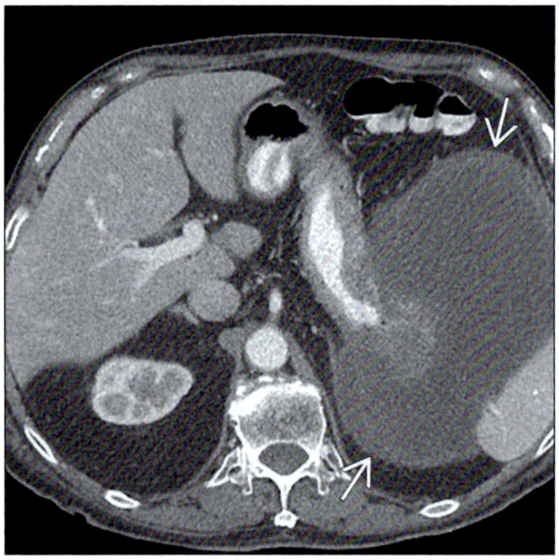

Axial CECT shows a large, hypoattenuating mass in the left upper abdomen ➡ originating from the greater curvature of the stomach.

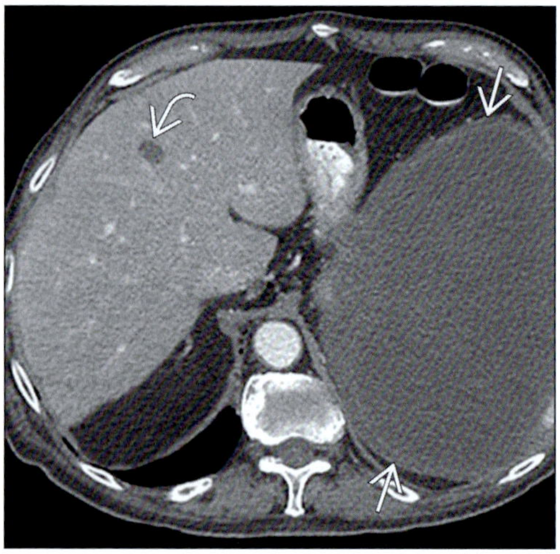

Axial CECT shows a large, hypoattenuating mass ➡ arising from the gastric wall, and a hypodense lesion within segment IV of the liver ↪ with internal attenuation of 24 HU.

CLINICAL SCENARIO

History
- 80-year-old man with gastric gastrointestinal stromal tumor (GIST)

IMAGE INTERPRETATION

Pitfalls
- Can be mistaken for simple or complex cyst

Actual Diagnosis
- Solitary cystic metastasis, secondary to GIST

Clues to Correct Diagnosis
- Enhancing solid component or mural nodule
- Ill-defined inner margins and irregular enhancing septa
- Multifocality and hyperattenuation (hemorrhage or mucin)
- History of malignancy leading to cystic metastases

BACKGROUND

General
- Some types of malignancies: Colon adenocarcinoma (particularly mucinous), neuroendocrine tumors, and GIST

Epidemiology
- Rate varies with type of primary neoplasm
- With colorectal, rate of synchronous metastasis is around 1.5%; of these, 1.8% are purely cystic
- In GIST, cystic changes can occur in untreated metastasis or develop after imatinib therapy

Relevant Physiology
- Cystic metastases tend to form via 3 mechanisms
  - Growth beyond vascular supply
  - Mucin production (e.g., colorectal or ovarian)
  - Therapy (e.g., GIST after imatinib [Gleevec])

Relevant Pathology
- Grossly: Necrotic debris and hemorrhagic clots
- Microscopically: Cancer cells are usually found in periphery, on outer wall; necrotic cells on inner wall

IMAGING FEATURES

US
- Hypoechoic; posterior acoustic enhancement; often thick irregular walls, septations, and fluid-fluid levels

CT
- NECT: Hypoattenuating
- Possible mural nodules, septations, and fluid-fluid levels
- CECT: Center remains unenhanced; occasional peripheral and septal enhancement

MR
- T1WI: Hypointense; can be hyperintense to liver if hemorrhagic (e.g., colorectal), proteinaceous (e.g., ovarian), or containing melanin (melanoma)
- T2WI: Hyperintense to liver
- T1WI C+: Occasional peripheral enhancement

PET/CT
- Most of active metastases are FDG avid
  - Minority of untreated GIST metastases are not FDG avid

Key Teaching Points
- Cystic metastasis can be misinterpreted as benign cystic lesion
- Diagnosis: Usually by biopsy or treatment response
- PET shows increased uptake of active cystic metastases

RELATED REFERENCES

1. Qian LJ et al: Spectrum of multilocular cystic hepatic lesions: CT and MR imaging findings with pathologic correlation. Radiographics. 33(5):1419-33, 2013
2. Del Poggio P et al: Cystic tumors of the liver: a practical approach. World J Gastroenterol. 14(23):3616-20, 2008

LIGATED ABERRANT RIGHT HEPATIC DUCT

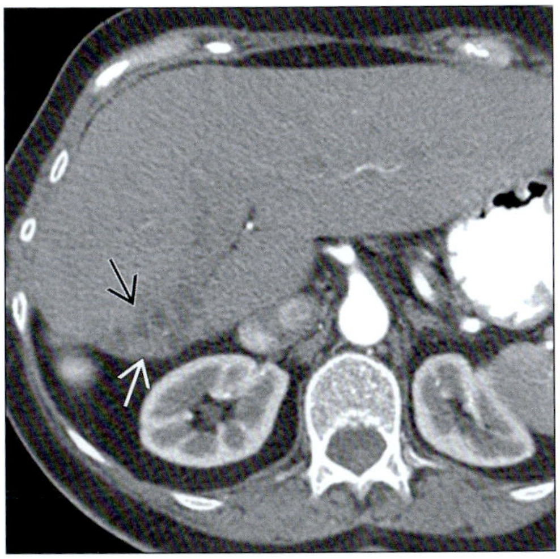

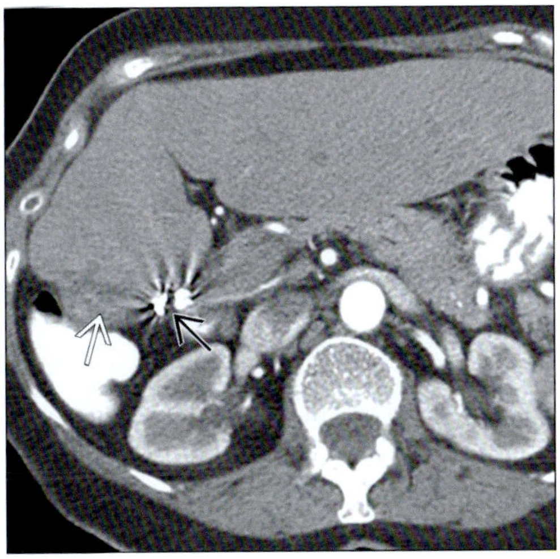

(Left) *Axial CECT shows scattered thin curvilinear enhancement* → *in the lesion relates to biliary ductal wall enhancement. Minimal residual enhancing normal liver tissue* → *is seen adjacent to lesion.* ***(Right)*** *Axial CECT in the same patient at a level slightly below shows a surgical clip* → *adjacent to hypoattenuating lesion in posterior right hepatic lobe. Thin curvilinear enhancement* → *is again seen. Focal hypoattenuation in left lobe corresponds to unopacified portal vein on subsequent images.*

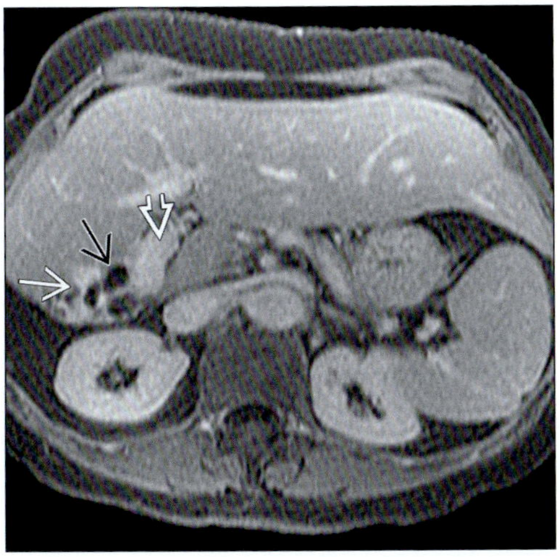

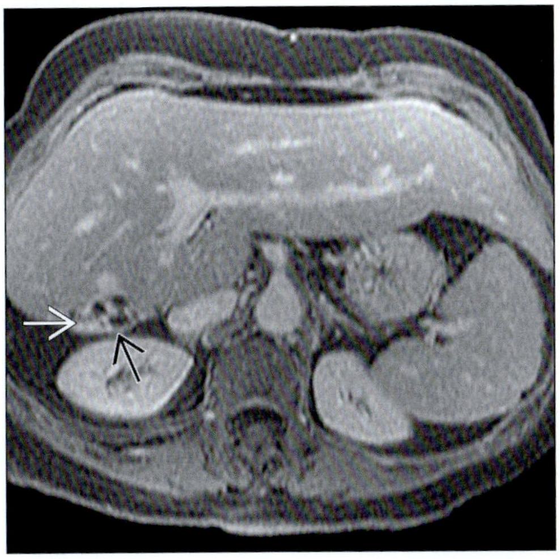

(Left) *Axial T1WI C+ MR in the portovenous phase shows serpentine dilated packed biliary ducts* →*. No soft tissue mass is present. Parenchymal atrophy is evident. The biliary ductal wall and stromal tissue* → *enhance. Adjacent portal vein* → *is patent.* ***(Right)*** *Axial T1WI C+ MR in the portovenous phase shows serpentine dilated packed biliary ducts* →*. The wedge shape of the lesion is apparent. The biliary ductal wall and stromal tissue enhance* →*.*

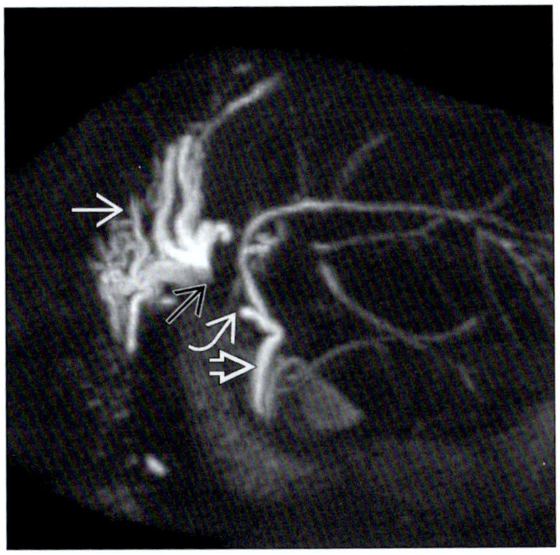

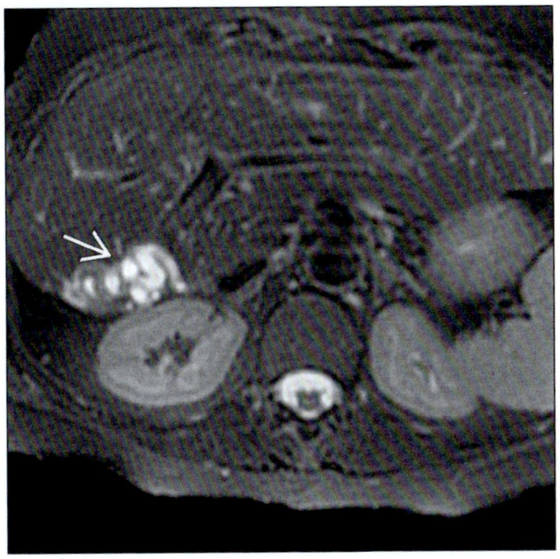

(Left) *MRCP shows packed dilated segmental biliary ducts* →*. There is abrupt cut-off medially* →*, with the right hepatic duct* → *inserting more inferiorly into a low position of the CBD. The remainder of the biliary tree is normal, including the common bile duct* →*. The gallbladder is surgically absent.* ***(Right)*** *Axial T2WI MR shows serpentine dilated packed biliary ducts* →*.*

HEPATIC RADIATION INJURY

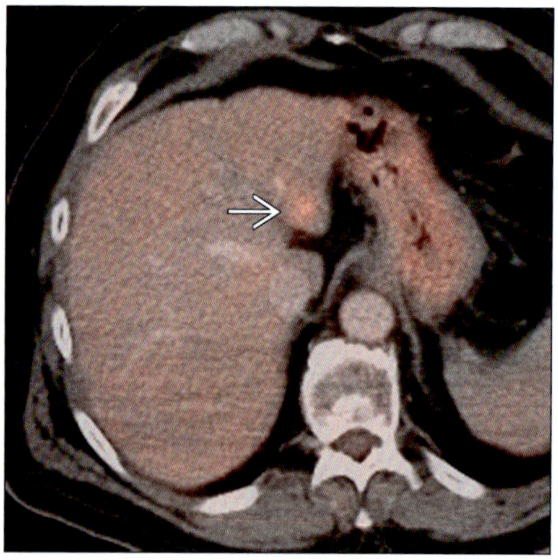

Axial PET/CT shows a subtle area of increased metabolic activity ➔ involving the posterior aspect of the left lobe of the liver.

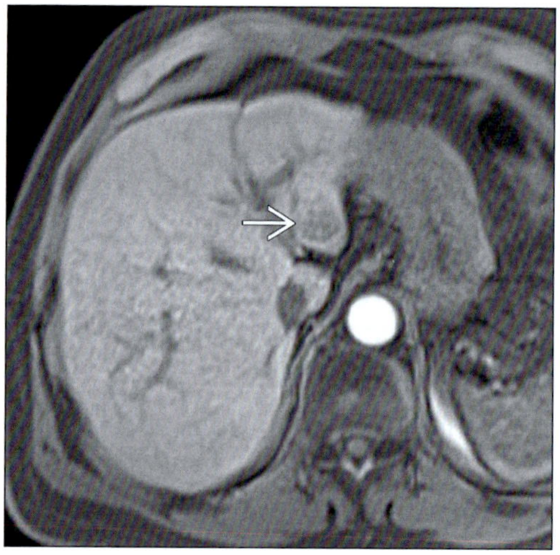

Axial T1WI C+ FS MR shows a rounded area of decreased signal intensity ➔ corresponding to the area of increased metabolic activity on PET/CT.

CLINICAL SCENARIO

History

- 65-year-old man with history of gastroesophageal junction carcinoma who received neoadjuvant radiotherapy
- PET/CT was obtained for preoperative staging

IMAGE INTERPRETATION

Pitfalls

- Left lobe hypermetabolic lesion can be mistaken for metastatic disease

Actual Diagnosis

- Hepatic radiation injury

Clues to Correct Diagnosis

- Straightforward diagnosis when imaging abnormality is segmental within radiation port
- Challenging diagnosis when abnormality is mass-like
  - Typical location within radiation port
  - Becomes less distinct and eventually resolves on follow-up

BACKGROUND

General

- Radiation therapy in patients with tumors of distal esophagus or gastroesophageal junction → inflammation and necrosis in adjacent liver parenchyma → radiation-induced liver damage

Relevant Pathology

- Initial histologic changes consist of occlusion of small hepatic veins, hyperemia, and diminished cellularity
  - Most striking at 1-3 months after external beam radiation therapy
- Imaging appearances of irradiated liver parenchyma likely reflect increased water content and impaired perfusion

IMAGING FEATURES

General

- Segmental areas of abnormal liver
  - Correspond to radiation port
  - Linear interface with normal liver parenchyma

US

- Hypo- or hyperechogenicity

CT

- Decreased attenuation
- Less enhancement than adjacent parenchyma in both arterial and portal venous phases
- Portal venous or delayed phase hyperenhancement several months after radiation injury
  - Likely due to impaired outflow of blood
- Ring-enhancing lesions have also been described

MR

- T1WI: Decreased signal intensity
- T2WI: Increased signal intensity
- Less enhancement than adjacent parenchyma in both arterial and portal venous phases

PET/CT

- Variable metabolic activity in irradiated liver
  - Increased or decreased activity

RELATED REFERENCES

1. Iwasa S et al: Ring-enhancing lesion associated with radiation-induced liver disease. J Clin Oncol. 31(14):e243-4, 2013
2. Maturen KE et al: Imaging effects of radiation therapy in the abdomen and pelvis: evaluating "innocent bystander" tissues. Radiographics. 33(2):599-619, 2013
3. Iyer RB et al: PET/CT and hepatic radiation injury in esophageal cancer patients. Cancer Imaging. 7:189-94, 2007
4. Nishino M et al: Uterine contractions evaluated on cine MR imaging in patients with uterine leiomyomas. Eur J Radiol. 53(1):142-6, 2005

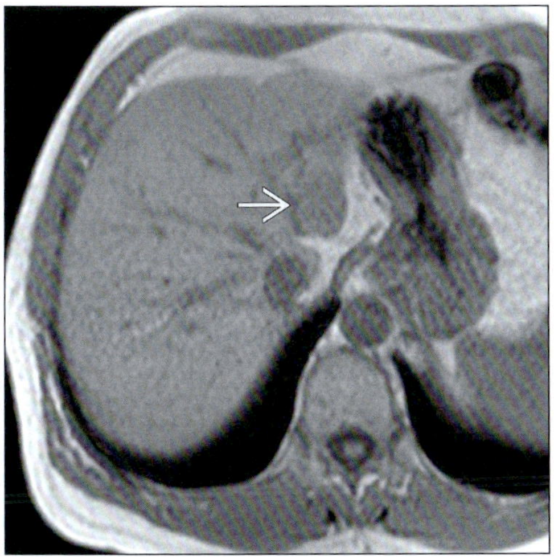

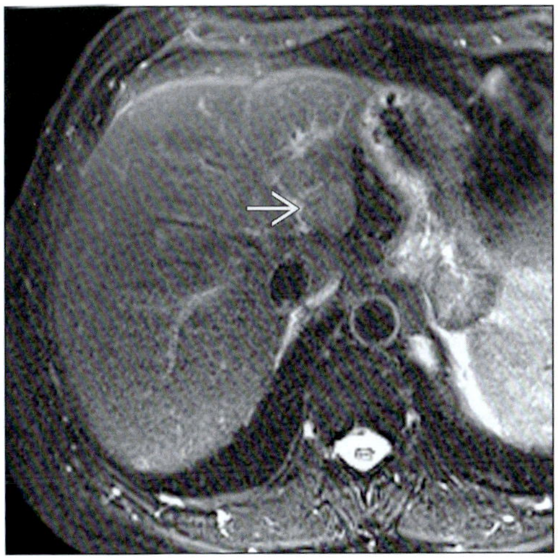

(Left) *Axial in-phase T1WI MR shows a rounded area of decreased signal intensity → in the posterior aspect of the left lobe within the radiation port in this patient with a history of distal esophageal carcinoma.* ***(Right)*** *Axial T2WI FS MR shows a rounded area of subtle increased signal intensity →.*

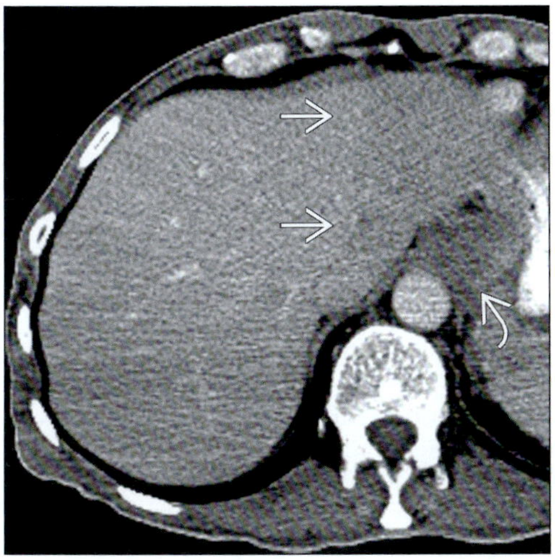

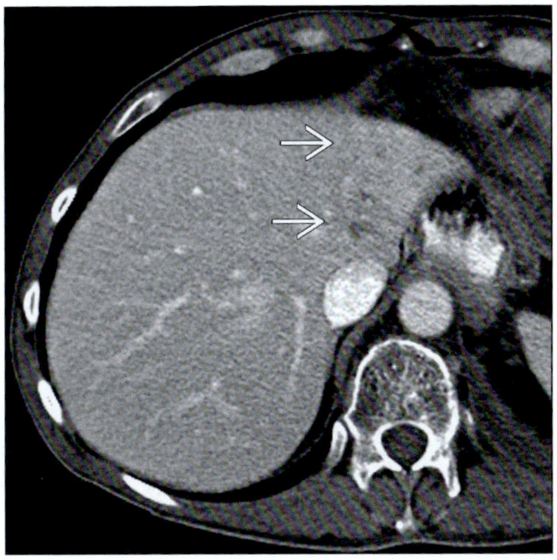

(Left) *Axial CECT shows a segmental area of decreased attenuation → involving the left lobe of the liver 6 weeks following radiation treatment of gastroesophageal carcinoma ↷. Note the linear interface between the abnormal low attenuation of the left lobe and normal liver.* ***(Right)*** *Axial CECT obtained 9 months later shows increased attenuation → of the irradiated left lobe. Note also interval decrease in the size of the left lobe.*

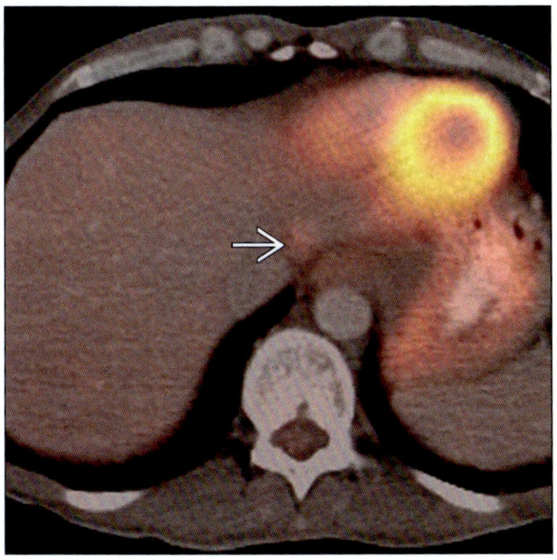

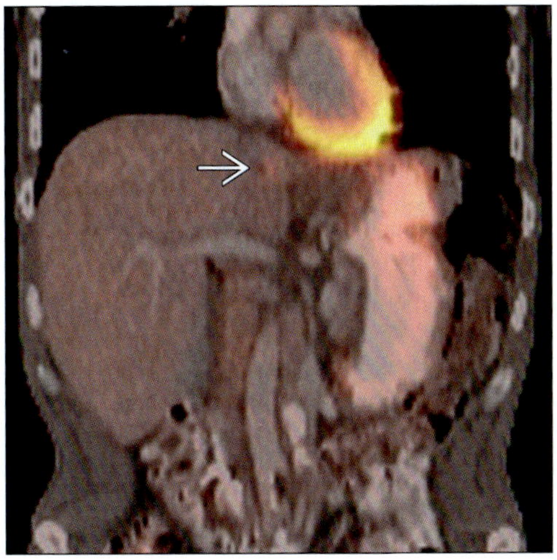

(Left) *Axial PET/CT shows a subtle area of increased metabolic activity → within the posterior aspect of the left lobe of the liver following radiation therapy of lower esophageal carcinoma.* ***(Right)*** *Coronal PET/CT shows a subtle area of increased metabolic activity → within the posterior aspect of the left lobe of the liver following radiation therapy of lower esophageal carcinoma.*

EARLY POST LIVER TRANSPLANT PITFALLS

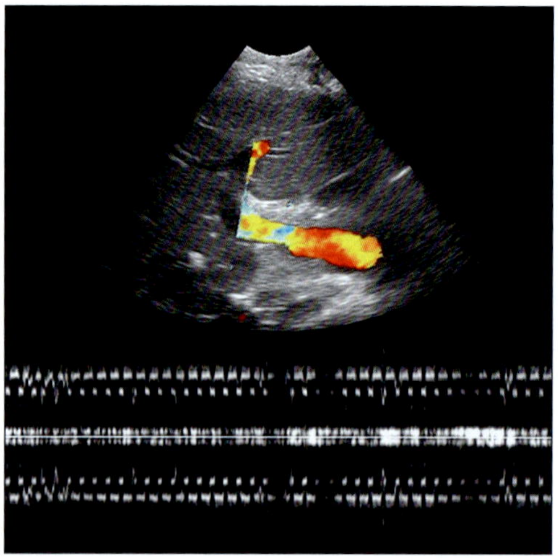

Color Doppler ultrasound examination demonstrates absent hepatic arterial color flow with Doppler tracing demonstrating only noise without arterial signal.

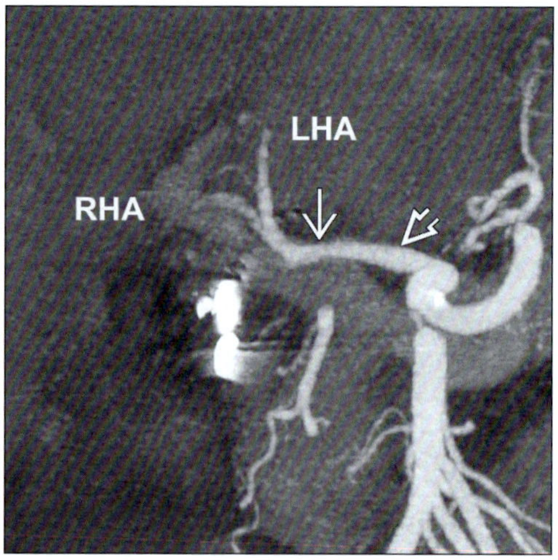

Maximum intensity projection image of CT angiography demonstrates patent proper ➡ and common hepatic arteries ⇨ as well as right and left hepatic arteries.

CLINICAL SCENARIO

History

- 54-year-old man with history of longstanding liver cirrhosis, presenting for ultrasound evaluation 2 days after orthotopic liver transplantation (OLT) surgery

Relevant Laboratory Tests

- Abnormally elevated liver function tests

IMAGE INTERPRETATION

Pitfalls

- Could be misinterpreted as hepatic arterial occlusion

Actual Diagnosis

- Normal postoperative findings

Clues to Correct Diagnosis

- Patent hepatic artery on CT or MR angiography
- In immediate postoperative period, increased resistance or even absent flow in hepatic artery is to be expected

BACKGROUND

General

- Variety of early postoperative US findings usually resolve within a few days
- Normalization of cold ischemia followed by reperfusion and manipulation of liver from point of donor extraction to recipient transplantation
- Liver function tests (LFTs) can be abnormal even in uncomplicated transplants; therefore, ↑ LFTs in early postoperative period are not helpful to correlate with imaging findings

IMAGING FEATURES

Findings

- Liver parenchyma
  - "Starry sky" appearance
    - Accentuation of portal vein walls due to ↓ parenchymal echogenicity can be seen due to stasis of fluid in extracellular spaces and reperfusion edema
    - May be 2° to vasospasm, tissue edema, ↑ portal flow, advanced donor age, and prolonged cold ischemia
  - Focal ↑ echogenicity and heterogeneity, possibly due to contusion &/or hemorrhage
- Hepatic artery
  - Absent flow could be seen on Doppler US
  - Velocity may be increased due to decreased vessel diameter
    - During 1st few days after OLT, ↑ velocity can be considered normal transient
    - Can occur due to a persistent ↑ arterial inflow from portal hypertension or luminal narrowing caused by anastomotic edema
    - Elevated resistive index (RI) may be a normal transient postoperative phenomenon and can occur in nearly 50% of patients, resolving in a few days
    - Tardus parvus waveform, particularly with normal hepatic function, should be closely followed up rather than misdiagnosed as arterial stenosis
- Portal vein
  - Velocity may be increased due to surrounding edema and other causes → turbulent or pulsatile flow on Doppler US
- Hepatic veins
  - May lose normal triphasic and demonstrate an abnormal monophasic pattern
- Transient findings resolve after few days post OLT
  - Close US follow-up to confirm resolution
    - If not resolved, CECT or MR should be performed

RELATED REFERENCES

1. Sanyal R et al: Orthotopic liver transplantation: reversible Doppler US findings in the immediate postoperative period. Radiographics. 32(1):199-211, 2012
2. García-Criado A et al: Doppler ultrasound findings in the hepatic artery shortly after liver transplantation. AJR Am J Roentgenol. 193(1):128-35, 2009

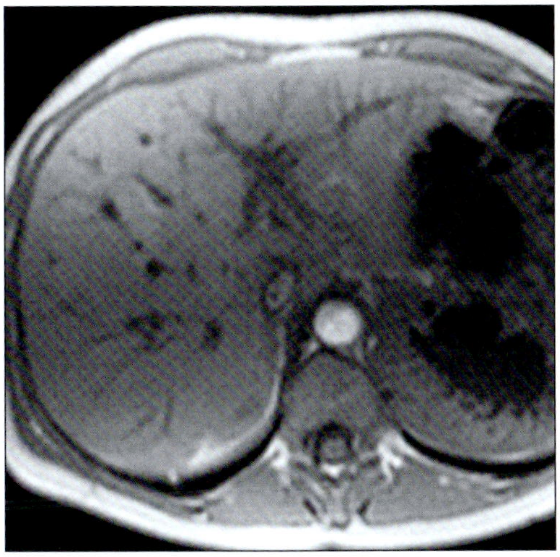
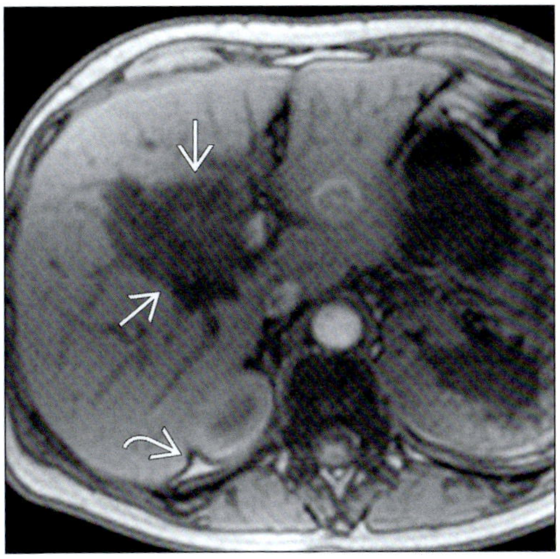

(Left) *Axial in-phase T1WI MR demonstrates homogeneous liver signal intensity with no evidence of liver masses.* ***(Right)*** *Axial out-of-phase T1WI MR shows a geographic area of signal dropout ➔ in the central liver compared to the in-phase T1WI MR, indicative of intracellular lipid content. Note "India ink" artifact at liver and renal borders ↷.*

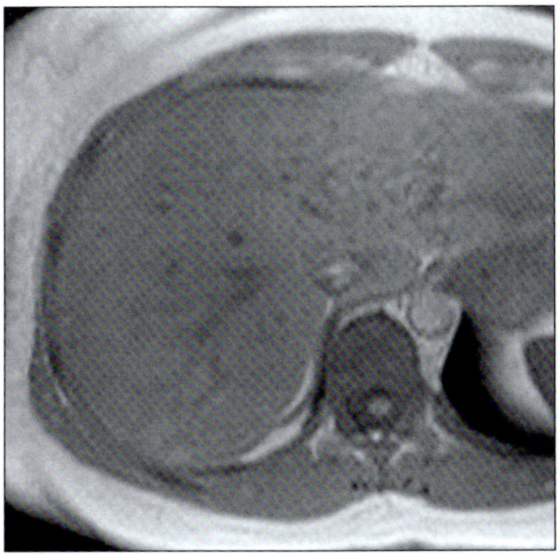
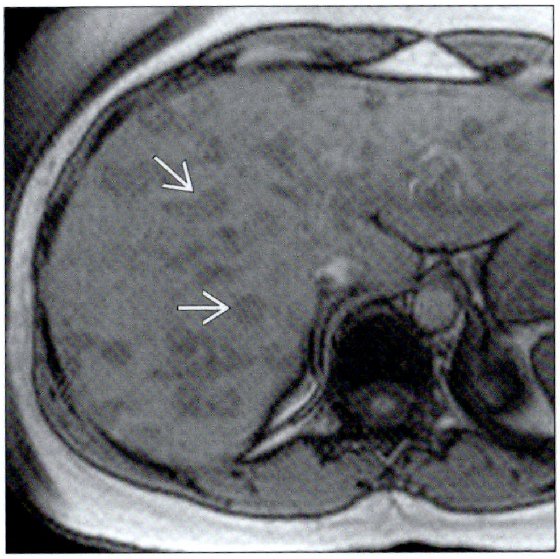

(Left) *Axial in-phase T1WI MR shows a different patient with a history of breast carcinoma who underwent MR for further evaluation of numerous hypodense lesions on CT (not shown) with a presumable diagnosis of metastases. This image demonstrates homogeneous liver signal intensity without focal lesions.* ***(Right)*** *Axial out-of-phase T1WI MR in the same patient demonstrates numerous focal areas ➔ with drop of signal intensity compared to in-phase T1WI MR, diagnostic of multiple areas of focal fatty infiltration.*

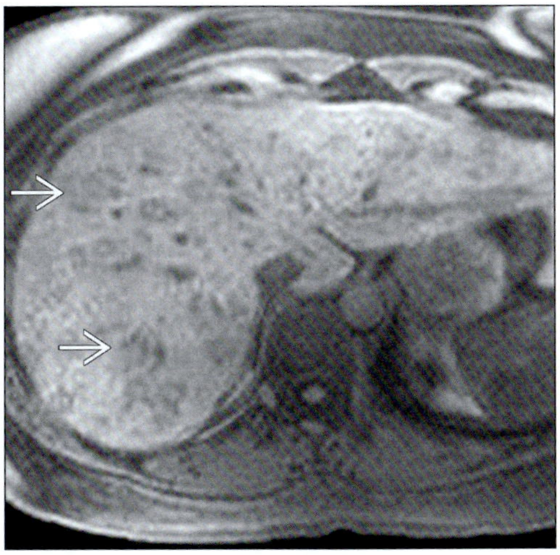
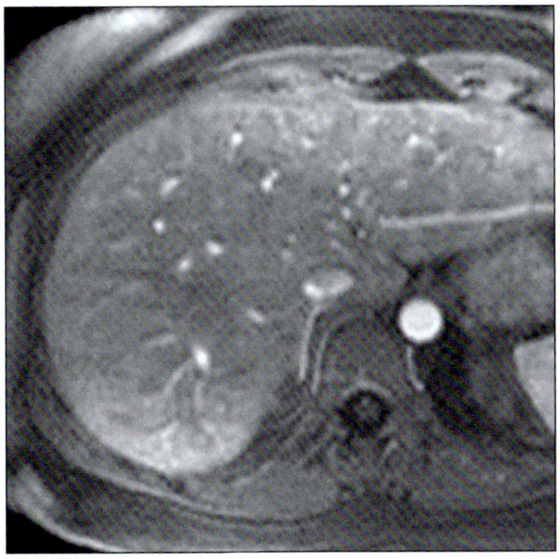

(Left) *Axial precontrast T1WI MR in the same patient with a history of breast carcinoma demonstrates the lesions again with relative hypointensity compared to the surrounding liver parenchyma ➔.* ***(Right)*** *Axial post-contrast T1WI MR shows no significant post-contrast enhancement of the aforementioned lesions.*

NODULAR FATTY SPARING

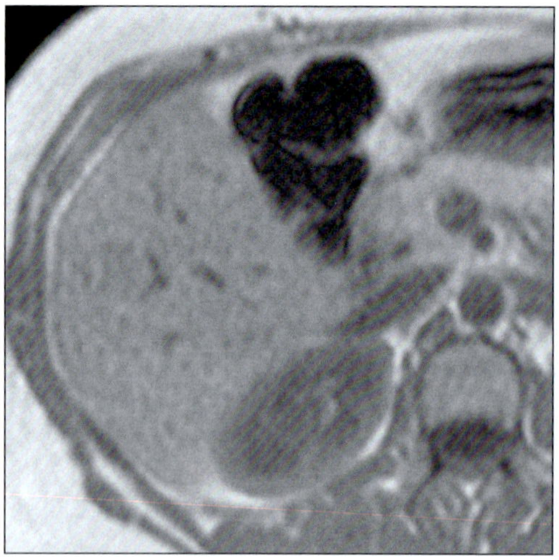

Axial in-phase MR shows homogeneous liver parenchyma. No focal lesions are seen.

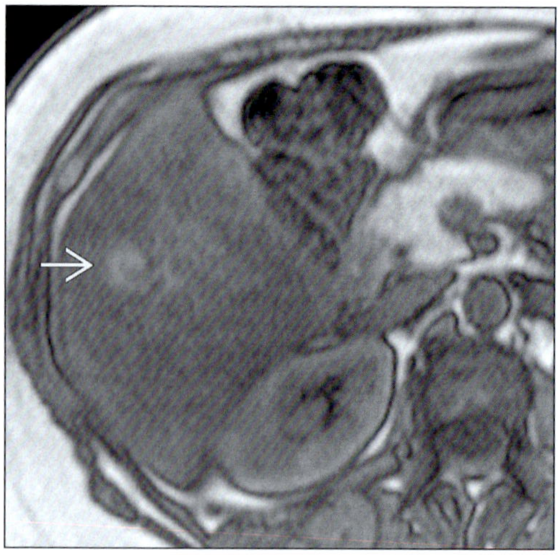

Axial opposed-phase T1WI MR in the same patient shows diffuse loss of liver parenchymal signal and a well-defined nodule ➔ of relatively high signal intensity.

CLINICAL SCENARIO

History

- 67-year-old man with history of colon cancer presented for staging

IMAGE INTERPRETATION

Pitfalls

- Well-defined liver nodule(s) in background of diffuse hepatic steatosis may be mistaken for metastatic deposit(s) or other focal liver lesion(s)

Actual Diagnosis

- Nodular fatty sparing in patient with hepatic steatosis

Clues to Correct Diagnosis

- Nodular fatty sparing is typically accompanied by segmental areas of fatty sparing
- Nodules are not seen on in-phase T1WI and best seen on opposed-phase T1WI
- Nodules are barely seen or slightly hypointense on T2WI
  - Metastases, however, are almost always hyperintense

Differential Diagnosis

- Fatty sparing can occur around focal lesions such as hemangiomas and metastases
  - Characteristic imaging features of focal lesion may be apparent within area of fatty sparing
  - DWI can be used to reveal metastases obscured by focal fatty sparing

BACKGROUND

General

- Focal fatty sparing usually has geographic configuration and occurs at characteristic locations within liver
  - Segments IV and V near gallbladder fossa
  - Around porta hepatis
- Nodular fatty sparing is rare

IMAGING FEATURES

US

- Nodular areas of decreased echogenicity within liver displaying diffuse increased echogenicity

CT

- Nodules of increased attenuation, similar to splenic enhancement, against background of diffuse decreased hepatic attenuation

MR

- T1WI
  - In-phase: No lesions are seen
  - Opposed-phase: Islands of high signal intensity against background of low signal intensity
    - Due to diffuse liver parenchymal signal loss resulting from diffuse steatosis
- T2WI
  - Lesions are barely seen or slightly hypointense relative to fatty infiltrated liver parenchyma
  - Lesions are not seen on T2WI FS
- T1WI C+ FS
  - Homogeneous enhancement, similar in degree to splenic enhancement

PET/CT

- Focal FDG uptake masquerading as hepatic metastasis has been described

RELATED REFERENCES

1. Purandare NC et al: Focal fat spared area in the liver masquerading as hepatic metastasis on F-18 FDG PET imaging. Clin Nucl Med. 33(11):802-5, 2008
2. Tom WW et al: Hepatic pseudotumor due to nodular fatty sparing: the diagnostic role of opposed-phase MRI. AJR Am J Roentgenol. 183(3):721-4, 2004

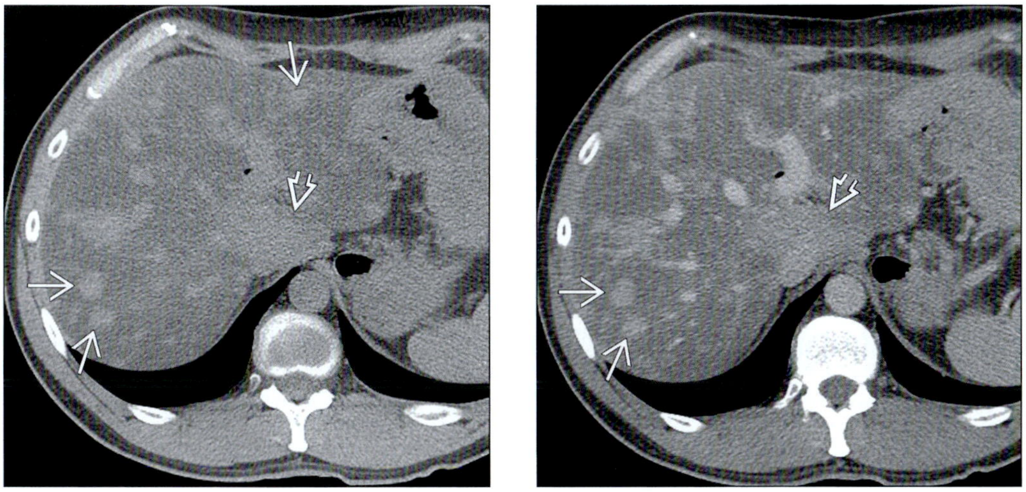

***(Left)** Axial NECT in a 59-year-old man with history of colon cancer shows a diffuse decrease in hepatic attenuation (0-10 HU) with multiple well-defined, rounded nodules ➡. There is also increased attenuation within the caudate lobe ⇨. **(Right)** Axial CECT in the same patient shows enhancing liver nodules ➡ and caudate lobe ⇨. The degree of enhancement is similar to that of the spleen. Because of the history, the possibility of metastatic disease was suggested.*

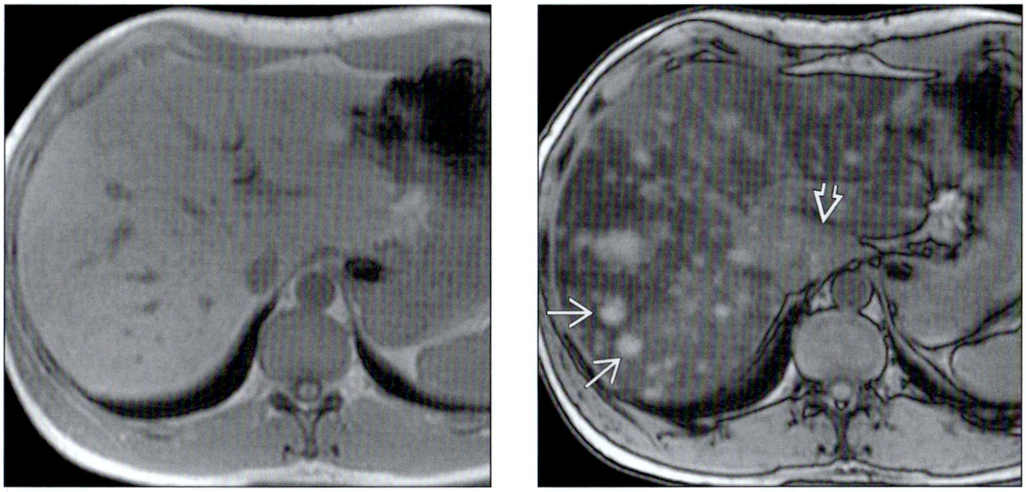

***(Left)** Axial in-phase T1WI MR in the same patient shows homogeneous liver parenchyma. No focal lesions are seen corresponding to the CT abnormalities. **(Right)** Axial opposed-phase T1WI MR in the same patient shows diffuse loss of signal compared with in-phase image due to diffuse hepatic steatosis. Islands of normal hepatic tissue that are spared from fatty infiltration are seen as well-defined nodular ➡ and segmental ⇨ areas against a background of low signal intensity.*

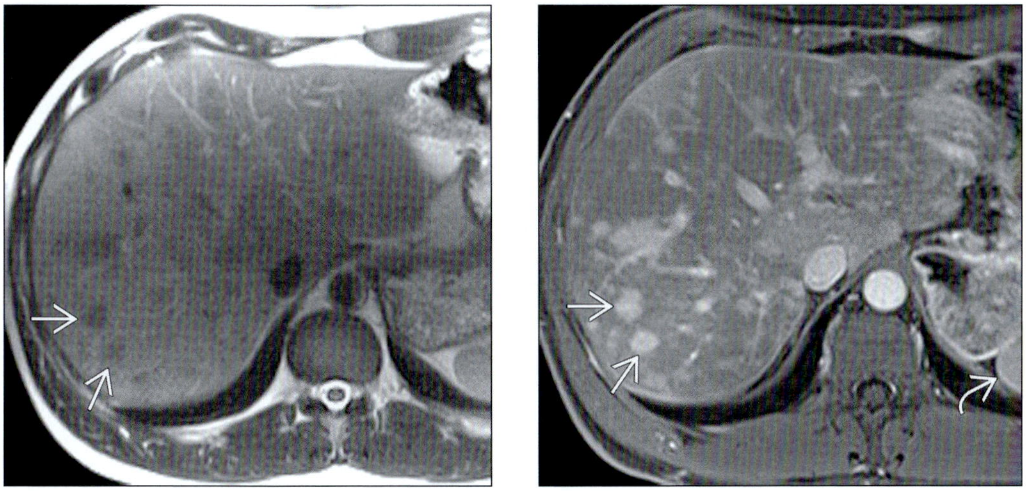

***(Left)** Axial T2WI MR in the same patient shows areas of nodular fatty sparing as nodules ➡ of low signal intensity. Metastases, on the other hand, should be expected to have high signal intensity. **(Right)** Axial T1WI C+ FS MR in the same patient shows enhancing nodular liver lesions ➡. The degree of enhancement is similar to that of the spleen ↪.*

PERIVASCULAR HEPATIC STEATOSIS

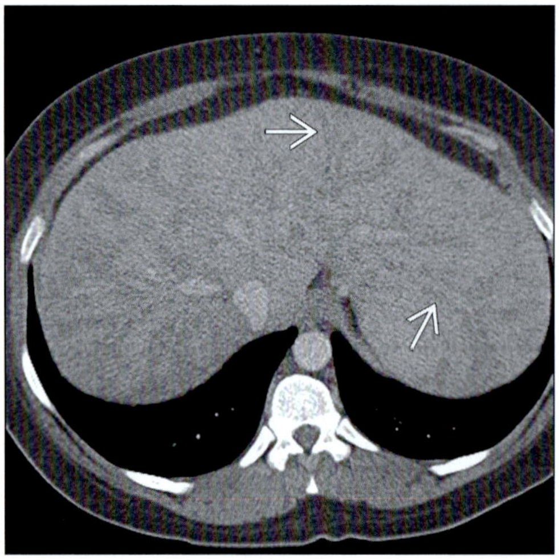

Axial CECT in a 47-year-old woman who presented with abdominal pain shows branching hypoattenuating areas ➡ surrounding the hepatic vein branches and involving both the right and left lobes.

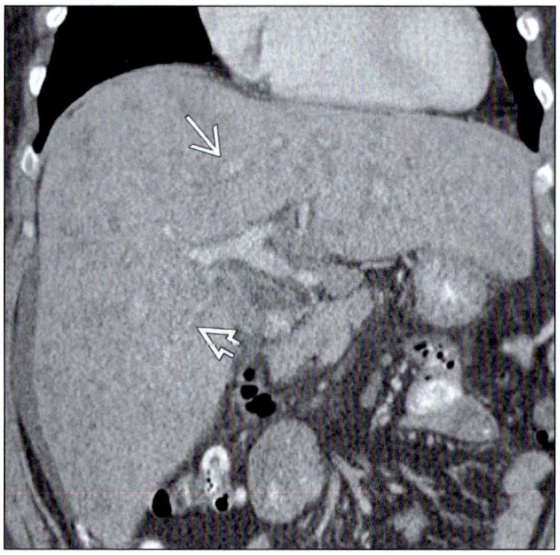

Coronal CECT in the same patient shows branching hypoattenuating areas surrounding the hepatic vein branches ➡ as well as the portal vein branches ⇨. Areas of low attenuation measured around 30 HU.

CLINICAL SCENARIO

History

- 34-year-old woman with history of excessive alcohol intake presented with severe abdominal pain and jaundice

Relevant Laboratory Tests

- Markedly elevated liver function tests

IMAGE INTERPRETATION

Pitfalls

- Perivascular areas of low attenuation of liver showing tram-like configuration for vessel segments parallel to imaging plane, and a ring-like or round configuration for vessel segments perpendicular to imaging plane
  - Can be seen around hepatic veins &/or portal veins
- This pattern can be confused with other vascular and neoplastic conditions that may affect the liver, e.g., Budd-Chiari syndrome

Actual Diagnosis

- Perivascular hepatic steatosis in alcoholic cirrhosis

Clues to Correct Diagnosis

- Measurement of HU in perivascular areas shows attenuation < 40 HU
- Pattern of hepatic steatosis in a perivascular distribution is characteristic of alcoholic cirrhosis

BACKGROUND

Relevant Pathology

- Pathogenesis of perivascular steatosis is not known
- Pattern has been described mainly in alcoholic cirrhosis
  - In our experience, this pattern can progress to diffuse hepatic steatosis
  - Pattern has also been described in
    - HIV
    - Patients undergoing intrahepatic islet cell transplantation

IMAGING FEATURES

US

- Perivascular hyperechogenicity of liver in comparison with kidney, attenuation of ultrasound beam by liver, and poor visualization of intrahepatic structures

CT

- NECT
  - Perivascular areas of absolute attenuation < 40 HU and relative attenuation at least 10 HU < spleen
- CECT
  - Perivascular areas of absolute attenuation < 40 HU

MR

- Perivascular areas of signal drop on opposed-phase T1WI compared to in-phase T1WI

PET/CT

- Areas of perivascular steatosis should not have increased metabolic activity

RELATED REFERENCES

1. Décarie PO et al: Fatty liver deposition and sparing: a pictorial review. Insights Imaging. 2(5):533-538, 2011
2. Hamer OW et al: Fatty liver: imaging patterns and pitfalls. Radiographics. 26(6):1637-53, 2006
3. Hamer OW et al: Imaging features of perivascular fatty infiltration of the liver: initial observations. Radiology. 237(1):159-69, 2005
4. Markmann JF et al: Magnetic resonance-defined periportal steatosis following intraportal islet transplantation: a functional footprint of islet graft survival? Diabetes. 52(7):1591-4, 2003

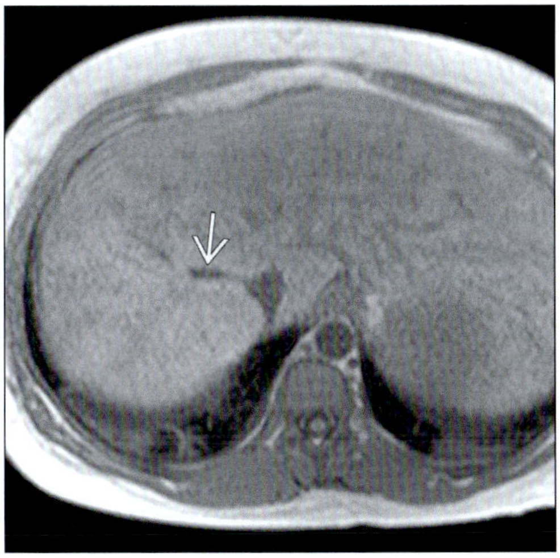

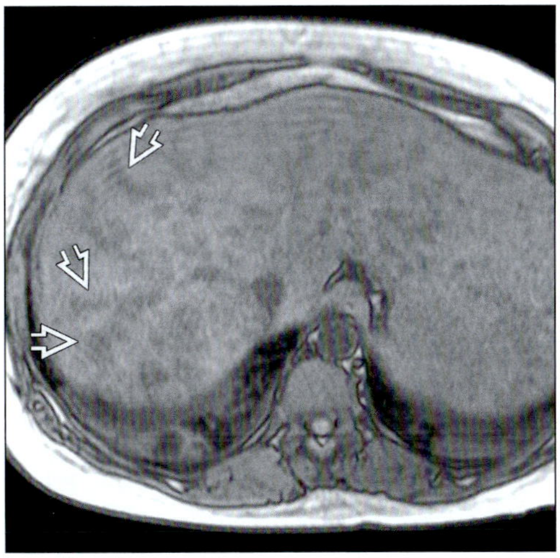

(Left) *Axial in-phase T1WI MR in a 34-year-old woman with history of alcoholism shows more or less homogeneous liver parenchymal signal intensity, no focal masses. The liver appears slightly voluminous with small attenuated hepatic vein* ➔. ***(Right)*** *Axial opposed-phase T1WI MR in the same patient shows branching low signal intensity structures* ➲ *in a perivascular distribution. The signal drop on opposed-phase images compared to in-phase images is due to the presence of fat.*

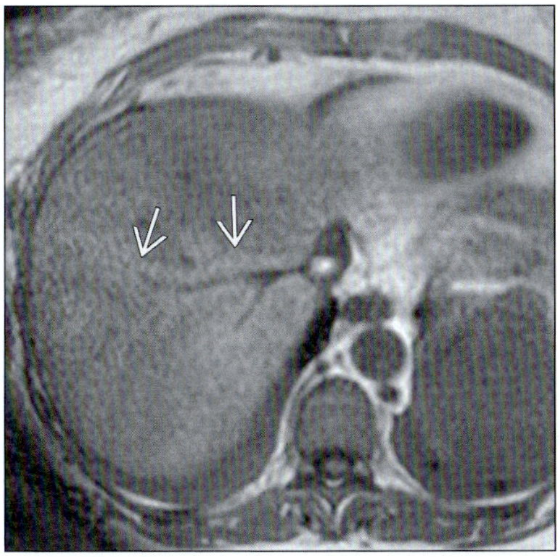

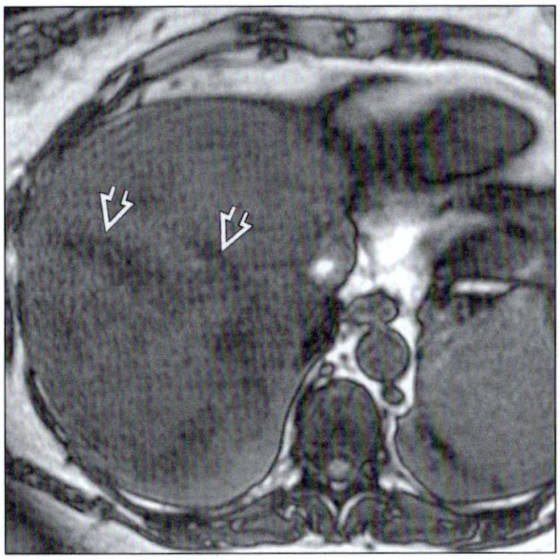

(Left) *Axial in-phase T1WI MR in a 58-year-old man with abdominal pain and history of excessive alcohol intake shows areas of subtle increased signal intensity around the hepatic veins* ➔. ***(Right)*** *Axial opposed-phase T1WI MR in the same patient shows signal drop in the perivascular areas of high signal intensity on the in-phase images* ➲*, consistent with fatty infiltration.*

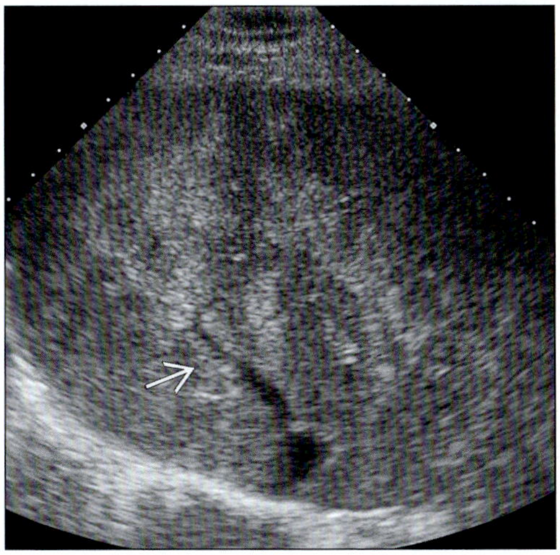

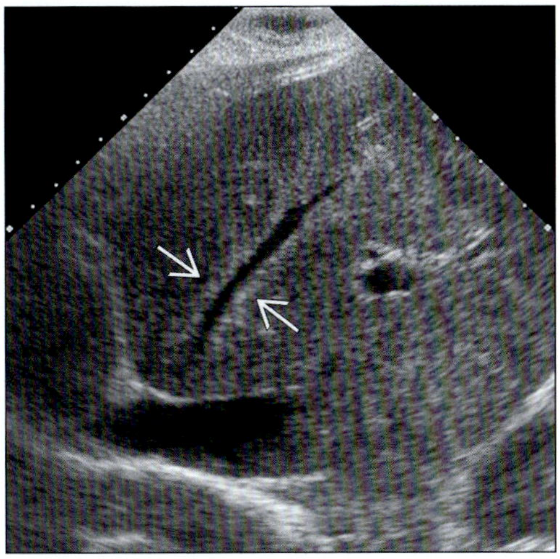

(Left) *Axial grayscale abdominal US in a 48-year-old woman with history of alcoholism who presented with liver failure shows heterogeneous liver echogenicity with stripes of increased echogenicity centered around the vascular structures* ➔. ***(Right)*** *Sagittal grayscale abdominal US in the same patient shows increased echogenicity centered around the hepatic vein* ➔.

DIFFUSE METASTASIS

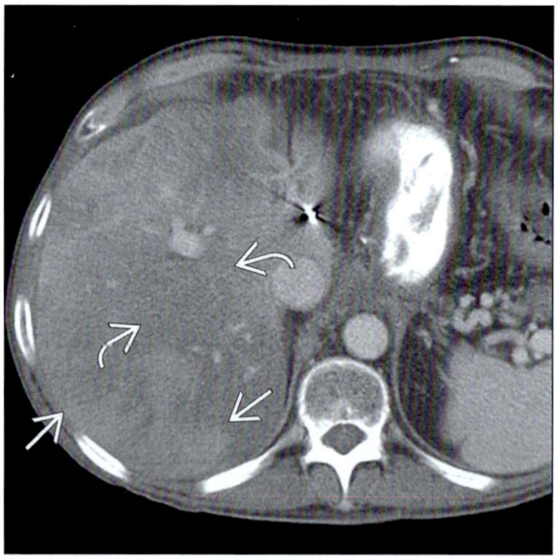

Axial CECT shows geographic and focal regions of decreased attenuation ➨ throughout the liver with coalescent areas of peripheral relatively increased density ➔.

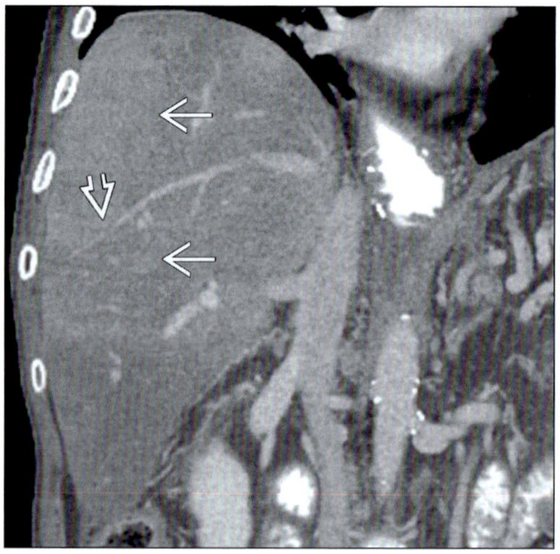

Coronal CECT shows coalescent peripheral hyperdense areas ➔, with mild irregularity of peripheral hepatic veins ➨. Mild bulge is present along the superolateral aspect of the right hepatic lobe.

CLINICAL SCENARIO

History

- 49-year-old man with gastric carcinoma

IMAGE INTERPRETATION

Pitfalls

- Steatosis limits evaluation for hepatic masses
- Diffuse metastases can mimic diffuse fatty infiltration

Actual Diagnosis

- Coalescent peripheral hepatic metastases superimposed on diffuse central fatty infiltration

Clues to Correct Diagnosis

- Normal vessels are not seen coursing through tumor
- Fatty infiltration and fatty sparing have typical distribution
- Bulging of liver capsule suggests presence of tumor

BACKGROUND

Relevant Physiology

- Steatosis: Excessive accumulation of triglycerides within hepatocytes, can occur focally or diffusely
- Metastases seed to liver from gastric cancer via portal circulation

IMAGING FEATURES

US

- Steatosis
  - Echogenic, only apparent when amount of fat reaches 15-20% of liver volume
- Metastases
  - Focal metastases are most commonly hypoechoic
  - Infiltrative metastases may be difficult to detect

CT

- Steatosis
  - Geographic distribution typically within segment IV anteriorly, adjacent to vessels, ligaments, & fissures
  - Vessels coursing through are not displaced (no mass effect)
  - NECT: Decreased attenuation compared to spleen (normally, liver is 8-10 HU > spleen)
  - Focal fatty sparing: Segment V or gallbladder fossa
- Diffuse hepatic metastases
  - Confluent tumor distorts vessels and bile ducts
  - Hepatic metastases can be iso-, hypo-, or hyperdense

MR

- Modality of choice
- Hepatic steatosis: Characteristic drop of signal on out-of-phase compared to in-phase T1WI
- Hepatic metastases: No drop of signal on out-of-phase compared to in-phase
  - T2WI: Increased signal intensity
  - T1WI C+: Improves detection of liver metastases
  - DWI: Restricted diffusion is present in metastases

PET/CT

- Hepatic steatosis: Normal FDG uptake
- Hepatic metastases: Increased FDG activity

Key Teaching Points

- Diffuse and focal fatty infiltration can mimic hepatic metastases and vice versa
- Diffuse fatty liver limits evaluation of hepatic masses
- Vessels are not distorted as they travel through hepatic steatosis in comparison to tumor
- Fatty infiltration and sparing have typical distribution
- MR can be helpful in inconclusive cases

RELATED REFERENCES

1. Abele JT et al: Effect of hepatic steatosis on liver FDG uptake measured in mean standard uptake values. Radiology. 254(3):917-24, 2010
2. Boll DT et al: Diffuse liver disease: strategies for hepatic CT and MR imaging. Radiographics. 29(6):1591-614, 2009

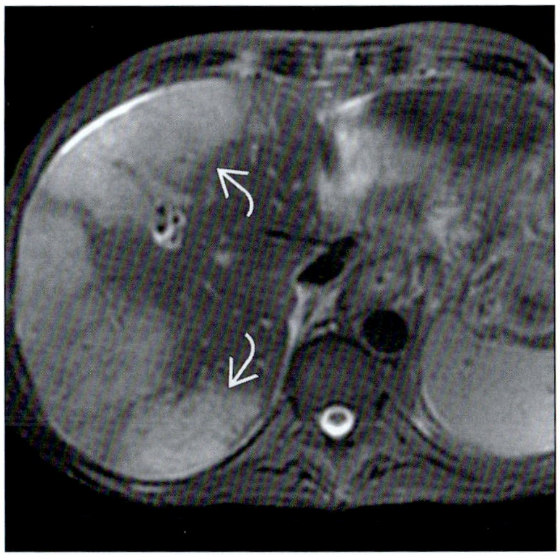

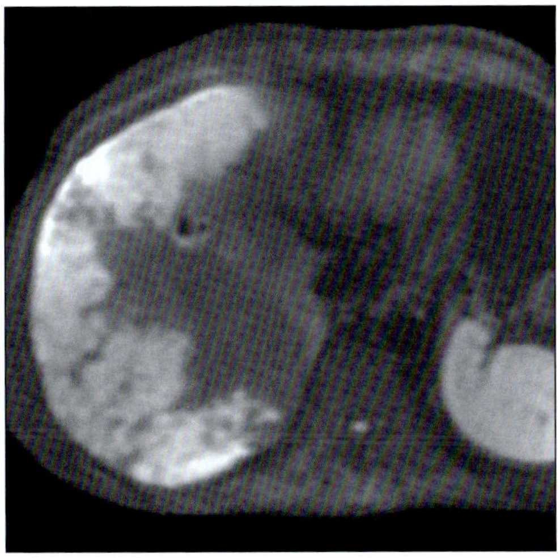

(Left) *Axial T2WI MR demonstrates confluent areas of increased signal intensity involving the peripheral right hepatic lobe, representing hepatic metastases.* ***(Right)*** *Axial DWI MR demonstrates confluent areas of increased signal intensity, indicating restricted diffusion in the same region, representative of hepatic metastases. (Corresponding ADC images not shown.)*

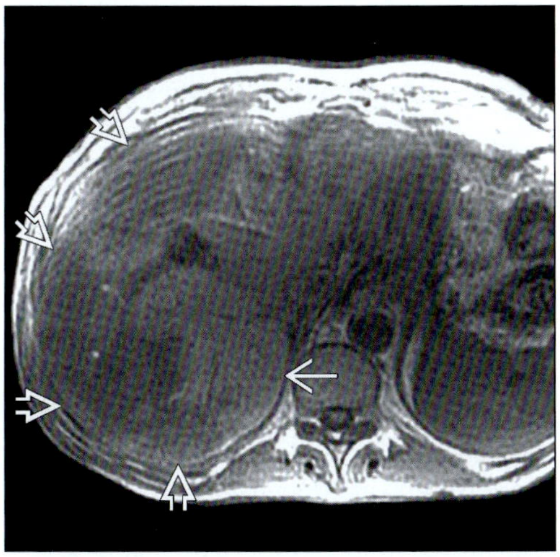

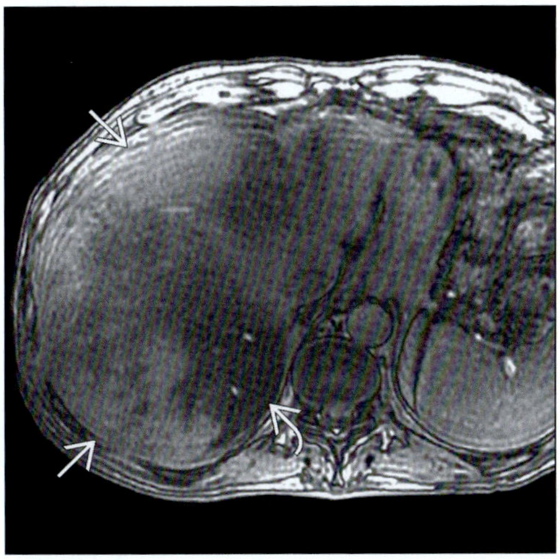

(Left) *Axial in-phase T1WI MR demonstrates heterogeneous liver with geographic areas. The central regions appear relatively hyperintense compared to the peripheral hypointense regions of the liver.* ***(Right)*** *Axial out-of-phase T1WI MR demonstrates central drop of signal intensity on out-of-phase compared to in-phase, compatible with diffuse fatty infiltration. The peripheral regions do not demonstrate this signal drop.*

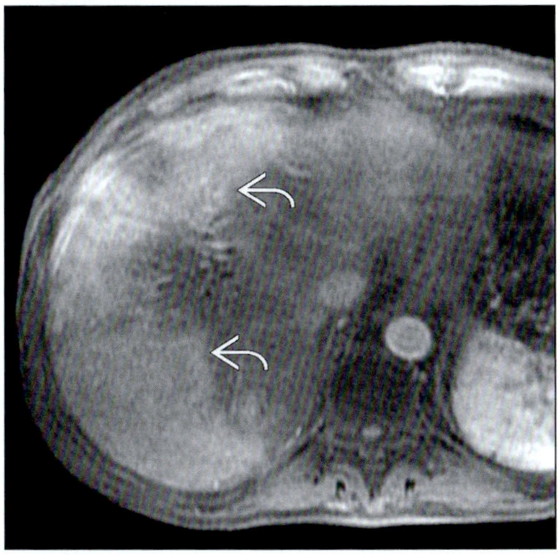

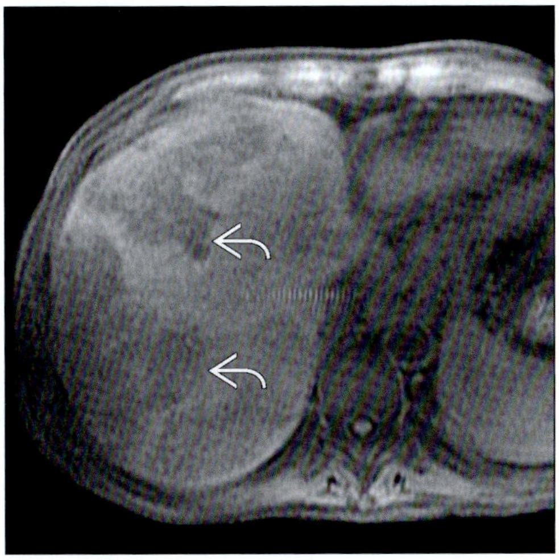

(Left) *Axial T1WI C+ FS MR in arterial phase post IV administration of gadoxetate disodium [Eovist]) demonstrates intense enhancement of large coalescent areas in the periphery of the right hepatic lobe.* ***(Right)*** *Axial T1WI C+ FS MR (20-minute delayed post IV administration of gadoxetate disodium [Eovist]) shows hypointensity (washout) of the arterially enhanced areas, compatible with infiltrative metastases.*

TRANSIENT HEPATIC ATTENUATION DIFFERENCE

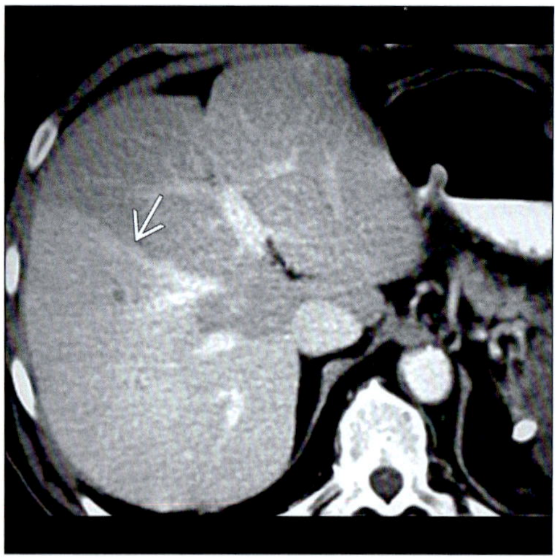

Axial CECT in arterial phase demonstrates an enhancing, smoothly marginated, large wedge-shaped area ➡ representing THAD.

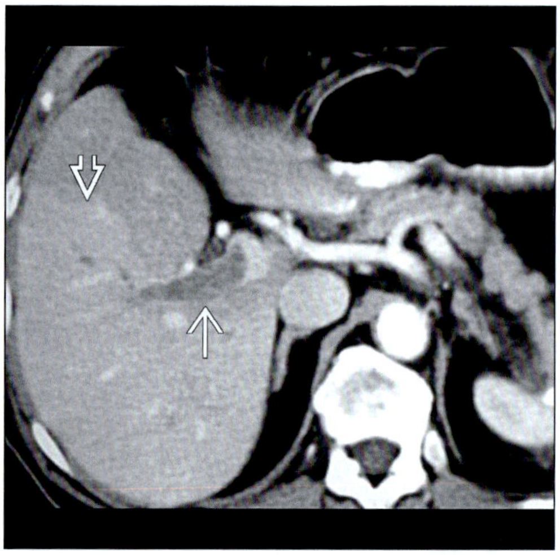

Axial CECT in portal venous phase shows nonenhancement of the right portal vein, which is filled by a thrombus ➡, causing the THAD ⇨. Note the decreased enhancement of THAD.

CLINICAL SCENARIO

History

- 73-year-old woman undergoing MR to rule out liver abnormality seen on CT

IMAGE INTERPRETATION

Pitfalls

- Can be mistaken for other enhancing focal liver lesions
- If seen on CECT or MR, extensive search must be made for underlying obstructive mass or portal vein thrombus

Actual Diagnosis

- On CT, transient hepatic attenuation difference (THAD)
- On MR, transient hepatic intensity difference (THID)

Clues to Correct Diagnosis

- Wedge-shaped subcapsular area of enhancement on arterial phase, which usually has subsegmental distribution
  - Demonstrates fading and subsequently becomes isoattenuating on portal venous phase

BACKGROUND

Relevant Physiology

- Liver is supplied by 2 sources of blood: Portal vein (PV) (75%) and hepatic artery (HA) (25%)
- Phenomenon results from compensatory ↑ in arterial flow when portal flow ↓
  - Also loss of diluting effect of nonenhanced portal venous blood at level of hepatic lobule

Pathogenesis

- THID/THAD without focal lesion secondary to
  - Portal hypoperfusion due to PV branch compression or thrombosis → segmental (wedge-shaped with straight border)
  - Flow diversion caused by arterioportal shunt or by an anomalous blood supply → multisegmental THAD
  - Inflammation of biliary vessels or adjacent organs
  - Can also be polymorphous or diffuse
- THID/THAD with a focal lesion secondary to
  - Siphoning effect → lobar multisegmental shape

IMAGING FEATURES

US

- May be visualized on contrast-enhanced US
- Referred to as transient hepatic echogenicity differences

CT

- Increased enhancement on early arterial phase imaging that fades on subsequent images
- Distribution pattern can vary depending on underlying cause
- There may be associated liver lesions (e.g., metastasis, hemangioma, etc.) or background of liver disease from a variety of causes (e.g., cirrhosis or inflammation)

MR

- T1WI C+: Similar to CT with increased enhancement on early arterial phase imaging that fades on subsequent images
- T2WI: No corresponding signal abnormality

RELATED REFERENCES

1. Catalano O et al: Transient hepatic echogenicity difference on contrast-enhanced ultrasonography: sonographic sign and pitfall. J Ultrasound Med. 26(3):337-45, 2007
2. Colagrande S et al: Transient hepatic intensity differences: part 1, Those associated with focal lesions. AJR Am J Roentgenol. 188(1):154-9, 2007
3. Colagrande S et al: Transient hepatic intensity differences: part 2, Those not associated with focal lesions. AJR Am J Roentgenol. 188(1):160-6, 2007
4. Colagrande S et al: Transient hepatic attenuation differences. AJR Am J Roentgenol. 183(2):459-64, 2004

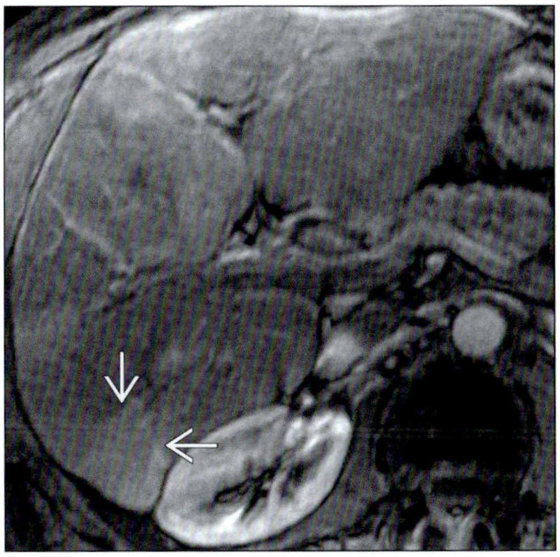
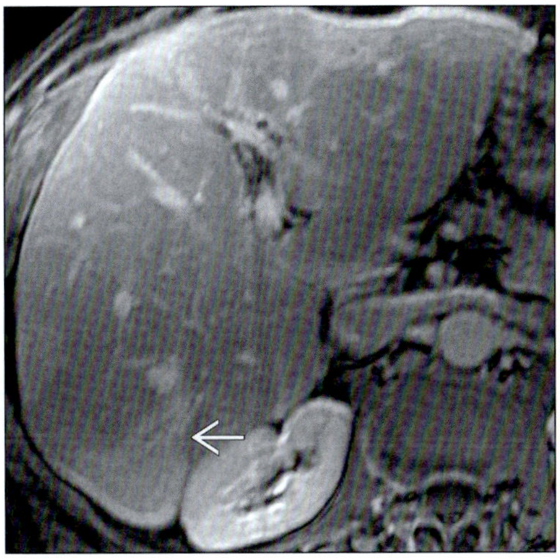

(Left) *Axial T1WI C+ MR in arterial phase demonstrates a wedge-shaped area of enhancement ➔ in the subcapsular region of the posterior segment of the right hepatic lobe.* ***(Right)*** *Axial T1WI C+ MR in delayed phase shows decreased enhancement of the wedge-shaped region ➔ within the right hepatic lobe, although this still remains slightly hyperintense relative to liver parenchyma.*

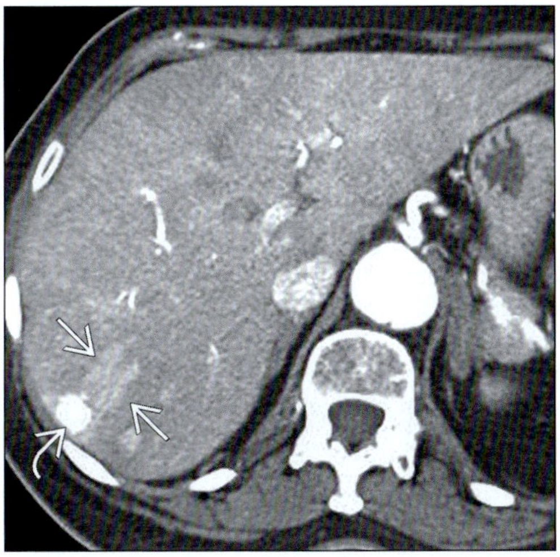
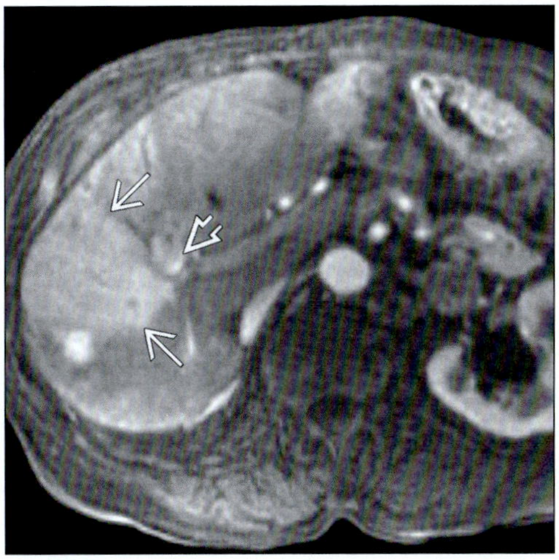

(Left) *Axial CECT in arterial phase in a 47-year-old man shows an enhancing, well-circumscribed lesion ➔ that demonstrated retention of enhancement in delayed phase (not shown), compatible with a small hemangioma. Associated wedge-shaped area of enhancement is noted, representing transient hepatic attenuation difference (THAD) ➔.* ***(Right)*** *Axial T1WI C+ MR in arterial phase in a 68-year-old woman with metastatic ovarian carcinoma demonstrates an enhancing metastasis ➔ causing THID ➔.*

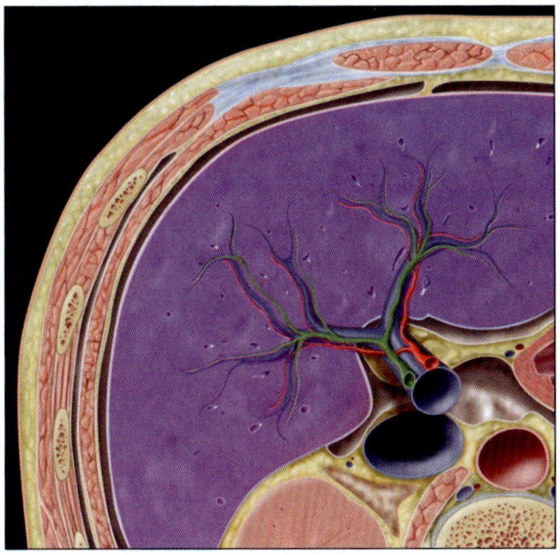
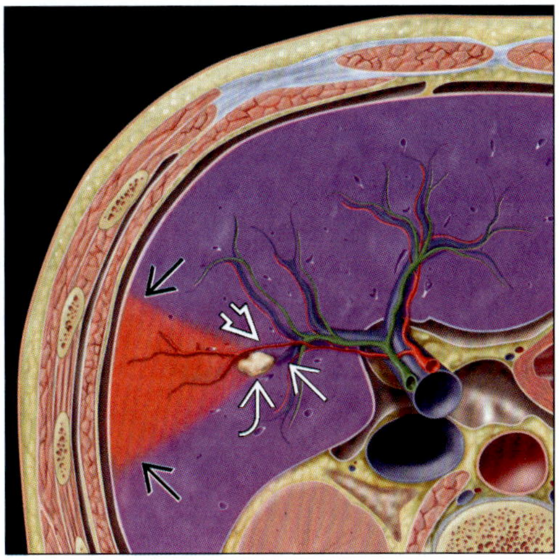

(Left) *Illustration of axial cross section of the liver demonstrates vascular blood supply of the liver; the majority is supplied by the portal vein (75%) more than the hepatic artery (25%).* ***(Right)*** *Illustration of axial cross section of the liver demonstrates a wedge-shaped area ➔, which is predominantly supplied by the patent hepatic arterial branch ➔. This represents THAD secondary to occlusion of a portal vein branch ➔ by a mass ➔.*

ABERRANT RIGHT GASTRIC VEIN DRAINAGE

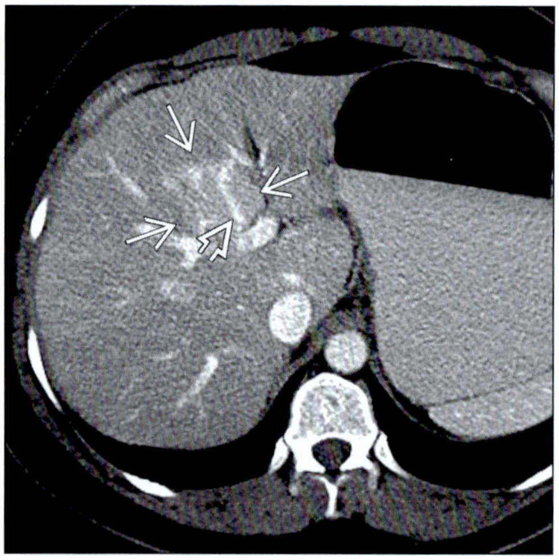

Axial CECT of the liver shows a mass-like area of enhancement ➡ involving the medial segment of the left lobe. An enhancing vessel ➡ is seen coursing through the area of enhancement.

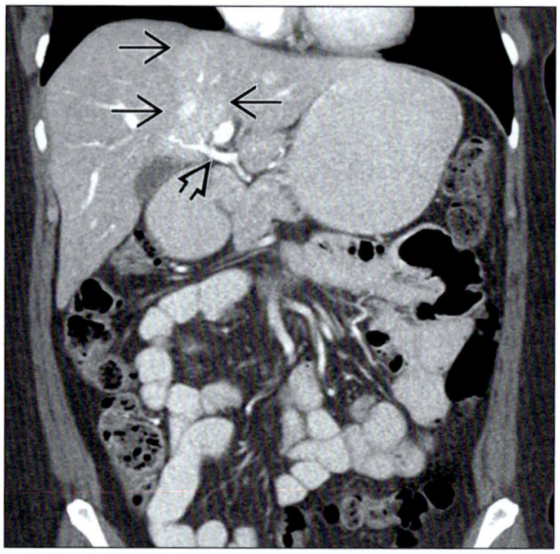

Coronal CECT shows a geographic area of enhancement ➡ involving the medial segment of the left lobe. A vessel ➡ is seen coursing into the liver parenchyma.

CLINICAL SCENARIO

History

- 53-year-old man with malignant melanoma of neck who is presenting for staging

IMAGE INTERPRETATION

Pitfalls

- Mass-like structure in segment IV of liver can be mistaken for enhancing mass, possibly metastatic in this patient with history of melanoma

Actual Diagnosis

- Pseudolesion due to aberrant right gastric vein (ARGV) draining directly into liver

Clues to Correct Diagnosis

- Typical location in posterior aspect of segment IV of liver
- Pseudolesion appears segmental and geographic
- ARGV can be seen coursing through area of relatively increased enhancement without obstruction or displacement

BACKGROUND

Relevant Anatomy

- Right gastric vein commonly drains into portal vein or splenic vein along lesser curvature of stomach
  - Aberrant gastric venous drainage occurs directly into liver

Relevant Physiology

- ARGV can cause pseudotumors in liver because it can cause focal area of fat sparing in fatty infiltrated liver
  - Substrates responsible for development of hepatic steatosis are delivered to liver through portal vein
- Different transit time of contrast in ARGV and portal vein can result in different degree of enhancement in segment supplied by ARGV compared to rest of liver

IMAGING FEATURES

US

- Focal area of sparing involving segment IV in fatty liver appears as low echogenicity relative to echogenic liver
- ARGV can be seen with color Doppler US

CT

- Focal area of increased enhancement can be seen posteriorly in segment IV, even in absence of fatty liver
  - Due to shorter contrast transit in gastric vein compared with portal vein
- Area of fatty sparing shows higher attenuation compared to rest of liver
- ARGV can be seen within area of fatty sparing and can be traced to lesser curvature of stomach

MR

- Area of fatty sparing shows no drop in signal on out-of-phase T1WI, whereas rest of liver shows signal drop compared to in-phase images
- Focal area of increased enhancement posteriorly in segment IV

PET/CT

- Normal metabolic activity of involved segment IV

RELATED REFERENCES

1. Seong NJ et al: Right gastric venous drainage: angiographic analysis in 100 patients. Korean J Radiol. 13(1):53-60, 2012
2. Yoon KH et al: Pseudolesion in segments II and III of the liver on CT during arterial portography caused by aberrant right gastric venous drainage. J Comput Assist Tomogr. 23(2):306-9, 1999
3. Matsui O et al: Focal sparing of segment IV in fatty livers shown by sonography and CT: correlation with aberrant gastric venous drainage. AJR Am J Roentgenol. 164(5):1137-40, 1995

HEMANGIOMA IN CIRRHOSIS

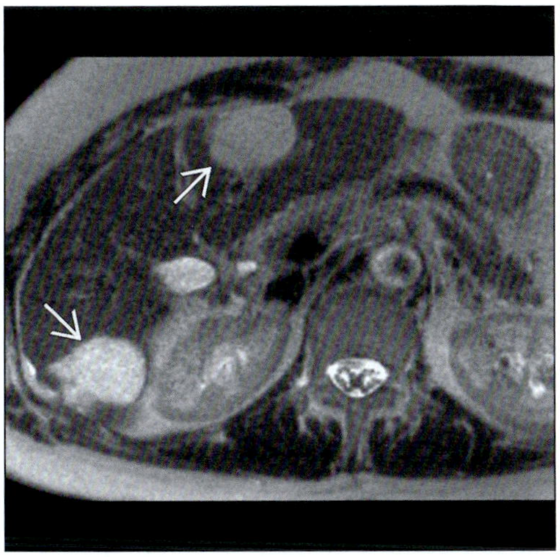

Axial T2WI MR demonstrates 2 well-circumscribed lesions ➔ within the left and right hepatic lobe exhibiting markedly high signal intensity.

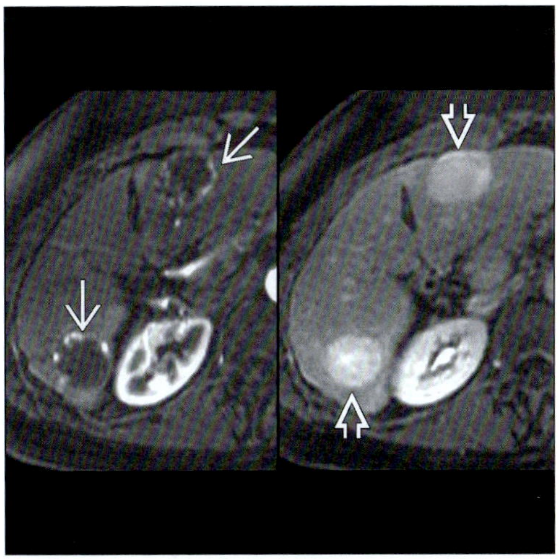

Axial T1WI C+ MR demonstrates early peripheral discontinuous nodular enhancement of the lesions on arterial phase ➔ with complete filling on delayed phase ⇨, typical for hemangiomas.

CLINICAL SCENARIO

History

- 52 year old with chronic liver disease

IMAGE INTERPRETATION

Pitfalls

- Due to rarity in cirrhotic liver, hemangioma is easily misdiagnosed as more common entities

Actual Diagnosis

- Hemangioma in background of cirrhosis

Clues to Correct Diagnosis

- It is important to ensure typical features of hemangioma when seeing vascular enhancing lesions in chronic liver disease patients
  - Retention of contrast on delayed phase

BACKGROUND

Epidemiology

- Hemangioma is most common benign hepatic neoplasm
- However, very rare incidence in advanced cirrhosis (2% of advanced cirrhosis in transplant specimens)

Relevant Pathology

- Hemangiomas are well-circumscribed benign tumors
- Variably sized vascular spaces lined by flat endothelial cells and myxoid or fibrous stroma

IMAGING FEATURES

US

- Well-circumscribed echogenic lesion with through transmission

CT

- NECT: Hypoattenuating
- Venous phase CECT: Peripheral nodular discontinuous enhancement
- Delayed phase CECT: Filling with contrast (centripetal extension with contrast)

MR

- Heterogeneous cirrhotic morphology of liver
- T1WI: Hypointense to liver
- T2WI: Hyperintense to liver
- T1WI C+ (venous phase): Peripheral nodular discontinuous enhancement
- T1WI C+ (delayed phase): Filling with contrast (centripetal extension with contrast)
- Enhancement should be more than that of liver parenchyma on delayed phase

Key Teaching Points

- Hemangioma is most common benign liver tumor
- Rare incidence in setting of advanced liver cirrhosis
- It is important, therefore, when detecting vascular enhancing lesions in liver in patients with chronic liver disease and considering diagnosis of hemangioma
  - Ensure typical features of hemangioma
  - Degree of enhancement appears more than that of liver parenchyma

RELATED REFERENCES

1. Elsayes KM et al: Focal hepatic lesions: diagnostic value of enhancement pattern approach with contrast-enhanced 3D gradient-echo MR imaging. Radiographics. 25(5):1299-320, 2005
2. Miller WJ et al: Malignancies in patients with cirrhosis: CT sensitivity and specificity in 200 consecutive transplant patients. Radiology. 193(3):645-50, 1994

HEMANGIOMA CHANGING MORPHOLOGY

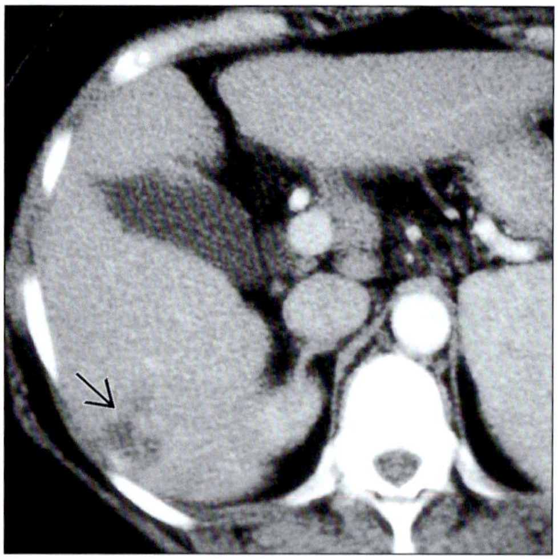

CECT in portal venous phase shows cirrhotic morphology of the liver (nodular outline, hypertrophied lateral segment of left lobe), with a well-defined lesion ➔ showing peripheral nodular enhancement.

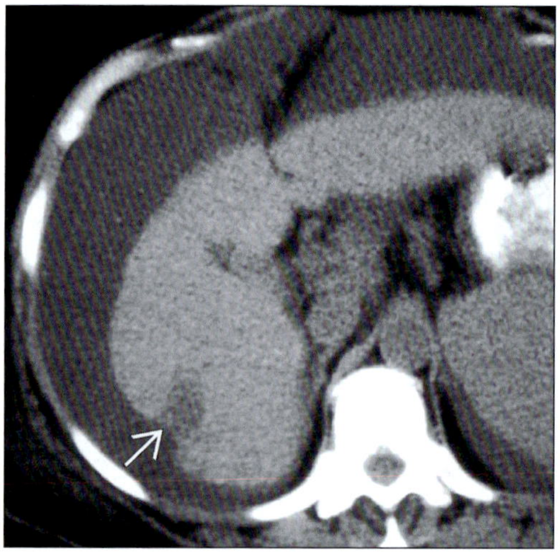

Follow-up NECT (18 months later) shows progressive diffuse liver scarring and shrinkage of liver volume, decreased size of the lesion ➔, and overlying capsular retraction, indicating scarring process.

CLINICAL SCENARIO

History

- 64-year-old man with chronic liver disease

IMAGE INTERPRETATION

Pitfalls

- Hemangioma changes morphology in cirrhotic liver; hence, it is important not to misdiagnose it as malignancy

Actual Diagnosis

- Hemangioma in cirrhotic liver

Clues to Correct Diagnosis

- Association with advanced cirrhosis
- Classic features of hemangioma on initial imaging
- Development of scarring and decrease in size on follow-up examination

BACKGROUND

Relevant Pathology

- Hypothesized that the rarity of hemangiomas in patients with advanced cirrhosis is due to fibrosis and scarring
- Fibrosis and scarring inherent in cirrhotic livers compress and collapse low-pressure systems in hemangioma
- Stasis occurs with thrombosis, eliminating the lesion and simulating fibrosis elsewhere in chronically scarred liver
- Not uncommon where hemangioma is initially seen, followed by shrinkage on follow-up examination

IMAGING FEATURES

US

- Well-circumscribed lesion with through transmission
- Changing morphology with shrinkage on follow-up examination with more advanced cirrhosis

CT

- Typical features of hemangioma on unenhanced, venous, and delayed phase
    - Low attenuation on NECT
    - Early peripheral nodular puddling
    - Centripetal extension of contrast on delayed phase
    - Enhancement pattern may deform on advanced cirrhosis
- Shrinking in size and morphology with developing scarring on follow-up imaging
    - Retraction of overlying capsule

MR

- Heterogeneous cirrhotic morphology of liver
- Typical features of hemangioma on unenhanced, venous, and delayed phases as well as T2WI
    - T1WI: Hypointense
    - T2WI: Hyperintense
    - T1WI C+: Typical enhancement may deform on advancing cirrhosis
- Shrinking in size and morphology with developing scarring on follow-up imaging

Key Teaching Points

- With advanced cirrhosis, hemangioma can change in morphology and decrease in size due to overlying scarring

RELATED REFERENCES

1. Galia M et al: Focal lesions in cirrhotic liver: what else beyond hepatocellular carcinoma? Diagn Interv Radiol. Epub ahead of print, 2014
2. de Caralt TM et al: Distortion of subcapsular hepatic hemangioma by hepatic cirrhosis. Can Assoc Radiol J. 50(2):137-8, 1999
3. Miller WJ et al: Malignancies in patients with cirrhosis: CT sensitivity and specificity in 200 consecutive transplant patients. Radiology. 193(3):645-50, 1994

HOT SPOT SIGN

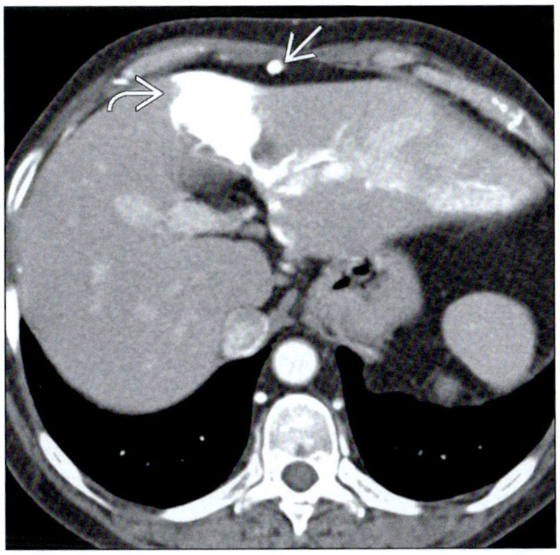

Axial CECT demonstrates intensely enhancing area ➯ within segment IV. Enhancing dilated structure anteriorly represents dilated paraumbilical vein ➔.

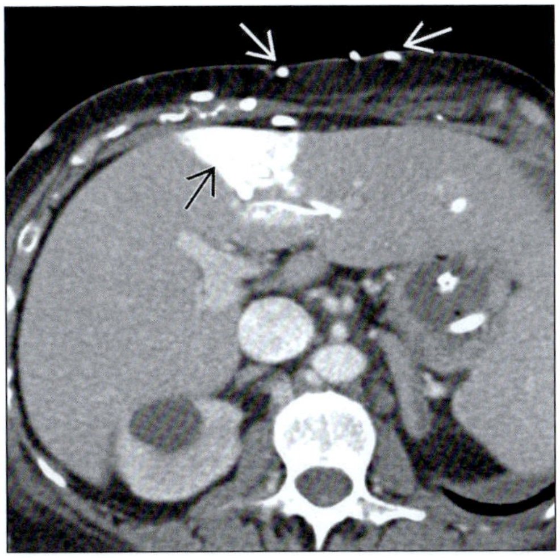

Axial CECT shows wedge-shaped area of intense enhancement in segment IV representing hepatic hot spot sign ➔. Note multiple dilated subcutaneous collaterals ➔.

CLINICAL SCENARIO

History

- 76-year-old woman with history of metastatic colorectal cancer

IMAGE INTERPRETATION

Pitfalls

- Wedge-shaped area of enhancement within segment IV mimics enhancing lesions, such as hepatic adenoma and hepatocellular carcinoma

Actual Diagnosis

- Hot spot sign due to superior vena cava (SVC) obstruction

Clues to Correct Diagnosis

- Early enhancement of segment IV in liver
- Multiple dilated tortuous anterior abdominal wall veins
- SVC occlusion
- Symptoms of dyspnea, facial swelling, headache, and pleural effusion

Key Point

- Presence of hot spot sign on abdominal CT or MR should prompt imaging of chest to identify cause of SVC obstruction

BACKGROUND

General

- Focal hot spot sign is thought to be due to portosystemic venous shunting between SVC and portal vein, causing intrahepatic areas of increased blood flow

Epidemiology

- SVC occlusion is most common cause
  - Caused by malignancies in 78-97% of cases; lung carcinoma and lymphoma are most common
  - Other causes include venous thrombosis due to indwelling catheters

Relevant Anatomy

- Anastomotic connection causing focal hot spot sign
  - Internal mammary vein to left portal vein via paraumbilical vein
- Other SVC obstruction collateral pathways
  - Azygous and hemiazygous veins
  - Lateral thoracic and vertebral veins
  - Thoracoepigastric and musculophrenic veins

IMAGING FEATURES

CT

- Arterial phase
  - Quadrate lobe may show area of intense enhancement ≥ that of aorta
- Portal venous phase
  - Partial washout, leaving area either hyperattenuating or isoattenuating

MR

- Early post-contrast enhancement in segment IV
- Isointensity on delayed phases

Tc-99m Sulfur Colloid Scans

- May show area of increased activity, or hot spot, in quadrate lobe

RELATED REFERENCES

1. Al-Makhzomi M et al: Abnormal liver uptake of (99m)Tc-macroaggregated albumin in a patient with superior vena cava syndrome. Am J Respir Crit Care Med. 187(9):1028, 2013
2. Katabathina VS et al: Imaging of oncologic emergencies: what every radiologist should know. Radiographics. 33(6):1533-53, 2013
3. Dickson AM: The focal hepatic hot spot sign. Radiology. 237(2):647-8, 2005

STARRY SKY APPEARANCE

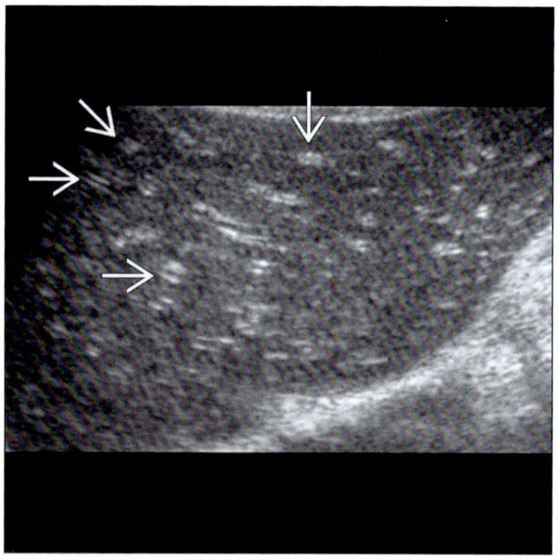

Transverse grayscale US shows centrilobular distribution of echogenic foci ➔ against a background of hypoechoic edematous liver parenchyma (starry sky appearance) due to acute viral hepatitis.

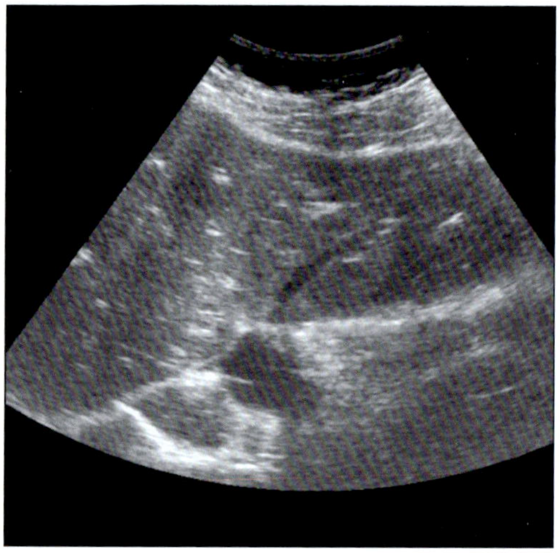

Transverse grayscale ultrasound examination in a 58-year-old woman with pain and jaundice demonstrates starry sky appearance secondary to cholestatic hepatitis.

CLINICAL SCENARIO

History

- 53-year-old man with RUQ pain, fever, and jaundice

IMAGE INTERPRETATION

Starry Sky Sign

- Classic for acute hepatitis
- Describes increased echogenicity around portal triads against background of hypoechoic liver parenchyma
- Nonspecific, seen with pathologies causing hepatocyte edema (e.g., Burkitt lymphoma, leukemia, toxic shock syndrome, fasting liver, & congestive hepatopathy)
- Seen in only 5% of acute hepatitis cases

BACKGROUND

General

- Acute hepatitis is a nonspecific inflammatory process of the liver, usually due to viral hepatitis
  - Other etiologies of hepatitis include autoimmune, alcohol, metabolic disorders, drug induced
- Self-limited, fulminant, or chronic hepatitis
- Imaging findings are nonspecific; thus, diagnosis usually based on clinical history, serology, and virology

Epidemiology

- Hepatitis A, B, and C are most common in USA
- Risk factors for HBV: High-risk sexual behavior and parenteral drug use (for HCV: Parenteral drug use and blood transfusion during 1980s)
- Worldwide prevalence of chronic HBV is 5%
- Chronic HBV → 50% of HCC worldwide

Relevant Physiology

- May be asymptomatic, but often presents with fever, RUQ pain, jaundice, hepatomegaly
- Diagnosis based on clinical findings, serology, virology

Relevant Pathology

- Acute hepatitis → edema of hepatocytes
- Leads to infiltration of different leukocyte types depending on chronicity of infection
- Stages of hepatitis → different severities of liver dysfunction, necrosis, fibrosis, & cirrhosis
- Chronic hepatitis B and C are risk factors for HCC

IMAGING FEATURES

General

- Nonspecific; hepatomegaly & periportal edema
- Imaging rules out other pathologies (e.g., extrahepatic cholestasis, diffuse metastases, cirrhosis)

US

- Starry sky centrilobular pattern described above
- Gallbladder wall thickening (especially in hepatitis A) due to inflammation and edema
- Contrasts with chronic hepatitis, which results in heterogeneous increased echogenicity of liver parenchyma

CT

- Hepatomegaly and heterogeneous enhancement
- Hypoattenuating bands parallel to portal vessels represent periportal edema

MR

- T2WI: Hyperintense bands parallel to portal vessels represent periportal edema
- T2WI: Irregular areas of parenchymal hyperintensity

RELATED REFERENCES

1. El-Serag HB: Epidemiology of viral hepatitis and hepatocellular carcinoma. Gastroenterology. 142(6):1264-1273, 2012
2. Abu-Judeh HH: The "starry sky" liver with right-sided heart failure. AJR Am J Roentgenol. 178(1):78, 2002
3. Tchelepi H et al: Sonography of diffuse liver disease. J Ultrasound Med. 21(9):1023-32; quiz 1033-4, 2002

TARGET LESION

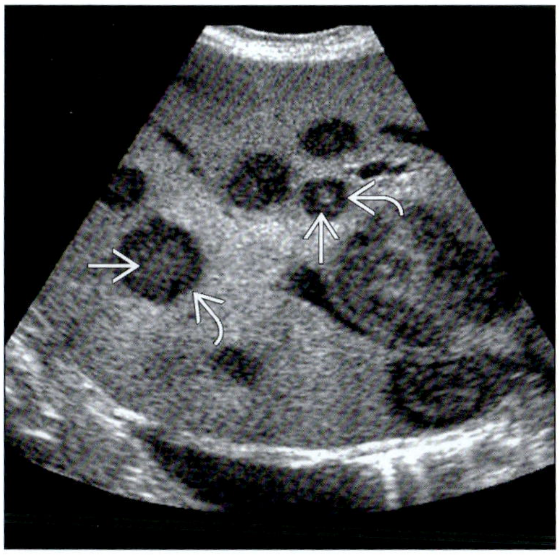

Transverse grayscale ultrasound of the liver reveals multiple target-like lesions. The lesions demonstrate central hyperechogenicity ➔ with a peripheral hypoechoic rim ➔.

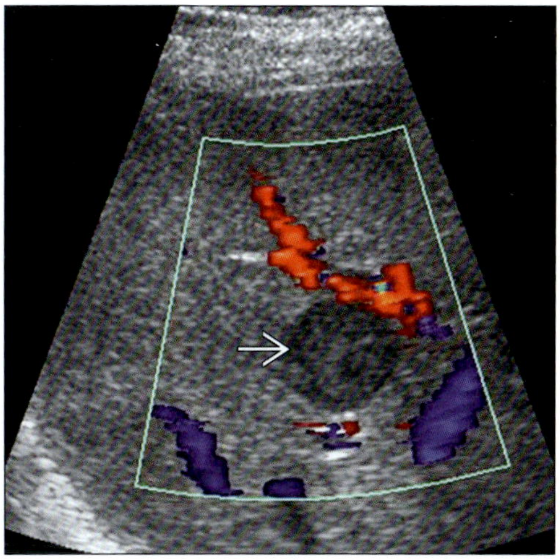

Color Doppler ultrasound of the liver reveals the target-like lesion ➔ with no evidence of abnormal color flow.

CLINICAL SCENARIO

History

- 45 year old with fever and right upper quadrant pain

IMAGE INTERPRETATION

Target Lesion

- Central echogenicity surrounded by hypoechoic rim
- Can be classic for abscess in proper clinical and laboratory settings
- Nonspecific: Can be seen in other conditions such as HCC, adenoma, and metastases

BACKGROUND

General

- Liver abscess is rare in healthy individuals
- Polymicrobial etiology in > 80% of cases in US
- Comorbidities: Diabetes or other immunocompromised
- Amebic abscess accounts for 10% of cases
- Fungal abscess (usually *Candida*) < 10% of cases
- Size: Few mm to > 10 cm; larger abscesses are usually of portal origin and smaller abscesses are usually of biliary origin
- Pyogenic abscess is usually treated by percutaneous drainage and antibiotics

Epidemiology

- Frequency: 8-16/100,000 hospitalized patients
- Causes of death: Sepsis, multiorgan & liver failure
- ↑ incidence with diverticulitis & ascending cholangitis
- Right lobe > left lobe

Relevant Physiology

- Biliary tract is most common source of pyogenic abscess
- Obstruction of bile flow (stones, cholangitis, malignancy) allows for bacterial proliferation
- Portal bed infection leads to septic thrombophlebitis
- Septic emboli get trapped by hepatic sinusoids and become nidus for microabscess formation

IMAGING FEATURES

US

- Variable appearance
  - Can be hypoechoic with minimal internal echoes
  - Target-like appearance with central echogenicity due to organizing fluid
  - Echogenic foci with posterior artifact 2° to gas
  - May contain septations

CT

- Well-circumscribed, low-attenuation lesions (0-50 HU)
- May contain gas or air-fluid levels
- Small abscesses may coalesce to form a large multiloculated lesion
- CECT: Occasional peripheral and septal enhancement
- Occasional associated segmental perfusion abnormality

MR

- T1WI: Typically hypointense (fungal infection may show mild hyperintensity)
- T2WI: Typically hyperintense (occasional hypointense septations) with hyperintense perilesional edema
- DWI: Increased signal intensity (restricted diffusion)
- T1WI C+: Occasional peripheral enhancement
  - Subcentimeter abscesses may show homogeneous enhancement

Nuclear Medicine

- Typically hot on gallium & WBC scans

RELATED REFERENCES

1. Alsaif HS et al: CT appearance of pyogenic liver abscesses caused by Klebsiella pneumoniae. Radiology. 260(1):129-38, 2011
2. Benedetti NJ et al: Imaging of hepatic infections. Ultrasound Q. 24(4):267-78, 2008

WATER LILY SIGN

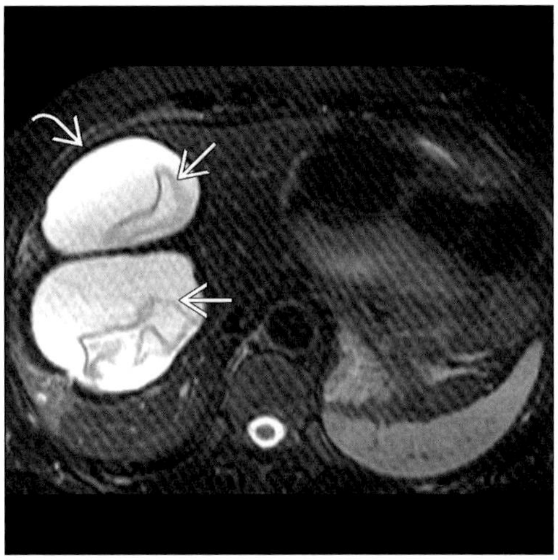

Axial T2WI MR of the liver shows a right hepatic lobe well-defined cystic mass ➡ with a "floating membrane" ➡ within the cavity, which is referred as the water lily sign.

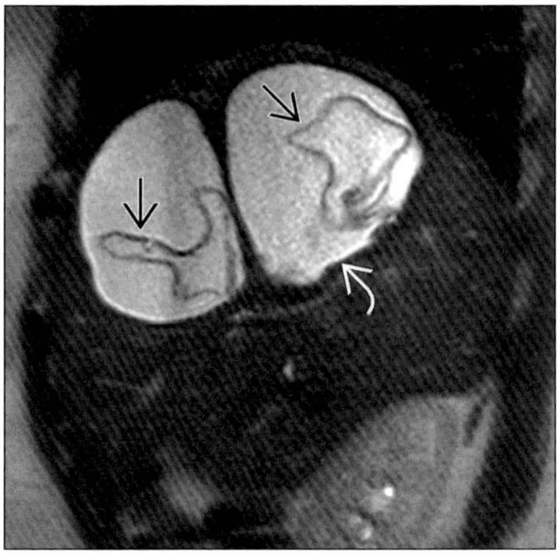

Sagittal T2WI MR shows the large, well-circumscribed cystic lesion ➡ with a wavy low signal intensity "floating membrane" ➡ within the cavity, which is referred as the water lily sign.

IMAGE INTERPRETATION

Appearance & Explanation

- Water lily sign is seen in hydatid infections when detachment of endocyst membrane → floating membranes within pericyst

Differential Diagnosis

- Main diagnostic possibilities for complex cystic masses
  - Biliary cystadenoma, abscess, cysts, amebic cysts, & calcifying lesions in liver (these do not have water lily sign)

BACKGROUND

Clinical Presentation

- Clinical severity is related to cyst size and location
- Most frequent sites are liver (mostly right lobe), lungs, muscles, bones, kidneys, brain, spleen, or heart
- Liver hydatid cyst may be asymptomatic in many cases or may present with an abdominal mass, abdominal pain, fatigue, weight loss, or jaundice
  - Cough, dyspnea, and chest pain if in lungs
  - Rupture of liver cysts in up to 58% of cases → pain, flushing, anaphylactic reaction, fever, & sepsis

Epidemiology

- Caused by *Echinococcus granulosus* (most common), *Echinococcus multilocularis* (most virulent), & *Echinococcus vogeli* (rarest)
- Tapeworms are zoonoses from dogs, cattle, & (most commonly) sheep
- Human is infected by ingesting at larval stage
- Endemic to Middle East, Africa, Iceland, Australia, & southern parts of South America but very rare in USA

Pathology

- Cysts usually have 3 components: Pericyst (inflammatory tissue of host origin), exocyst, endocyst (scolices [larval stage of parasite] and laminated membrane are produced here)
- Cyst classification
  - Type I: Simple cyst with no internal architecture
  - Type II: With daughter cyst(s)
    - Type IIa: Round daughter cysts at periphery
    - Type IIb: Larger, irregular daughter cysts occupying most of mother cyst
    - Type IIc: Oval masses with scattered calcifications & occasional daughter cysts
  - Type III: Calcified cyst (dead cyst)
  - Type IV: Complicated cyst (e.g., ruptured cyst)

IMAGING FINDINGS

Plain Radiography

- Occasional rim calcification in liver cyst or lung cavity

US

- Usually echogenic 2° to daughter cysts or membranes
- Daughter cysts can be either echogenic or anechoic
- Fragments may be seen in common bile duct

CT

- Fluid-filled masses, may have septations
  - May be multiple daughter cysts
- Wall may be calcified or enhance with contrast
- Inner layer of cyst may separate from outer layer → serpentine structure inside cyst (water lily sign)
- Multilocular cysts may have a honeycomb pattern

MR

- Multivesicular alveolar echinococcal lesions
- Best modality for characterizing cyst components
- T2WI: Areas of ↑ signal intensity (SI) correspond to small cystic or necrotic components, & areas of ↓ SI correspond to fibrotic or collagenous components

RELATED REFERENCES

1. Gwee A et al: The water lily sign. J Pediatr. 162(6):1294, 1294, 2013
2. Hamid R et al: Hydatid cyst of liver: Spontaneous rupture and cystocutaneous fistula formation in a child. J Indian Assoc Pediatr Surg. 17(2):73-4, 2012

PERIPHERAL WASHOUT

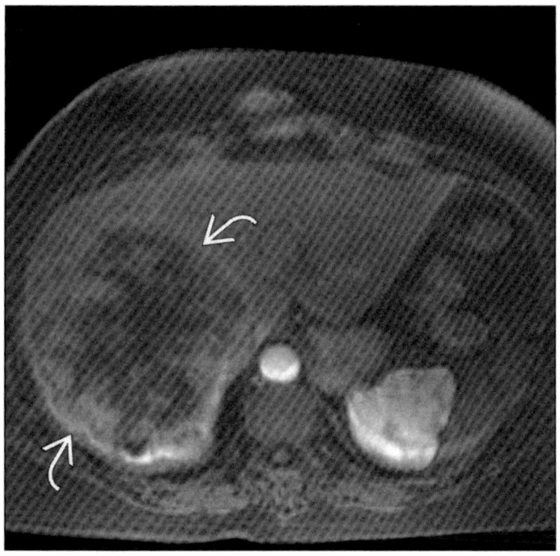

Axial T1WI C+ MR in arterial phase demonstrates a large, heterogeneously enhancing mass within the right hepatic lobe with peripheral enhancement ➔ and without significant enhancement in the center.

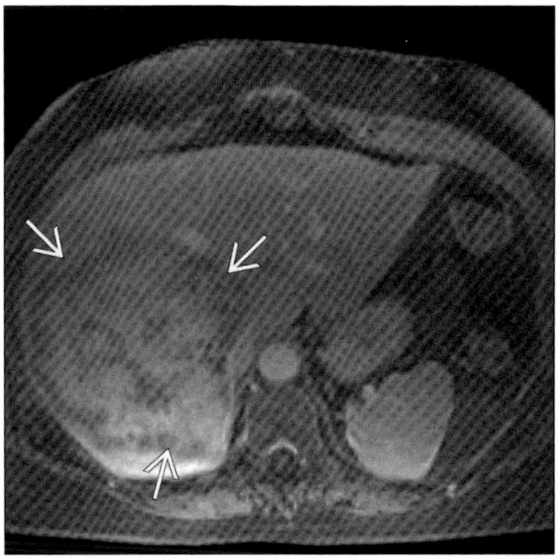

Axial T1WI C+ MR in delayed phase demonstrates central enhancement of the lesion with a hypointense peripheral rim ➔, so-called peripheral washout.

CLINICAL SCENARIO

History
- 53-year-old man with history of colon adenocarcinoma

IMAGE INTERPRETATION

Pitfalls
- Focal hepatic lesions can be mistaken for benign liver lesions such as hemangiomas

Actual Diagnosis
- Metastatic deposit secondary to colon adenocarcinoma

Clues to Correct Diagnosis
- Peripheral washout is a specific sign for malignancy
- History of primary malignancy

BACKGROUND

Explanation
- Characterized by peripheral zone of decreased enhancement in some malignant lesions
- Can be explained by difference in vascularity and contents between periphery and center of tumor
  - Tumor overgrowing blood supply → ischemia, necrosis, and degeneration in center of lesion
  - Peripheral rim contains growing tumor margins with neovascularity

Significance
- Specific sign for differentiation between malignant and benign focal hepatic lesions
  - Seen only in malignant lesions
  - Absence of this sign in benign lesion can be explained by homogeneity of tissue characteristics of benign lesions

Differential Diagnosis
- Peripheral washout sign has been reported to occur in
  - Metastases 2° to carcinoid, colon carcinoma, breast carcinoma, and gastric carcinoma
  - Primary malignancy: Hepatocellular carcinoma and cholangiocarcinoma

IMAGING FEATURES

General
- Peripheral washout sign has been described to occur in 10-minute delayed phase of contrast-enhanced MR
- Based on our experience, this sign was also observed in delayed phase of CECT and in delayed post-contrast phases obtained < 10 minutes after IV contrast administration

MR
- T1WI: Variable signal of whole lesion, but more likely hypointense
- T2WI: Variable signal intensity of whole lesion, but more likely hyperintense
- T1WI C+
  - Peripheral rim (average 3.5 mm in thickness) typically enhances in early phase, then washes out in delayed phase
  - Center does not enhance in early phase, then enhances in delayed phase

PET/CT
- Increased FDG uptake of lesion

RELATED REFERENCES

1. Kanematsu M et al: Imaging liver metastases: review and update. Eur J Radiol. 58(2):217-28, 2006
2. Elsayes KM et al: Focal hepatic lesions: diagnostic value of enhancement pattern approach with contrast-enhanced 3D gradient-echo MR imaging. Radiographics. 25(5):1299-320, 2005
3. Mahfouz AE et al: Peripheral washout: a sign of malignancy on dynamic gadolinium-enhanced MR images of focal liver lesions. Radiology. 190(1):49-52, 1994

CENTRAL DOT SIGN

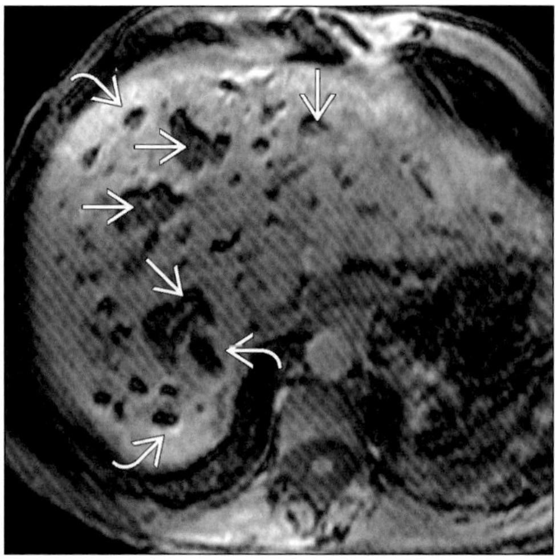

Axial T1WI C+ MR shows multiple hypointense lesions ➲ seen scattered in both hepatic lobes. Some appear tubular in morphology with tiny enhancing dots seen within some as a central dot ➔.

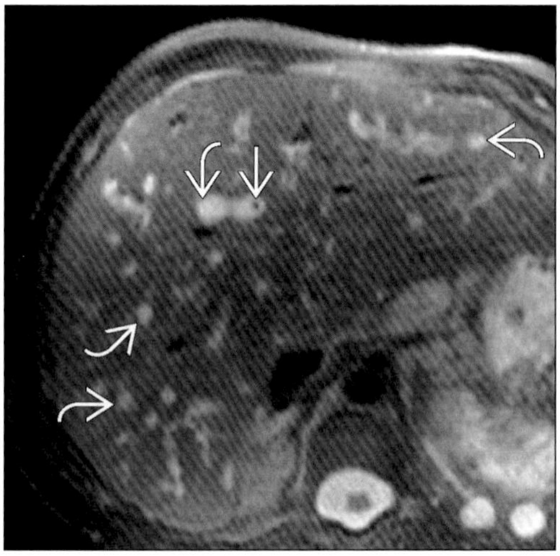

Axial T2WI demonstrates numerous lesions with high signal intensity ➲ and some lesions that have a central dot with a hypointense signal ➔.

CLINICAL SCENARIO

History

- 44-year-old woman with several-day history of right upper quadrant pain

IMAGE INTERPRETATION

Classic Sign

- Central dot sign is classic for Caroli disease

BACKGROUND

General

- Caroli disease is a rare autosomal-recessive condition
- Congenital cystic dilatation of intrahepatic bile ducts

Epidemiology

- Very rare (1/1,000,000)

Relevant Anatomy

- Although Caroli disease generally involves entire liver, it may be segmental or lobar

Relevant Pathology

- Multifocal cystic dilatation of intrahepatic biliary tree
- Central dot sign correlates to small portal venous branch protruding into dilated intrahepatic bile ducts
- 2 forms of Caroli disease have been described
  - Type 1: Less common "pure" form
  - Type 2: More complex form, associated with other ductal plate abnormalities such as hepatic fibrosis
- Often, patients clinically present with bouts of recurrent fever and right upper quadrant pain
- Complications
  - Bile stagnation, which leads to cholangitis and formation of calculi, which may result in biliary obstruction and jaundice
  - Cholangiocarcinoma has been reported to complicate Caroli disease in 7% of cases

IMAGING FEATURES

General

- Central dot sign is classic for Caroli disease

CT

- Multiple saccular dilatations of intrahepatic bile ducts
- Can be seen as numerous cystic lesions on axial sections
- Central dot sign in center of cystically dilated biliary tree
- Can detect complications of Caroli

US

- Multiple anechoic cysts, with possible central echogenic portal venous branch

PET/CT

- Multiple cystically dilated tubes appear photopenic

MR

- T1WI: Low signal intensity saccular structures demonstrating low signal intensity
- T2WI: High signal intensity tubular/saccular structures communicating with intrahepatic biliary ducts, with occasional central low signal intensity dots
- T1WI: Occasional central dot which enhances
- MRCP is most sensitive and specific
  - Will show abnormal cystic dilatation of intrahepatic bile ducts

RELATED REFERENCES

1. Lefere M et al: Caroli disease: review of eight cases with emphasis on magnetic resonance imaging features. Eur J Gastroenterol Hepatol. 23(7):578-85, 2011
2. Vachha B et al: Cystic lesions of the liver. AJR Am J Roentgenol. 196(4):W355-66, 2011
3. Yonem O et al: Clinical characteristics of Caroli's syndrome. World J Gastroenterol. 13(13):1934-7, 2007

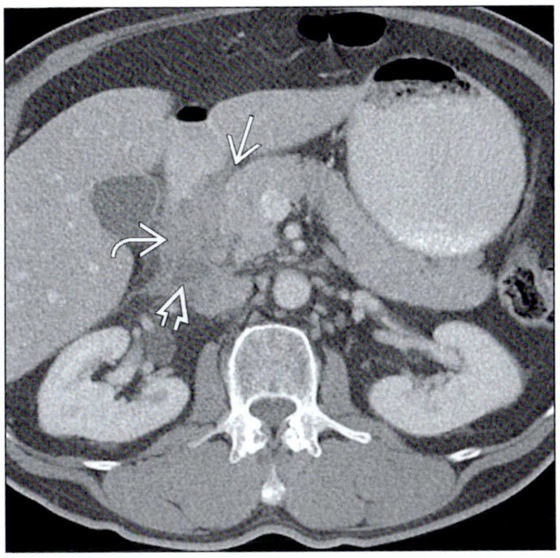

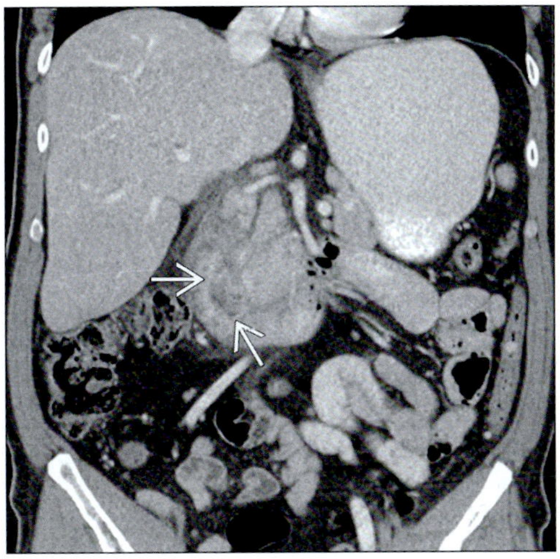

(Left) *Axial CECT in a 48-year-old man with history of alcohol abuse who presented with epigastric pain and abnormal liver function tests shows a relatively hypoenhancing, band-like mass* ↪ *involving the pancreaticoduodenal groove* ➔ *with some cystic changes* ⇨. ***(Right)*** *Coronal CECT in the same patient shows a relatively hypoenhancing, band-like mass* ➔ *in the pancreaticoduodenal groove.*

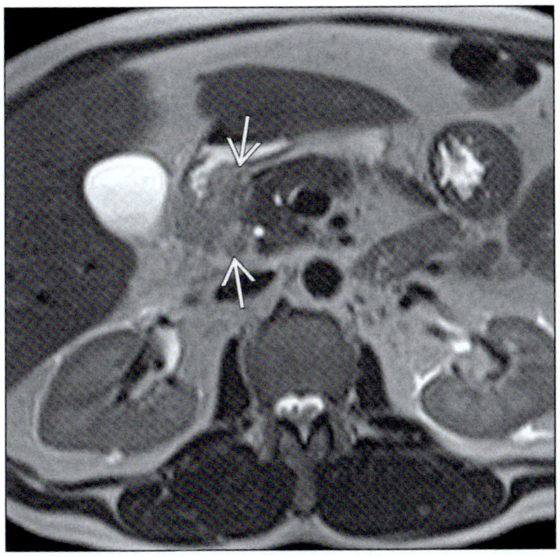

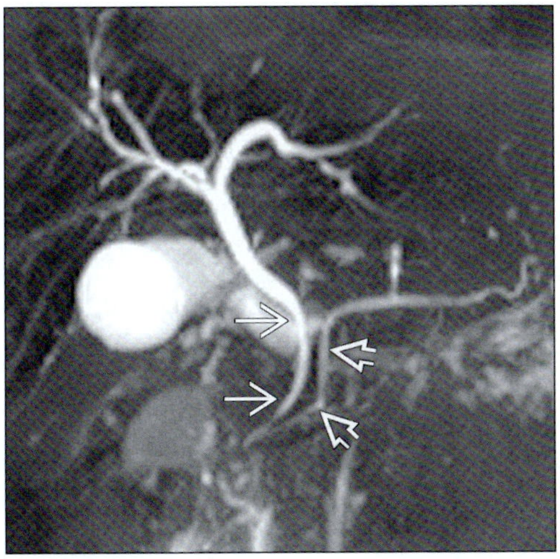

(Left) *Axial T2WI MR in the same patient shows a sheet-like area of subtle increased signal intensity* ➔ *within the pancreaticoduodenal groove associated with mild thickening of the duodenal wall.* ***(Right)*** *MRCP in the same patient shows smooth narrowing of the intrapancreatic portion of the common bile duct* ➔ *as well as the portion of the main pancreatic duct within the head of pancreas* ⇨.

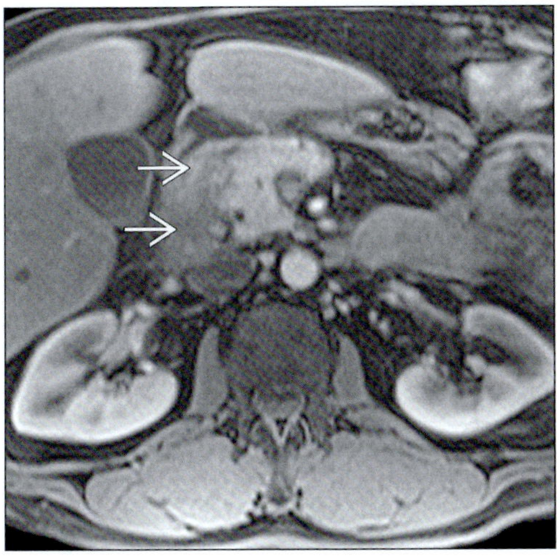

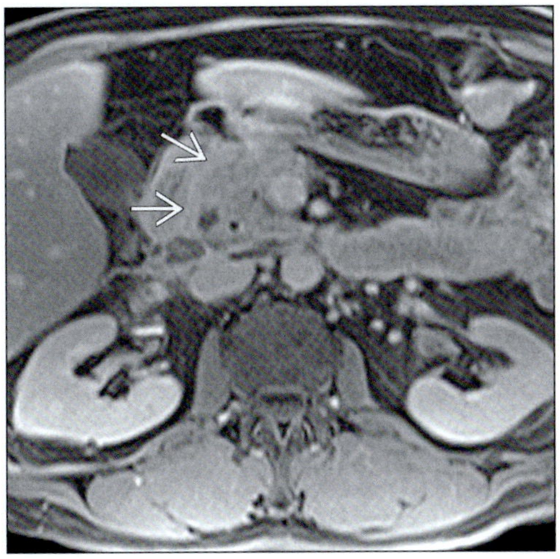

(Left) *Axial T1WI C+ FS MR during the arterial phase in the same patient shows a band-like area of low signal intensity at the pancreaticoduodenal groove* ➔ *with involvement of the adjacent aspect of the pancreatic head.* ***(Right)*** *Axial T1WI C+ FS MR 5 minutes after contrast administration in the same patient shows progressive enhancement of the abnormal fibrotic tissue at the pancreaticoduodenal groove* ➔.

INTRAPANCREATIC ACCESSORY SPLEEN

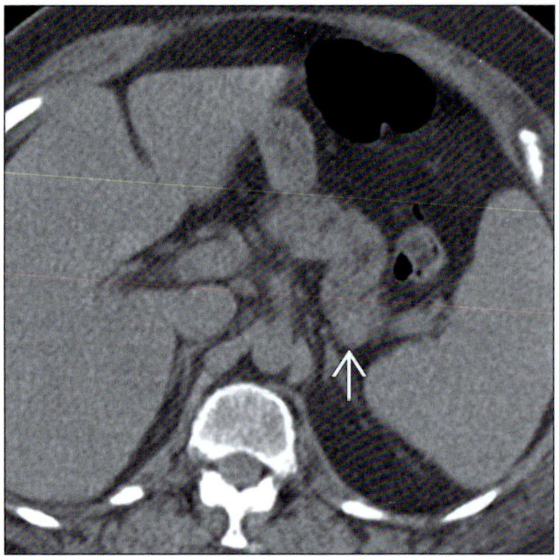

Axial NECT demonstrates a small ovoid mass ➡ within the pancreatic tail appearing slightly hyperdense compared to the liver parenchyma. The mass has a similar density to the splenic parenchyma.

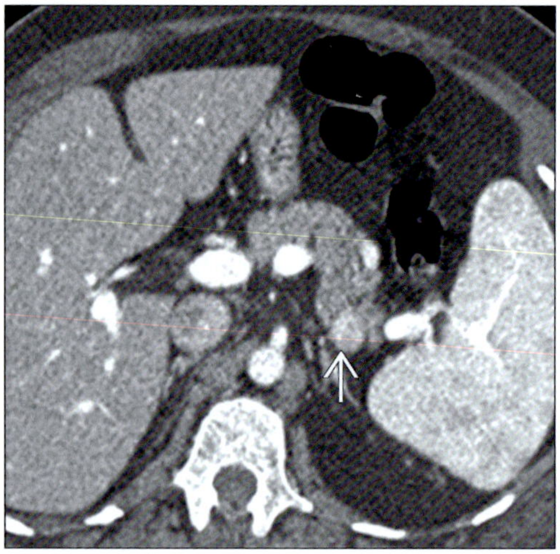

Axial CECT demonstrates a small ovoid mass ➡ within the pancreatic tail, which enhances significantly in the arterial phase, similar to spleen and higher attenuation than the liver parenchyma.

CLINICAL SCENARIO

History

- 45-year-old woman with Hodgkin lymphoma

IMAGE INTERPRETATION

Pitfalls

- Mimic neoplasm (e.g., neuroendocrine tumors [NET] and hypervascular mets)
- Incorrect diagnoses may result in unnecessary surgery
- Awareness of accessory spleen is important when intention is to remove all functional splenic tissue
- Accessory spleen may be FDG avid

Actual Diagnosis

- Intrapancreatic accessory spleen

Clues to Correct Diagnosis

- Follows enhancement pattern of spleen
- Typically located within 3 cm of distal pancreatic tail
- Tc-99m-labeled RBCs is most specific test

BACKGROUND

General

- Most common location is splenic hilum
  - 2nd most common location: Tail of pancreas (20%)
- Supplied by branches of splenic artery
- Varies from 1 mm to usually < 1.5 cm
- Usually asymptomatic, but may result in pain & nausea
- Rarely torse, rupture, bleed, or form cysts

Epidemiology

- Accessory spleens occur in 10-30% of autopsies

Relevant Physiology

- Failure of fusion of splenic anlage, which is located in dorsal mesogastrium, during 5th week of life
- Accessory spleen may hypertrophy after splenectomy
- Post splenectomy for hematologic disease, recurrence may occur in accessory spleen

Relevant Pathology

- Macroscopic: Fibrous capsule surrounds well-defined mass and separates it from surrounding pancreas
- Microscopic: Red pulp (vascular sinuses), white pulp (lymphoid follicles), and reticuloendothelial cells

IMAGING FEATURES

US

- Round, oval, homogeneously hypoechoic mass in left upper quadrant or within pancreas

CT

- NECT: Homogeneous and slightly hyperdense to liver
- CECT: Enhances (follows spleen on all phases)
  - Serpentine arterial enhancement on arterial phase, becomes homogeneous in portovenous phase

MR

- T1WI: Hypointense to normal pancreas and liver
- T1WI C+: Serpentine enhancement on arterial phase, becomes homogeneous in portovenous phase
- T2WI: Hyperintense to normal pancreas and liver
- DWI: May be helpful to distinguish from malignancy as it does not restrict diffusion

Nuclear Scintigraphy

- Tc-99m-labeled, heat-damaged RBCs: Best, most sensitive imaging test demonstrates increased activity
- Tc-99m sulfur colloid (SC): Sensitive for nodules > 2 cm
- Tc-99m SC is less sensitive than Tc-99m RBCs as 10% of SC is taken by spleen (vs. 90% of RBCs)

PET/CT

- Increased FDG activity

RELATED REFERENCES

1. Hagan I et al: Superior demonstration of splenosis by heat-denatured Tc-99m red blood cell scintigraphy compared with Tc-99m sulfur colloid scintigraphy. Clin Nucl Med. 31(8):463-6, 2006

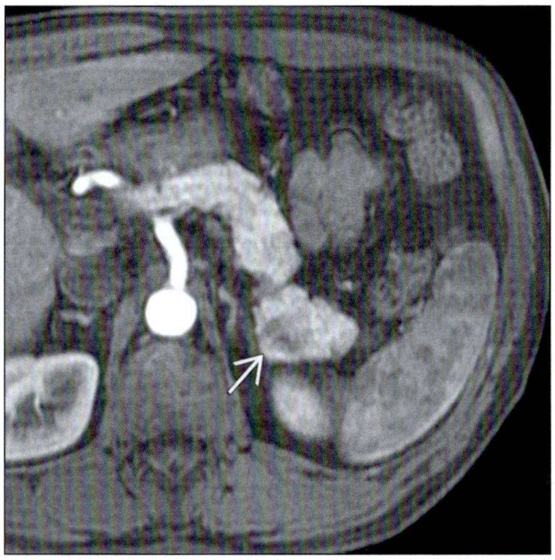

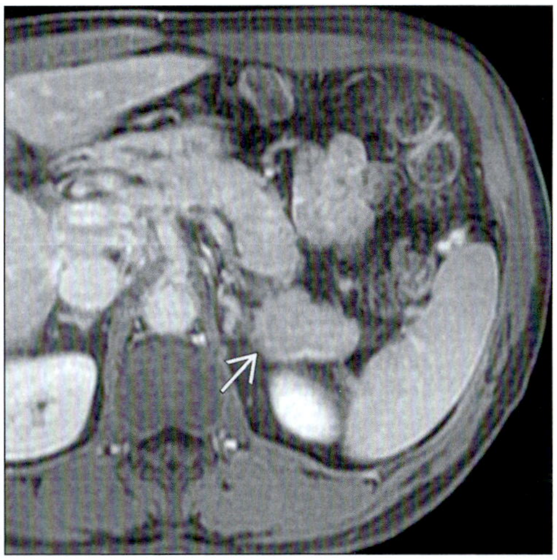

(Left) *Axial T1WI C+ FS MR during the arterial phase in the same patient shows a well-defined pancreatic tail mass →. The mass shows heterogeneous enhancement similar to that of the spleen.* ***(Right)*** *Axial T1WI C+ FS MR during the delayed phase in the same patient shows a poorly defined pancreatic tail mass →. The mass shows enhancement similar to that of the pancreas and spleen and is not well demarcated as in the other sequences.*

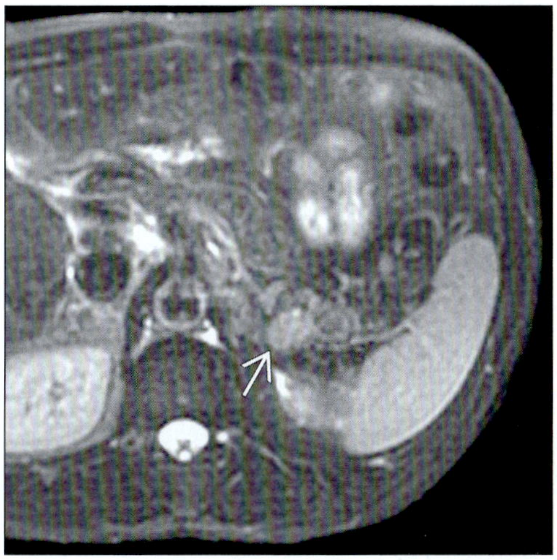

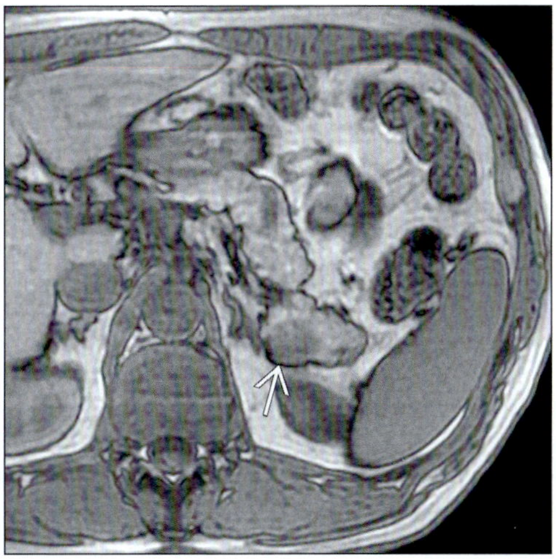

(Left) *Axial T2WI FS MR in the same patient shows a well-defined pancreatic tail mass →. The mass is hyperintense relative to the pancreas and has signal intensity similar to that of the spleen.* ***(Right)*** *Axial opposed-phase T1WI MR in the same patient shows a well-defined pancreatic tail mass →. The mass is hypointense relative to the pancreas and has signal intensity similar to that of the spleen.*

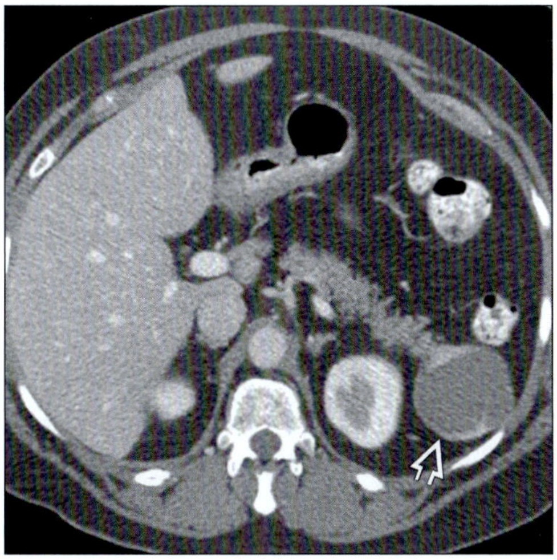

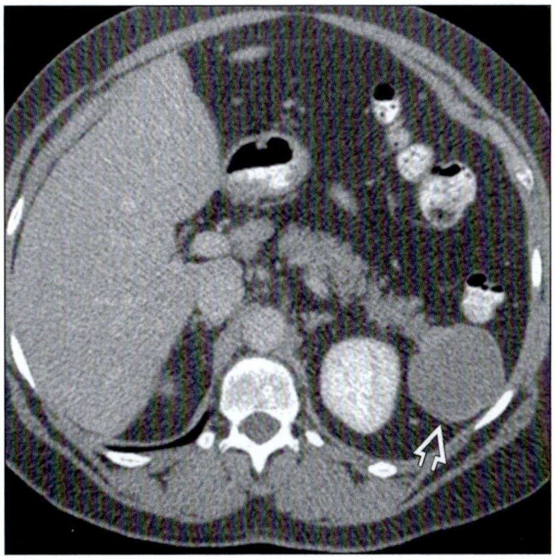

(Left) *Axial CECT (arterial phase) in a patient with a history of gastric carcinoma demonstrates a cystic mass ⇨ within the pancreatic tail with a thick enhancing wall. This mass was surgically proven to be an intrapancreatic accessory spleen containing a benign epithelial cyst.* ***(Right)*** *Axial CECT (delayed phase) in the same patient demonstrates the cystic mass ⇨ within the pancreatic tail with relatively less enhancement of its thick wall.*

PANCREATIC FOCAL FATTY INFILTRATION

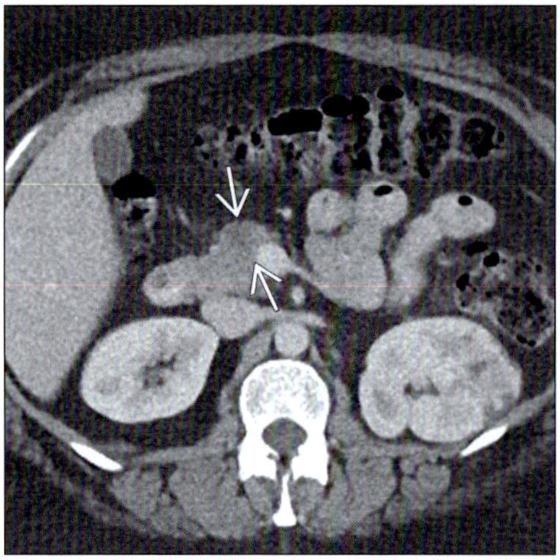

Axial CECT shows an ill-defined area of decreased attenuation ➔ within the pancreatic head that was concerning for pancreatic adenocarcinoma.

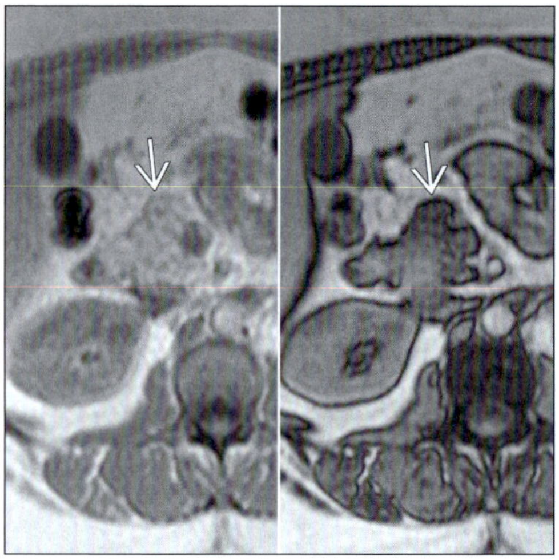

Axial in-phase (left) and opposed-phase (right) T1WI show loss of signal on the opposed-phase image compared to the in-phase image in the area of concern ➔.

CLINICAL SCENARIO

History

- 73-year-old man with incidentally noted low-attenuation lesion in pancreatic head on abdominal CT

IMAGE INTERPRETATION

Pitfalls

- Low-attenuation lesion of pancreas can be mistaken for pancreatic mass (particularly adenocarcinoma)

Actual Diagnosis

- Focal fatty infiltration of pancreas

Clues to Correct Diagnosis

- Focal fatty infiltration does not exhibit ancillary findings of pancreatic carcinoma (including mass effect, pancreatic ductal dilatation, vascular invasion, lymphadenopathy, etc.)
- Chemical shift MR imaging confirms presence of microscopic fat (true pancreatic tumors generally do not contain lipids)
  - Involved areas display reduction in signal intensity on opposed-phase compared to in-phase T1WI

BACKGROUND

General

- Fatty infiltration of pancreas is also known as pancreatic lipomatosis
- May be diffuse (common) or focal (less likely)
- Associated with older age, obesity, chronic pancreatitis, diabetes, cystic fibrosis, and steroid use

Relevant Physiology

- Occurs most frequently in anterior pancreatic head due to differences in fat content between ventral and dorsal pancreas

Relevant Pathology

- Process of fatty replacement is confined to pancreatic interstitium (no involvement of endocrine or exocrine glands)
- May contain macroscopic or microscopic fat

IMAGING FEATURES

General

- Focal lesion most frequently within anterior head of pancreas
- Not associated with mass effect or pancreatic ductal dilatation

US

- Hyperechoic compared to normal pancreatic parenchyma

CT

- Lesion with decreased attenuation within pancreas
- May exhibit characteristic fat attenuation if lesion contains macroscopic fat (not present with mild degree of focal fatty replacement)
- Mild enhancement of fatty areas (sometimes does enhance like true mass due to normal parenchyma within area of fatty infiltration)

MR

- Can appear iso- or hypointense relative to the rest of pancreas on T1WI & T2WI
- Moderate to marked signal loss in opposed-phase T1-weighted images compared to in-phase T1-weighted images

RELATED REFERENCES

1. Low G et al: Multimodality imaging of neoplastic and nonneoplastic solid lesions of the pancreas. Radiographics. 31(4):993-1015, 2011
2. Kim HJ et al: Focal fatty replacement of the pancreas: usefulness of chemical shift MRI. AJR Am J Roentgenol. 188(2):429-32, 2007

SOLID SEROUS CYSTADENOMA

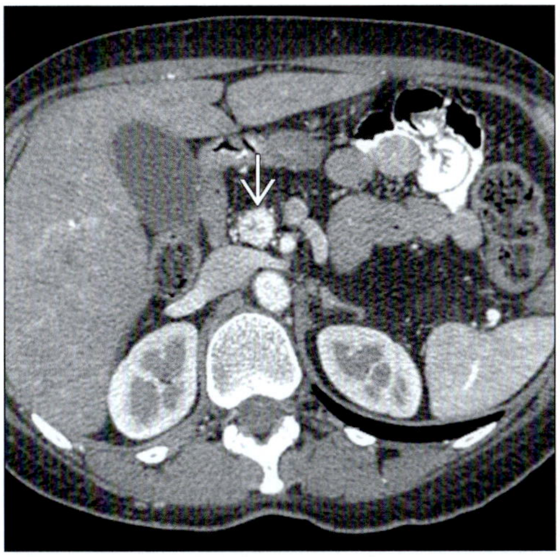

Axial CECT demonstrates a well-circumscribed, enhancing 1.5 cm lesion ➡ in the pancreatic head, with a central low-attenuation focus.

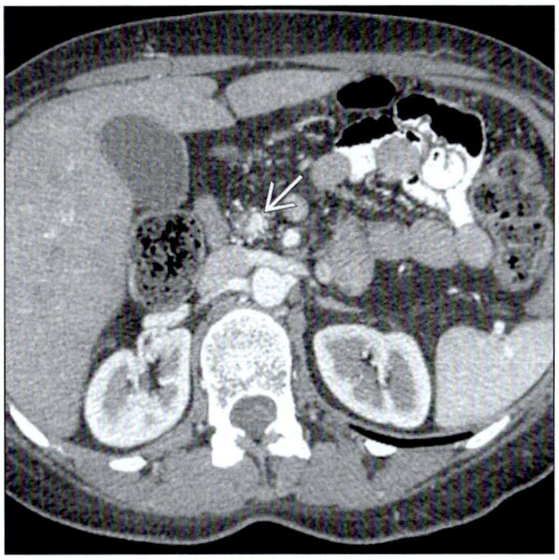

Axial CECT at a lower level demonstrates the inferior aspect of the enhancing lesion ➡ within the pancreatic head.

CLINICAL SCENARIO

History

- 45-year-old woman with right upper quadrant pain
- CT is performed for further characterization of pancreatic mass incidentally noted on US

IMAGE INTERPRETATION

Pitfalls

- Enhancing solid variant of serous cystadenoma (SCA) can simulate the more common neuroendocrine tumor (NET), which typically presents as enhancing solid mass

Actual Diagnosis

- Solid variant of serous cystadenoma

Clues to Correct Diagnosis

- Too rare to be included in common differential diagnoses of enhancing pancreatic mass
  - However, central scar (if present) should raise suspicion of solid SCA
- Absent hormonal abnormalities (characteristic for functioning NET, although nonfunctioning NET are not associated with hormonal disturbances)

BACKGROUND

Epidemiology

- SCA is most common in females > 60 years; F:M = 3:1

Pathology

- SCA is thought to derive from centroacinar cells or epithelial cells of small pancreatic duct
- Most are benign; malignant transformation is rare
- Grossly microcystic appearance (> 6 cysts, each < 2 cm)
- Stellate (sometimes calcified) central scar (10-30%)
- Types: Microcystic, macrocystic, mixed (micro- and macrocystic) and solid variant

Differential Diagnosis

- Most common differential diagnoses for enhancing solid mass: NET and vascular metastases (2° to RCC)

IMAGING FEATURES

US

- SCA is most commonly cystic
- Variable echogenicity
- Rare solid SCA presented here appeared hypoechoic

CT

- SCA: Most are multicystic (> 6 cysts, each < 2 cm)
- Central stellate scar/calcification (10-30%)
- Rare solid SCA appear solid enhancing
- Precontrast low attenuation: Described for solid variant

MR

- More common cystic type appears cystic, but solid rare variant is
  - T1WI: Hypointense
  - T2WI: Relatively hyperintense
  - Post-contrast T1WI: Hyperenhancement

Teaching Point

- Solid variant of SCA is rare
- Typically appears as solid enhancing mass
- Can simulate the more common NET
- Very difficult diagnosis to make prospectively
- Central scar (uncommon), raises possibility of SCA
- Absent hormonal disturbances excludes functioning NET, but NET can be nonfunctioning

RELATED REFERENCES

1. Kim HJ et al: CT of serous cystadenoma of the pancreas and mimicking masses. AJR Am J Roentgenol. 190(2):406-12, 2008
2. Yamamoto T et al: A case of solid variant type of pancreatic serous cystadenoma mimicking islet cell tumor. Clin Imaging. 28(1):49-51, 2004

RUPTURED PANCREATICODUODENAL ARTERY ANEURYSM

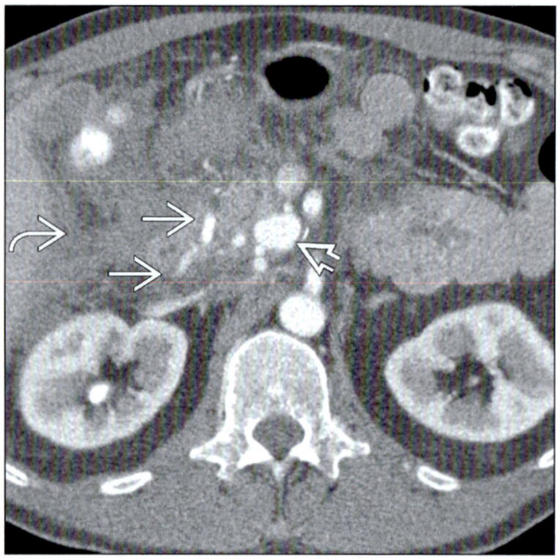

Axial CECT shows dilatation of the pancreaticoduodenal (PD) arcade ➡ with a sizable aneurysm ⇨. There is a large amount of high-attenuation retroperitoneal fluid ↪.

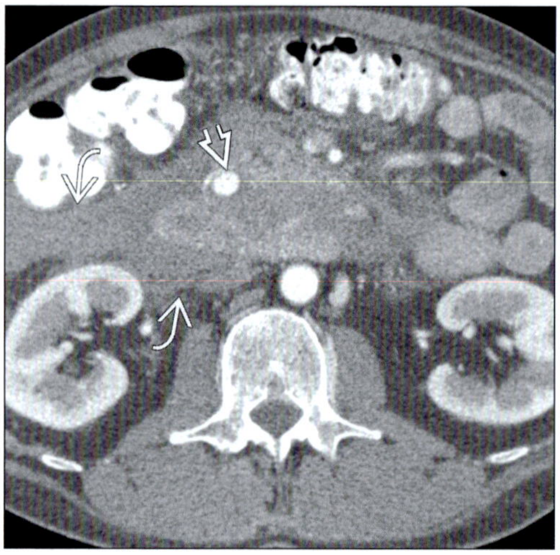

Axial CECT in the same patient shows a 2nd aneurysm ⇨ along the PD arcade. There is a large amount of high-attenuation retroperitoneal fluid ↪.

CLINICAL SCENARIO

History

- 79-year-old man with severe abdominal pain and hypotension

IMAGE INTERPRETATION

Pitfalls

- Presence of retroperitoneal fluid may suggest possibility of pancreatitis and formation of pseudoaneurysms

Actual Diagnosis

- Retroperitoneal rupture of pancreaticoduodenal (PD) artery aneurysm resulting from median arcuate ligament compression of celiac artery origin

Clues to Correct Diagnosis

- Presence of dilated PD arterial arcade with multiple aneurysms
- Sagittal reformations should be performed to evaluate patency of celiac axis and superior mesenteric artery (SMA)

Key Teaching Point

- Always look for celiac artery stenosis when PD arcade aneurysm is found

BACKGROUND

General

- > 1/2 of true PD artery aneurysms are associated with celiac axis stenosis or occlusion
  - Causes include
    - Median arcuate ligament compression
    - Atherosclerotic osteal stenosis

Epidemiology

- True PD artery aneurysms are rare, accounting for ~ 2% of all visceral aneurysms

Relevant Physiology

- Development of PD artery aneurysms might be related to ↑ retrograde blood flow through PD arcades when there is stenosis or occlusion in celiac axis
- Aneurysm formation is generally preceded by enlargement of arcades to accommodate ↑ blood flow

Relevant Pathology

- ~ 60% of reported cases presented with rupture
  - Mortality rate of 21%
- Rupture is most commonly retroperitoneal
- Enlarging aneurysms can be considered unstable and probably have higher risk of rupture than stable aneurysms

IMAGING FEATURES

Plain Radiography

- Calcified aneurysms may appear as ring-shaped calcifications

US

- Aneurysms appear as anechoic structures with turbulent blood flow on color Doppler images

CT

- Aneurysms appear as enhancing structures with attenuation similar to that of aorta
- Peripheral calcifications may be seen

MR

- Signal voids with enhancement similar to that of aorta

RELATED REFERENCES

1. Armstrong MB et al: Pancreaticoduodenal artery aneurysm associated with median arcuate ligament syndrome. Ann Vasc Surg. 28(3):741, 2014
2. Takao H et al: Natural history of true pancreaticoduodenal artery aneurysms. Br J Radiol. 83(993):744-6, 2010

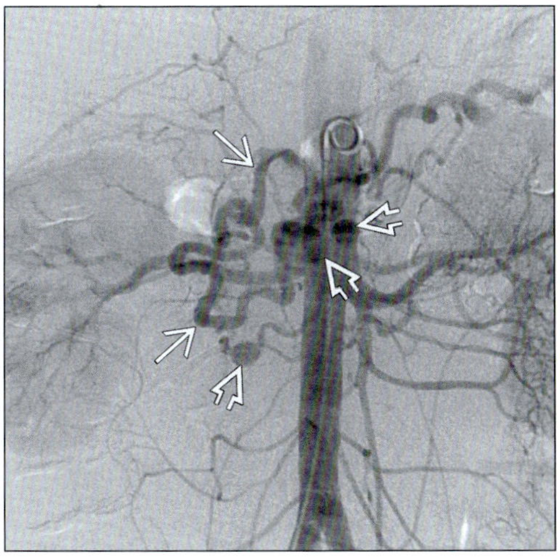

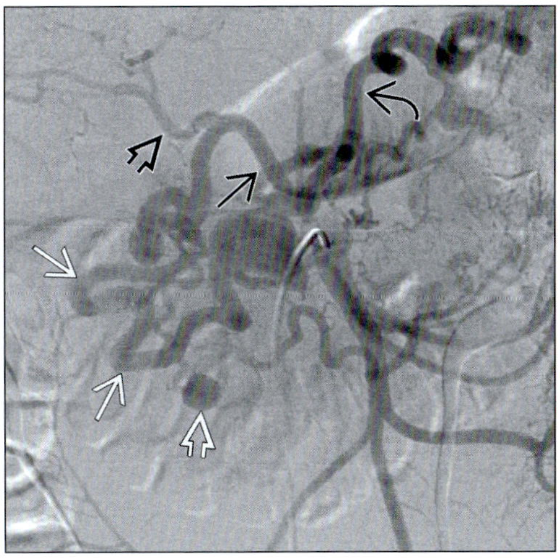

(Left) *Frontal view from an aortogram shows dilatation of the pancreaticoduodenal (PD) arcade ➔ with multiple aneurysms ➔.* ***(Right)*** *Frontal view from a selective superior mesenteric artery (SMA) angiogram in the same patient shows dilatation of the PD arcade ➔ with multiple aneurysms ➔. Note filling of the gastroduodenal ➔, hepatic ➔, and splenic arteries ➔ due to retrograde flow from the SMA through the PD arcade to the branches of the celiac axis.*

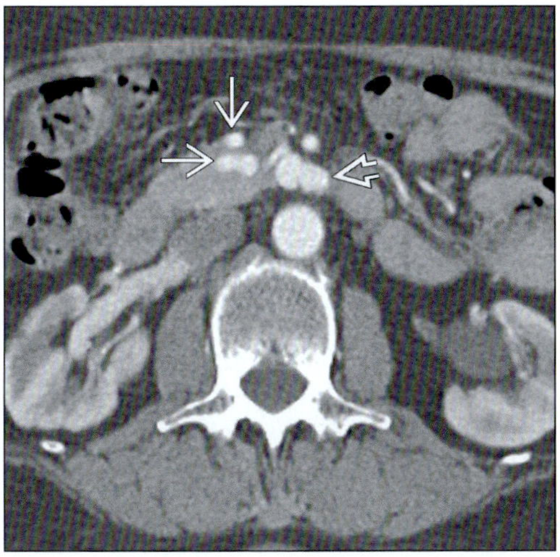

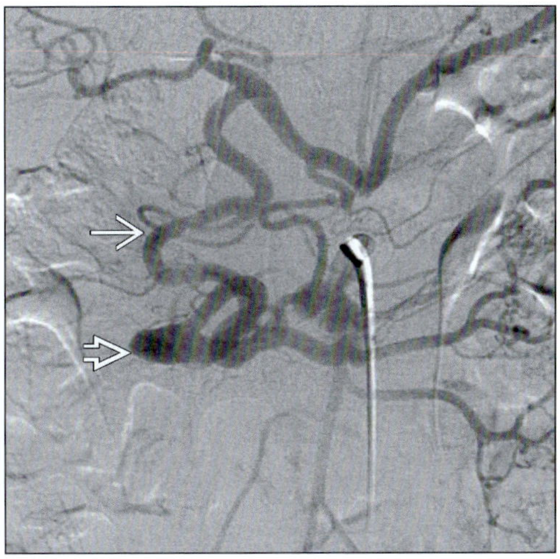

(Left) *Axial CECT in a 68 year old who presented with postprandial abdominal pain shows dilatation of the PD arcade ➔ with a sizable aneurysm ➔.* ***(Right)*** *Frontal view from a selective SMA angiogram in the same patient shows dilatation of the PD arcade ➔ with a sizable aneurysm ➔. Note filling of the celiac branches due to retrograde flow from the SMA through the PD arcade to the branches of the celiac axis.*

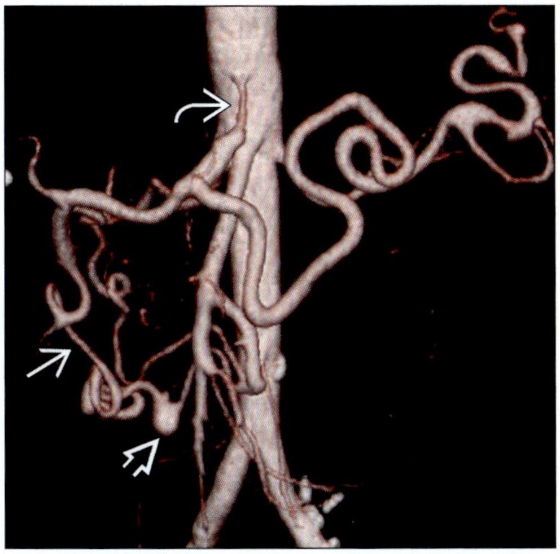

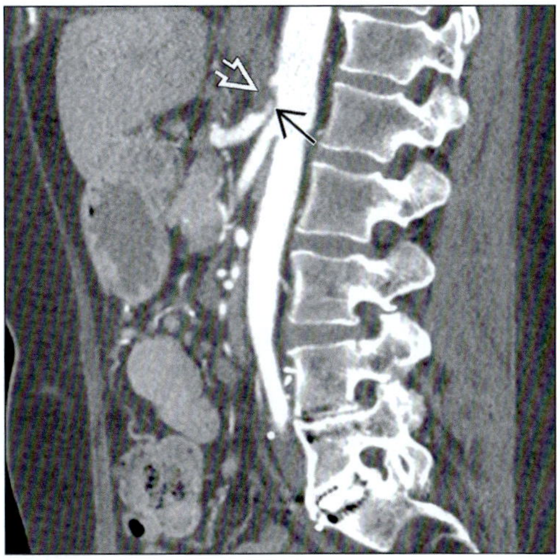

(Left) *3D reconstruction from CECT in the same patient shows dilatation of the PD arcade ➔ with a sizable aneurysm ➔. Note marked narrowing of the celiac artery ➔ due to median arcuate ligament (MAL) compression.* ***(Right)*** *Sagittal CECT in the same patient shows marked narrowing of the celiac artery ➔ due to MAL compression ➔. The MAL is the fibrous connection of the left and right diaphragmatic crura typically found at the level of T12-L1 just anterior to the aortic hiatus.*

DUCT-PENETRATING SIGN

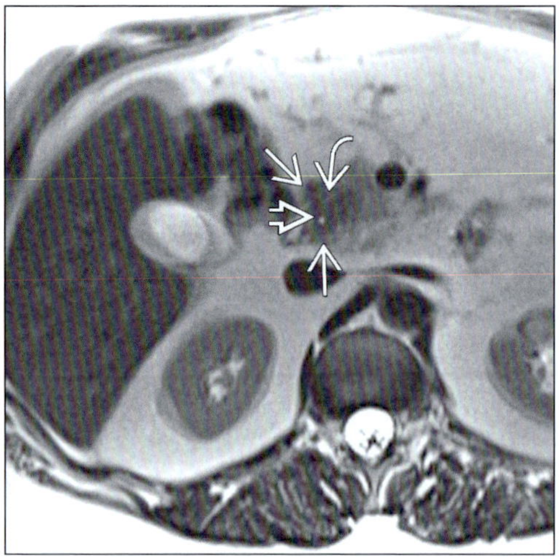

Axial T2WI shows an ill-defined mass-like lesion ➡ within the pancreatic head, surrounding the distal common bile duct ➡ and pancreatic duct ➡.

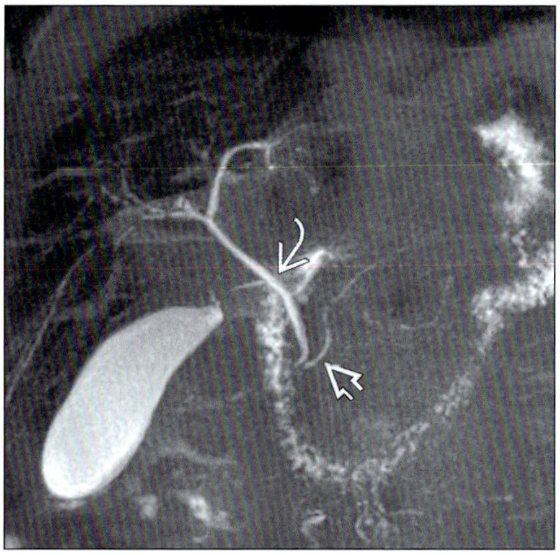

MIP MRCP image in the same patient shows a normal pancreatic duct ➡ through the area of abnormality without obstruction or dilatation. The common bile duct ➡ likewise shows normal tapering.

CLINICAL SCENARIO

History

- 55-year-old woman with chronic epigastric pain

IMAGE INTERPRETATION

Pitfalls

- A smoothly stenotic or normal main pancreatic duct (MPD) penetrating a mass
  - Focal inflammatory pancreatic head mass may be mistaken for pancreatic adenocarcinoma

Actual Diagnosis

- Focal chronic pancreatitis of pancreatic head

Clues to Correct Diagnosis

- Unobstructed MPD penetrating through area of abnormal signal
  - Duct may be completely normal or smoothly stenotic

Clinical Significance

- Duct-penetrating sign on MRCP has sensitivity of 85% and specificity of 96% for distinguishing inflammatory pancreatic mass from pancreatic carcinoma

BACKGROUND

General

- Chronic focal pancreatitis is a clinical entity characterized by focal inflammation of pancreas
  - Focal lesion or distortion of pancreas, which can be difficult to distinguish from adenocarcinoma
- Any etiology that causes chronic pancreatitis such as alcohol (most commonly) or autoimmune pancreatitis can cause chronic focal pancreatitis
- Symptoms and radiological appearance of focal chronic pancreatitis and adenocarcinoma may overlap

IMAGING FEATURES

General

- In this section, imaging features for focal chronic pancreatitis & duct-penetrating sign are discussed

US

- Limited in diagnosis of focal chronic pancreatitis due to factors such as body habitus and bowel gas
- Usually hypoechoic focal mass
- ± dilation of common bile duct and pancreatic duct

CT

- Mass-like focal enlargement of pancreas, which appears isoattenuating to adjacent parenchyma and spleen on pre-contrast imaging
- Hypoattenuating on venous phase relative to adjacent pancreas, an appearance almost identical to adenocarcinoma of pancreas
- Dilation of main pancreatic duct may be present, also an overlapping appearance with carcinoma
- If main pancreatic duct is not obstructed, it is more suggestive of focal chronic pancreatitis
- No extrapancreatic extension or vascular invasion
- Capsule-like rim virtually excludes adenocarcinoma

MR

- T1WI: Focal area of low signal intensity
- T2WI: Low signal intensity
- T1WI FS C+: Usually poor enhancement on early phases & progressive enhancement on delayed phases
- MRCP: Duct-penetrating sign (smoothly stenotic or normal MPD penetrating a mass) can distinguish focal chronic pancreatitis from malignancy

RELATED REFERENCES

1. Sun GF et al: Focal autoimmune pancreatitis: radiological characteristics help to distinguish from pancreatic cancer. World J Gastroenterol. 19(23):3634-41, 2013
2. Ichikawa T et al: Duct-penetrating sign at MRCP: usefulness for differentiating inflammatory pancreatic mass from pancreatic carcinomas. Radiology. 221(1):107-16, 2001

CHAIN OF LAKES SIGN

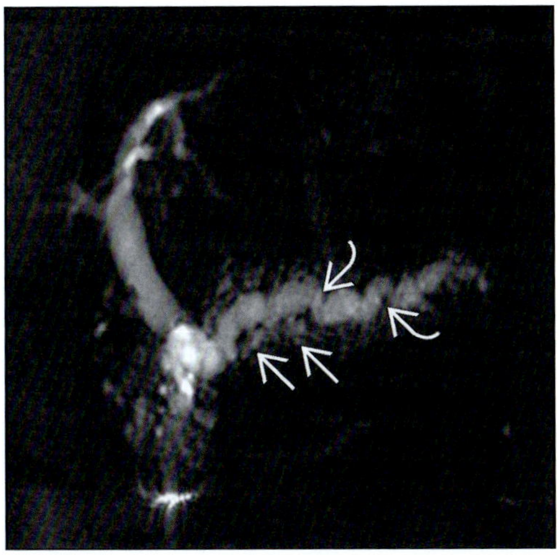

MRCP 3D reconstruction demonstrates a dilated main pancreatic duct with intervening segments of stenosis and ectasia of the side branches.

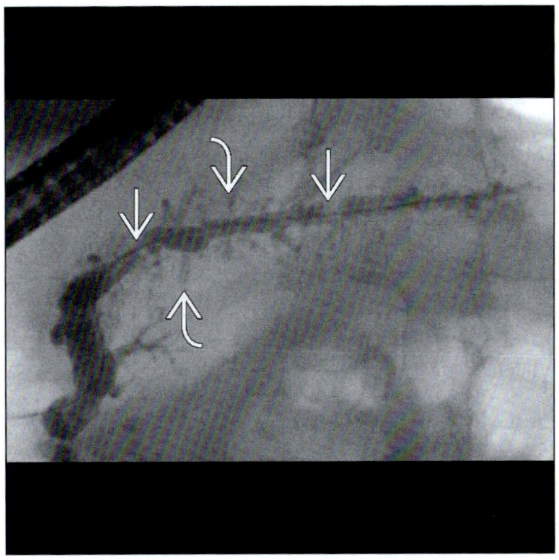

Frontal view of ERCP image demonstrates a dilated main pancreatic duct with intervening segments of stenosis and ectasia of the side branches.

CLINICAL SCENARIO

History

- 55-year-old man with chronic intermittent abdominal pain in setting of alcohol abuse

IMAGE INTERPRETATION

Clues to Correct Diagnosis

- Diffusely dilated main pancreatic duct with intervening segments of stenosis and side branch ectasia chain of lakes sign is classic for chronic pancreatitis

BACKGROUND

General

- Chronic inflammation → progressive damage → exocrine and endocrine dysfunction
- 3 types: Calcifying, obstructive, and inflammatory
- May present with steatorrhea, pain, or diabetes
- Inflammatory strictures → biliary obstruction and jaundice
- Increased risk for pancreatic cancer
- Surgery/endoscopy may be needed to treat complications, such as biliary strictures or symptomatic pseudocysts

Epidemiology

- M > F, middle-aged patients
- Most cases (70%) in USA are related to alcohol abuse

Relevant Physiology

- Basal hypersecretion of pancreatic enzymes
- Decrease in protease inhibitors
- Change in pancreatic secretions → calculi and protein plugs

Relevant Pathology

- Lymphocytic infiltration, fibrosis, and irregular loss of glandular tissue

IMAGING FEATURES

ERCP

- May demonstrate irregularly dilated main pancreatic duct with side branch duct ectasia chain of lakes
- Intraductal filling defects representing calculi

US

- Pancreatic calcifications
- Dilated main pancreatic duct
- Pancreatic parenchymal atrophy or enlargement
- Pseudocyst: Well-defined cyst without internal echoes or vascularity

CT

- Pancreatic calcifications
- Dilated main pancreatic duct
- Pancreatic parenchymal atrophy or enlargement
- Intrapancreatic or peripancreatic pseudocysts: Well defined, fluid attenuation, no internal enhancement
- May present as iso- or hypoattenuating, mass-like area

MR

- T1WI: Early findings: Low signal intensity of pancreas, parenchymal hypoenhancement, and delayed enhancement
- Late findings: Pancreatic atrophy or enlargement, dilated irregular main pancreatic duct, ductal calcifications and pseudocysts
- MRCP: Irregularly dilated main pancreatic duct with ectasia of side branch ducts (chain of lakes)

RELATED REFERENCES

1. Hansen TM, et al. Morphological and functional evaluation of chronic pancreatitis with magnetic resonance imaging. World J Gastroenterol.19(42):7241-6; 2013
2. Miller FH et al: MRI of pancreatitis and its complications: part 2, chronic pancreatitis. AJR Am J Roentgenol. 183(6):1645-52, 2004
3. Leyendecker JR, et al. MR cholangiopancreatography: spectrum of pancreatic duct abnormalities. AJR Am J Roentgenol.179(6):1465-71; 2002

DOUBLE DUCT SIGN

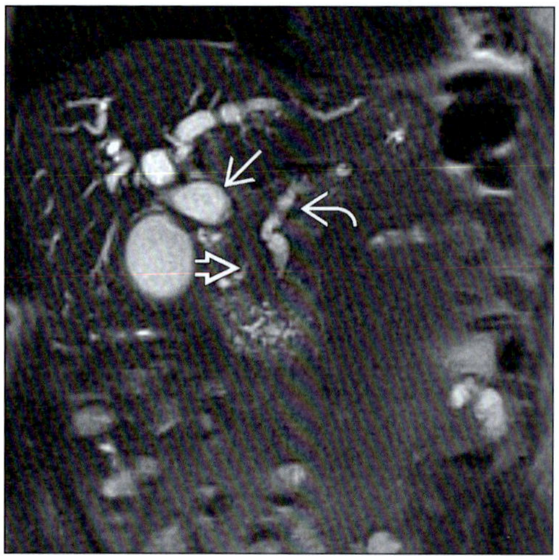

Coronal heavily T2-weighted (SSFSE) image demonstrates significant dilatation of the pancreatic duct ➔ and common bile duct ➡, secondary to a low signal intensity mass within the pancreatic head ⇨.

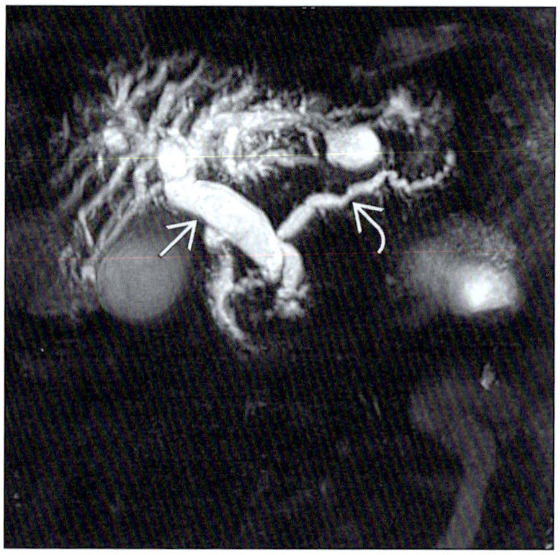

Coronal thick slab MRCP demonstrates double duct sign with significant dilatation of the pancreatic duct ➔ and common bile duct ➡, secondary to adenocarcinoma of the pancreatic head.

CLINICAL SCENARIO

History

- 70-year-old man with jaundice and weight loss

IMAGE INTERPRETATION

Classic Sign

- Simultaneous dilation of common bile duct (CBD) and pancreatic duct (double duct sign) is classic for adenocarcinoma of pancreatic head
- Less likely, this can occur with other obstructive pathologies, including focal chronic pancreatitis

BACKGROUND

General

- Pancreatic adenocarcinoma is most commonly seen in head (60%), followed by body (15%) and tail (5%)
- Clinical: Weight loss, pain, obstructive jaundice
- Elevated levels of CEA or CA19-9 may be present
- Treatment depends on stage
- Prognosis: Poor (5-year survival < 5%)

Epidemiology

- M > F, typical age > 50 years (peak in 7th decade)
- Genetic predisposition in 5-10% including *HNPCC*, *BRCA1* & *BRCA2*, ataxia-telangiectasia, & Peutz-Jeghers
- Other risk factors: Smoking, diabetes, obesity, and chronic pancreatitis

Relevant Physiology

- Obstruction of pancreatic duct and CBD occurs simultaneously from invasion of ampulla of Vater
- Spread of tumor: Commonly through lymphatics, direct, vascular, and perineural invasion

Relevant Pathology

- Gross: Poorly marginated, gray-white, firm mass
- Microscopic: Mucin production, tubular glands surrounded by stroma, marked atypia, and desmoplasia

IMAGING FEATURES

ERCP

- Often dilated pancreatic duct ± CBD dilation

Upper GI

- Wide duodenal C loop or inverted 3 sign: Distortion of medial wall of 2nd part of duodenum

US

- Heterogeneous ill-defined hypoechoic solid mass
- Endoscopic US: Often useful in guided tissue sampling
- Appearance is nonspecific with specificity of 53%

CT

- CECT is preferred modality for staging
- Typically hypoenhancing mass on arterial phase
- Distal pancreatic duct dilation and atrophy
- Double duct sign is often present

MR

- T1WI: Hypointense
- T2WI: Variable intensity
- T1WI C+: Hypoenhancing relative to normal pancreas
- MRCP: Double duct sign

PET/CT

- Focal FDG avidity
- Nonspecific, as benign etiologies such as pancreatitis may demonstrate FDG avidity
- May be helpful when CT findings are equivocal

RELATED REFERENCES

1. Ahualli J: The double duct sign. Radiology. 244(1):314-5, 2007
2. Brennan DD et al: Comprehensive preoperative assessment of pancreatic adenocarcinoma with 64-section volumetric CT. Radiographics. 27(6):1653-66, 2007
3. Tamm EP et al: Diagnosis, staging, and surveillance of pancreatic cancer. AJR Am J Roentgenol. 180(5):1311-23, 2003

SAUSAGE PANCREAS AUTOIMMUNE PANCREATITIS

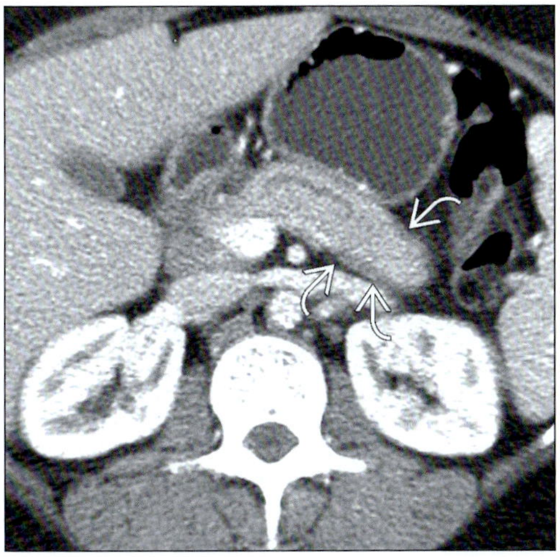

Axial CECT in a patient with autoimmune pancreatitis shows a peripheral hypoattenuation rim ➔ and minimal peripancreatic stranding.

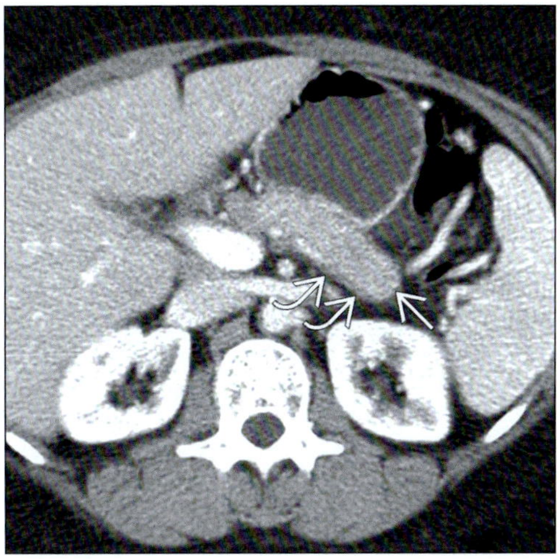

Axial CECT demonstrates mild diffuse enlargement of the pancreas: Sausage-like appearance ➔ with peripheral hypoattenuation rim ➔.

CLINICAL SCENARIO

History

- 55-year-old man with jaundice and abdominal pain

IMAGE INTERPRETATION

Appearance

- Mild smooth enlargement, sausage-like appearance with peripheral hypoattenuation rim and minimal peripancreatic stranding is consistent with autoimmune pancreatitis

BACKGROUND

General

- Subtype of chronic pancreatitis
- a.k.a. lymphoplasmacytic sclerosing pancreatitis
- Clinically present with obstructive jaundice, abdominal pain, diabetes, or weight loss
- Elevated serum IgG4
- Extrapancreatic manifestations include involvement of biliary tree, kidneys, retroperitoneum, arteries, mesentery lungs, and salivary glands

Epidemiology

- Mean age: 56 (range: 14-77 years)

Relevant Pathology

- Infiltration of lymphocytes and plasma cells and granulocytic epithelial lesions around medium-sized and large interlobular ducts
- Consequent destruction of duct epithelium and venules
- Intraductal calcifications are usually absent
- Abundant IgG4-positive plasma cells
- Typically responds to treatment with steroid therapy

Relevant Anatomy

- Diffuse involvement of pancreas is common
- When focal, it most commonly involves head of pancreas and distal common bile duct (CBD)

IMAGING FEATURES

US

- Diffusely or focally enlarged hypoechoic pancreas

CT

- Mild smooth enlargement, sausage-like appearance with peripheral hypoattenuation rim and peripancreatic stranding
- Loss of lobulated contour (featureless pancreas)
- NECT: Appears hypodense
- CECT: Hypoenhancing, with peripheral rim of hypoattenuation
- Calcifications and pseudocysts are not common

MR

- T1WI: Hypointense
- T2WI: Hyperintense
- T1WI C+: Hypoenhancement relative to surrounding pancreas parenchyma
- Hypointense peripheral rim in T1WI and T2WI
- MRCP: Diffuse or segmental narrowing of pancreatic &/ or CBD
  - Biliary involvement appears as thickening of CBD and occasionally thickening of hepatic ducts at confluence, mimicking Klatskin tumor

RELATED REFERENCES

1. Kawamoto S et al: Lymphoplasmacytic sclerosing pancreatitis (autoimmune pancreatitis): evaluation with multidetector CT. Radiographics. 28(1):157-70, 2008
2. Kamisawa T et al: MRCP and MRI findings in 9 patients with autoimmune pancreatitis. World J Gastroenterol. 12(18):2919-22, 2006
3. Klöppel G et al: Autoimmune pancreatitis: pathological findings. JOP. 6(1 Suppl):97-101, 2005

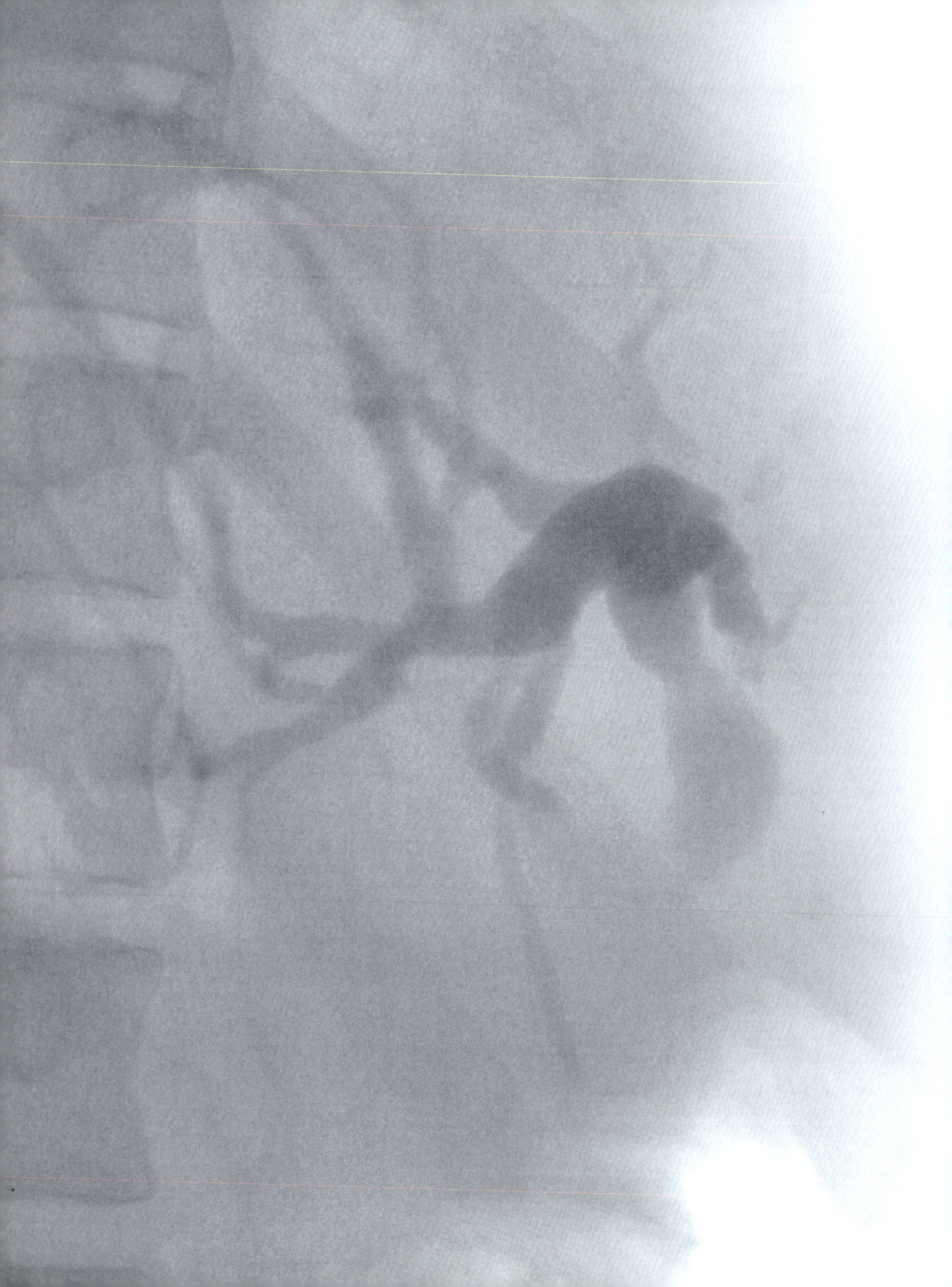

MRCP-RELATED PITFALLS

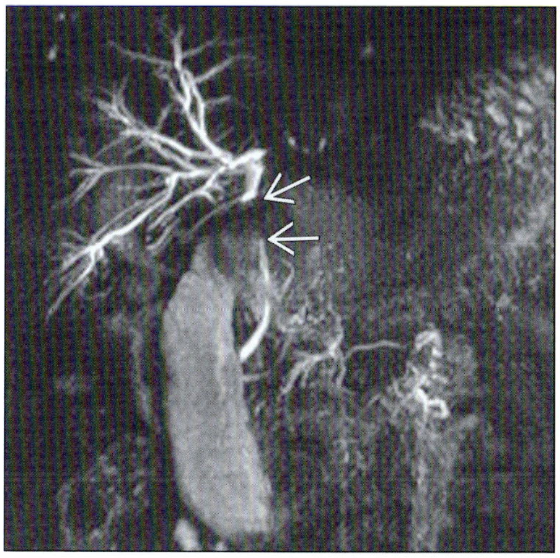

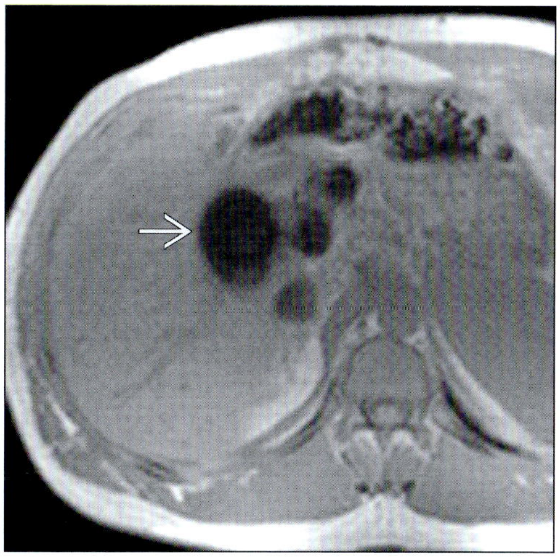

***(Left)** MRCP MIP image in a patient with a history of abdominal trauma resulting in partial hepatectomy and biliary leak shows a long segment of nonvisualized common hepatic duct* ➔. ***(Right)** Axial in-phase T1WI MR in the same patient shows a large susceptibility artifact* ➔ *resulting from surgical clips. The size of the artifact is characteristically larger on the in-phase images compared to opposed-phase images due to longer TE.*

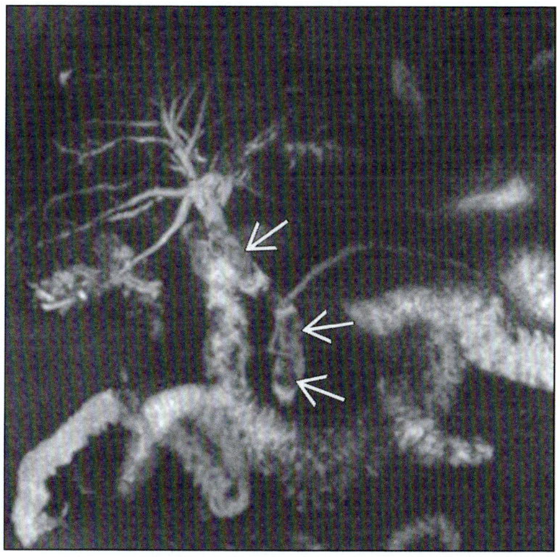

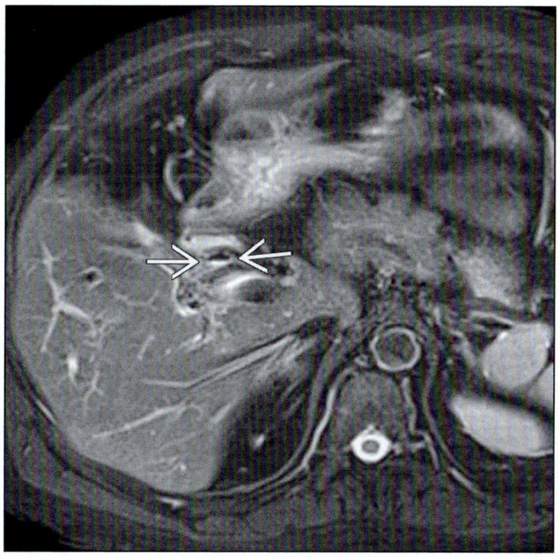

***(Left)** MRCP MIP image in a patient with a history of distal common bile duct stricture and repeated sphincterotomy shows multiple extrahepatic bile ducts filling defects* ➔ *resembling biliary stones.* ***(Right)** Axial T2WI MR in the same patient shows signal-void gas bubbles float ventrally to the T2-hyperintense bile, producing gas-fluid level* ➔.

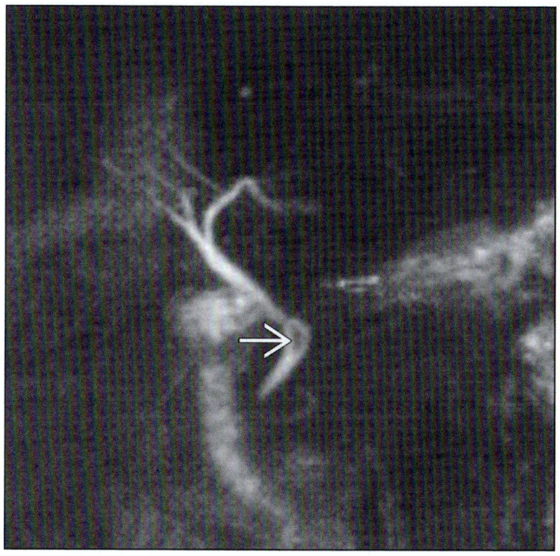

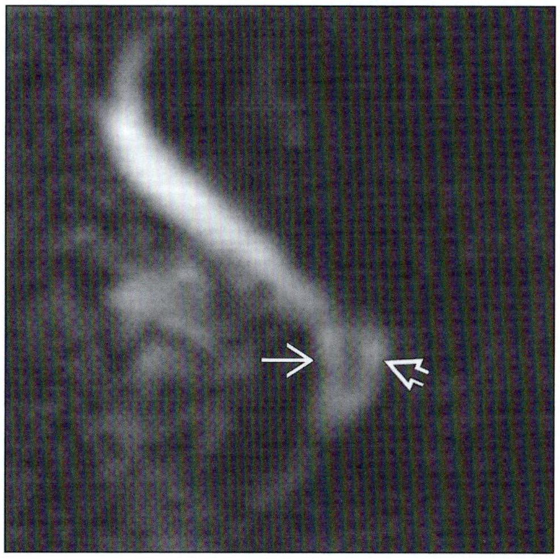

***(Left)** MRCP MIP image in a patient with a history of prior cholecystectomy and elevation of liver function tests shows an apparent extrahepatic bile duct filling defect* ➔ *resembling biliary stone.* ***(Right)** MRCP source image shows that the filling defect perceived on MIP image represents a gap between the distal common hepatic duct* ➔ *and a low-lying cystic duct stump* ⇨.

XANTHOGRANULOMATOUS CHOLECYSTITIS

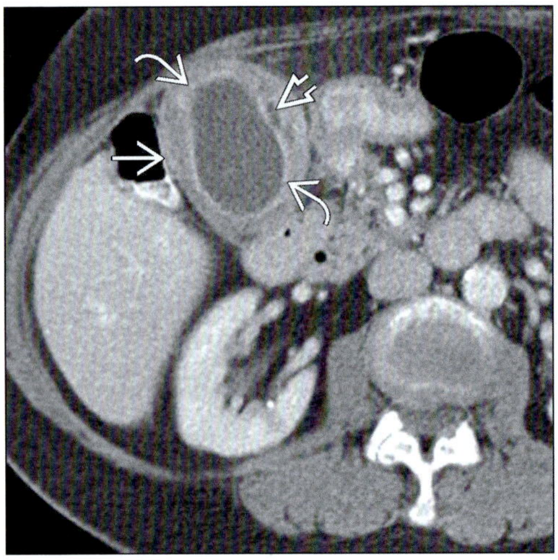

Axial CECT shows diffuse gallbladder wall thickening and intramural bands of decreased attenuation. Note the continuous enhancing mucosal line.

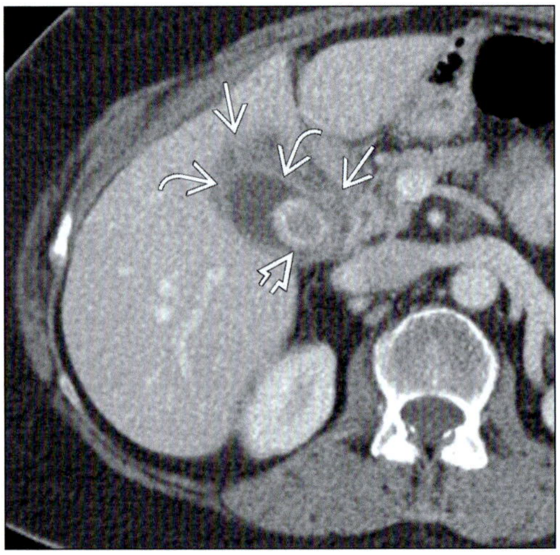

Axial CECT shows diffuse gallbladder wall thickening. Note the continuous enhancing mucosal line and the calcified gallstone.

CLINICAL SCENARIO

History

- 45-year-old woman with 2-week history of right upper quadrant abdominal pain

Relevant Laboratory Tests

- Normal white blood cell count

IMAGE INTERPRETATION

Pitfalls

- Can be mistaken for gallbladder (GB) carcinoma

Actual Diagnosis

- Xanthogranulomatous cholecystitis (XGC)

Clues to Correct Diagnosis

- 5 findings on CECT are predictive of XGC rather than carcinoma
  - Diffuse GB wall thickening
  - Continuous mucosal line
  - Intramural low-attenuation nodules &/or bands
  - Absence of hepatic invasion
  - Absence of intrahepatic bile duct dilatation

BACKGROUND

General

- Rare inflammatory disease of GB

Epidemiology

- 0.7% in USA and up to 10% in India and Japan among patients with symptomatic GB disease
- Most common age at presentation: 44-63 years
- M:F = 1:2-9

Relevant Pathology

- Focal or diffuse inflammatory process, with accumulation of lipid-laden macrophages, fibrous tissue, and acute and chronic inflammatory cells
- Results from extension of bile into GB wall from rupture of Rokitansky-Aschoff sinuses
  - Gallstones may have an important role in pathogenesis
- Fairly high incidence of complications occurring in > 30% of cases
  - GB perforation and hepatic abscesses
  - Fistulas into adjacent structures

IMAGING FEATURES

General

- Thickened GB wall (focal or diffuse) with gallstones

US

- Hypoechoic nodules or bands in GB wall

CT

- Intramural low-attenuation nodules or bands
- Continuous enhancing mucosal line

MR

- T1WI
  - Loss of signal on out-phase images compared to in-phase images due to presence of fat
- T2WI
  - Intramural lesions with markedly elevated T2 signal intensity
- Preservation of linear mucosal enhancement

PET/CT

- Increased metabolic activity on FDG PET
  - Not useful to differentiate carcinoma from XGC

RELATED REFERENCES

1. Zhao F et al: CT and MR features of xanthogranulomatous cholecystitis: an analysis of consecutive 49 cases. Eur J Radiol. 82(9):1391-7, 2013
2. Shuto R et al: CT and MR imaging findings of xanthogranulomatous cholecystitis: correlation with pathologic findings. Eur Radiol. 14(3):440-6, 2004

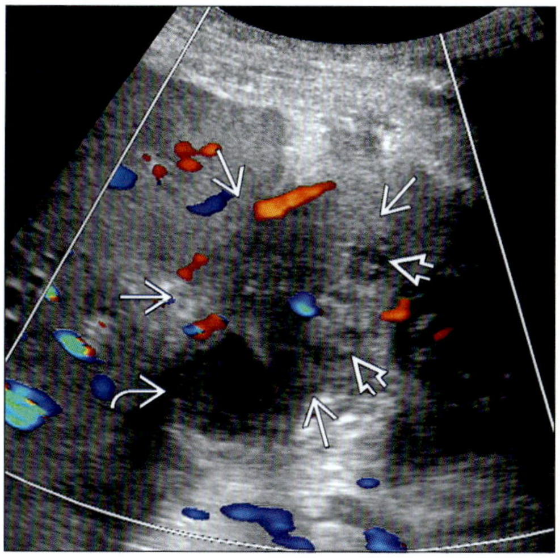

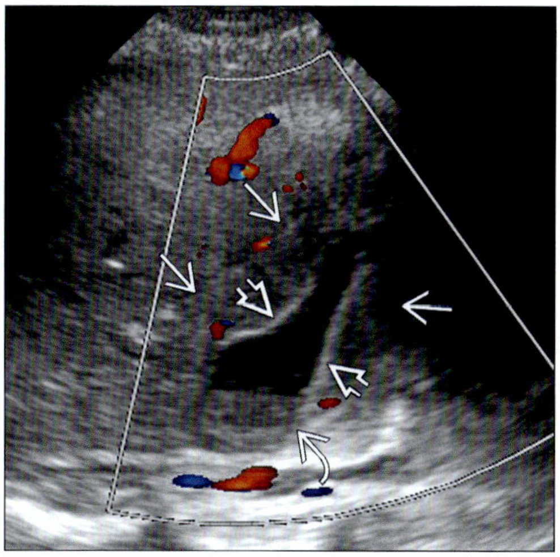

(Left) *Axial color Doppler US in a 56-year-old woman who presented with right upper quadrant abdominal pain for 1 month shows marked thickening of the gallbladder (GB) wall with multiple hypoechoic nodules. The lumen of the GB is not distended.* ***(Right)*** *Axial color Doppler US in the same patient shows marked diffuse thickening of the GB wall. The lumen of the GB is not distended. Note the intact echogenic mucosa.*

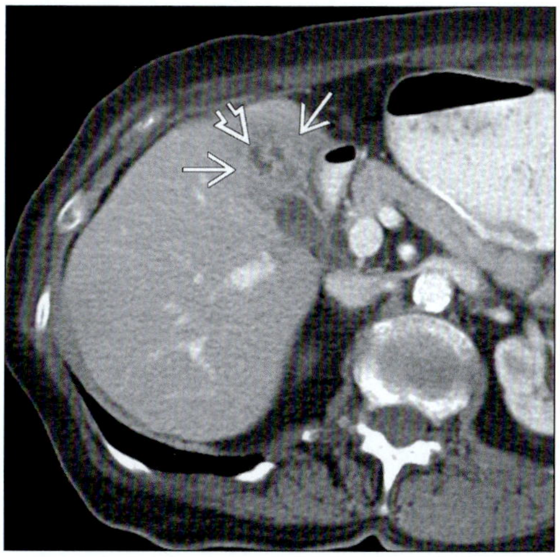

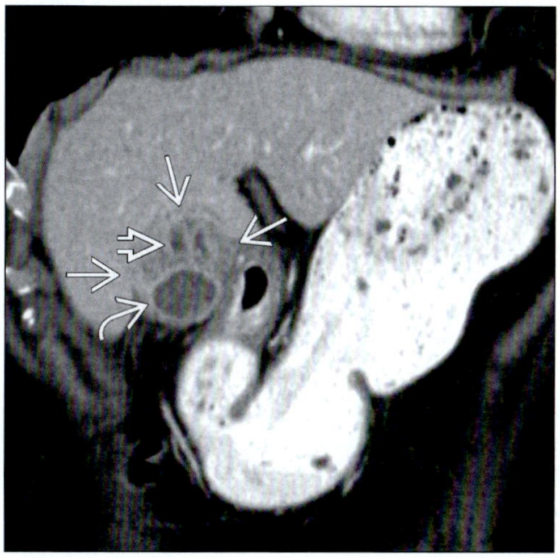

(Left) *Axial CECT in a 44-year-old woman who presented with right upper quadrant abdominal pain and normal WBC count shows thickening of the GB wall with multiple low-attenuation, cystic-appearing structures.* ***(Right)*** *Coronal CECT in the same patient shows thickening of the GB wall on the liver side with multiple low-attenuation, cystic-appearing structures. Note the intact enhancing mucosa.*

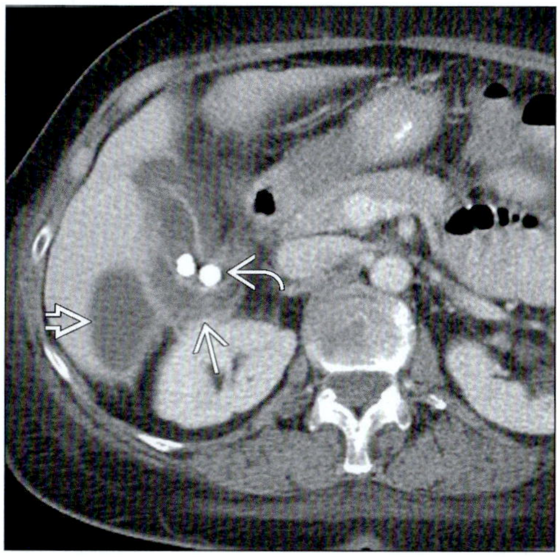

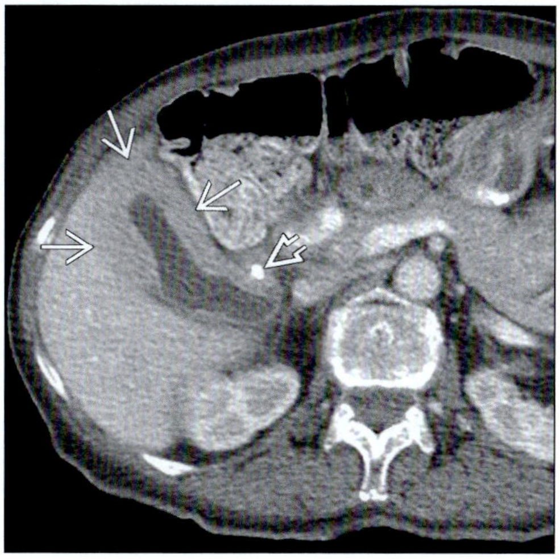

(Left) *Axial CECT in a 75-year-old woman who presented with clinical features of acute cholecystitis shows gallstones and an abscess adjacent to the GB as well as a subcapsular liver abscess. Percutaneous drainage of the abscesses was performed, and surgery was postponed due to other comorbidities.* ***(Right)*** *Axial CECT in the same patient 3 months later shows massive thickening of the GB wall and a stone impacted in the GB neck. Surgery confirmed xanthogranulomatous cholecystitis.*

GIANT BILIARY HAMARTOMA

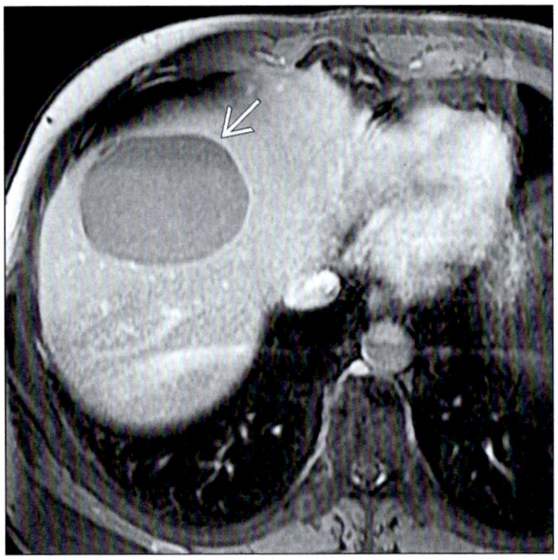

Axial T1WI C+ MR in delayed phase demonstrates a large, well-circumscribed lesion with a relatively low signal intensity and a uniform faint wall enhancement ➡.

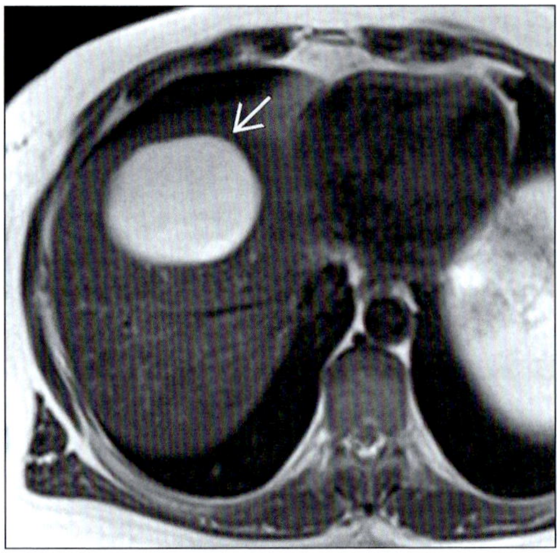

Axial T2WI MR demonstrates a large, well-circumscribed lesion with a high internal signal intensity, compatible with fluid content with a low signal intensity of the wall ➡.

CLINICAL SCENARIO

History
- History of vague abdominal pain

IMAGE INTERPRETATION

Pitfalls
- Can be mistaken for large simple cyst or biliary cystadenoma (leading to more aggressive management if misinterpreted as biliary cystadenoma)

Actual Diagnosis
- Giant biliary hamartoma (von Meyenburg complex)

Clues to Correct Diagnosis
- Well-circumscribed; no internal enhancement
- Hypointense T2 rim and thin rim of peripheral contrast enhancement (fibrous capsule)
- Occasionally hyperintense on T1WI, secondary to intracystic hemorrhage &/or proteinaceous fluid

BACKGROUND

General
- Benign biliary malformation categorized under spectrum of fibropolycystic diseases
- Arise from bile duct embryological remnant due to anomalous development of ductal plate
- Can be solitary or more commonly multiple, small

Epidemiology
- Biliary hamartoma occurs in 3% of population
- Large hamartomas are very rare, mostly occur secondary to intralesional hemorrhage

Relevant Anatomy
- Usually scattered in both lobes, especially in subcapsular region

Relevant Pathology
- Congenital bile duct malformations due to failure of embryonic involution
- Grossly, lesions are gray, uniform in size, and < 1.5 cm
- Microscopically, dilated, tortuous or branching bile ducts lined by a single layer of cuboidal cells and embedded in fibrocollagenous stroma

IMAGING FEATURES

General
- Often small (< 1.5 cm), innumerable, & uniform in size
- Very rarely, single large lesion, likely 2° to bleeding

US
- Can be hyper- and hypoechoic lesions with posterior acoustic enhancement

CT
- Multiple hypoattenuating with marginal faint enhancement
- Small lesions can be too small to be characterize by CT
- Large lesion demonstrates fluid attenuation; increased attenuation when complicated by hemorrhage

MR
- T1WI: Hypointense to adjacent liver parenchyma, could be hyperintense secondary to hemorrhage or proteinaceous material
- T2WI: Hyperintense with hypointense wall due to fibrous tissue
- T1WI C+: No internal enhancement with delayed enhancement of wall
- MRCP: No communication with biliary tree

RELATED REFERENCES

1. Martin DR et al: Giant and complicated variants of cystic bile duct hamartomas of the liver: MRI findings and pathological correlations. J Magn Reson Imaging. 31(4):903-11, 2010

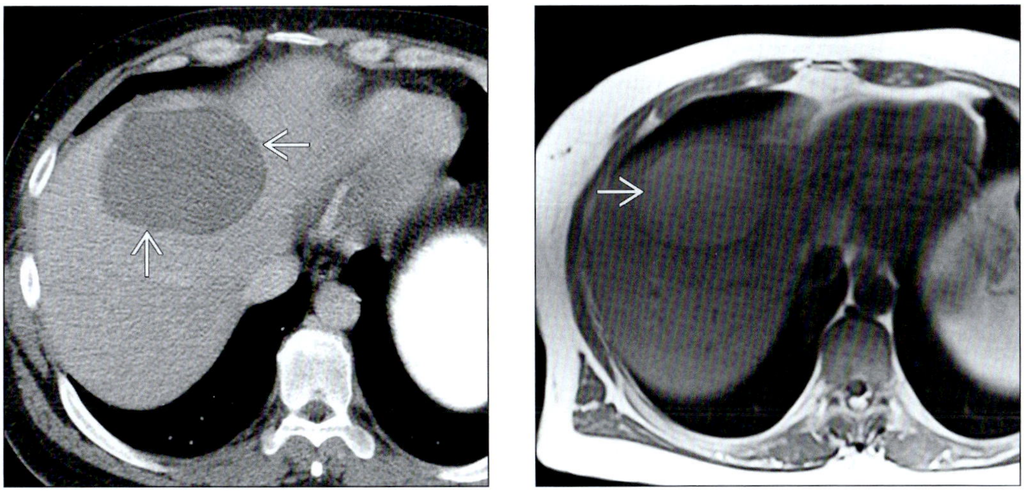

(Left) *Axial CECT demonstrates a large, well-circumscribed fluid attenuation with a faint peripheral enhancement* ➔. ***(Right)*** *Axial T1WI MR in-phase shows a large, well-circumscribed lesion that demonstrates an internal increased signal intensity* ➔ *secondary to hemorrhage.*

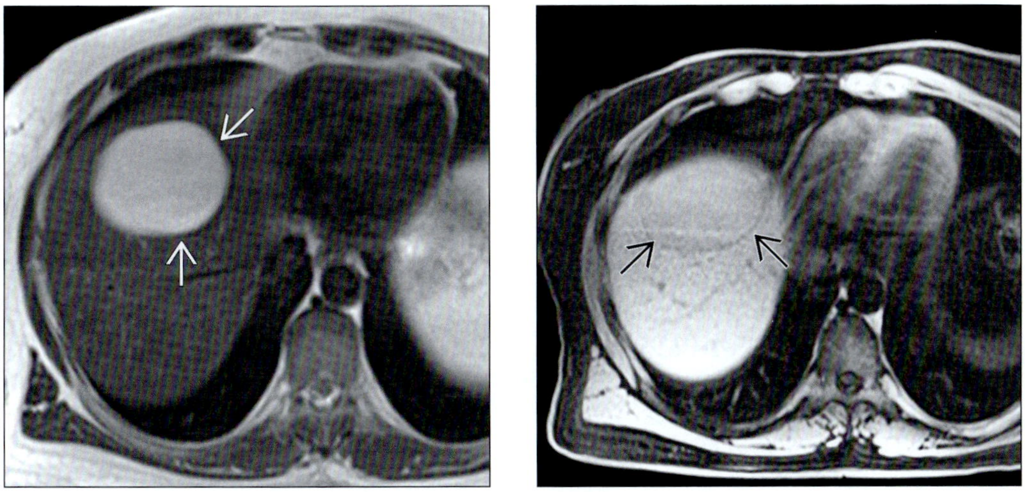

(Left) *Axial T2WI MR in the same patient demonstrates increased signal intensity of the lesion with a low signal intensity of its wall* ➔ *secondary to fibrous capsule.* ***(Right)*** *Axial T1WI FS MR demonstrates slightly increased signal intensity of the lesion secondary to hemorrhage with a low signal intensity of its wall* → *owing to the fibrous capsule.*

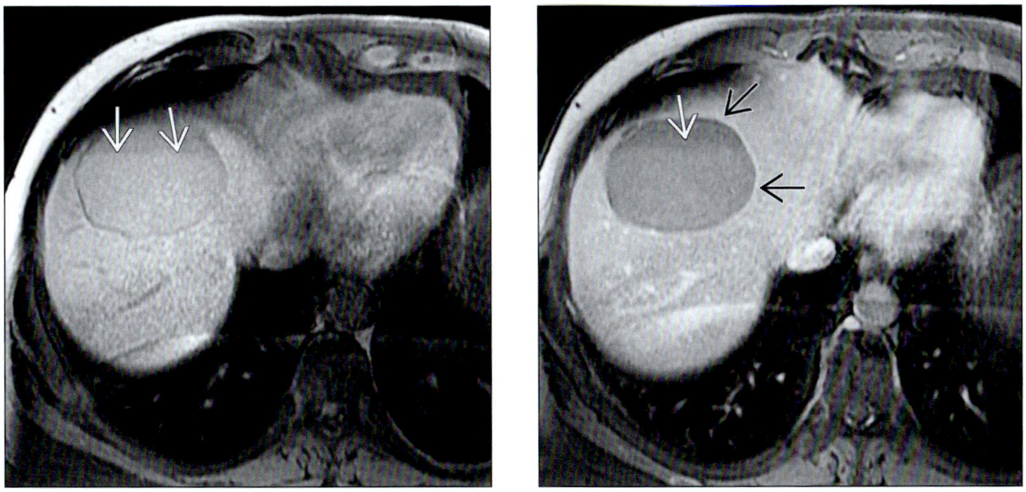

(Left) *Axial T1WI FS MR demonstrates slightly increased signal intensity of the lesion secondary to hemorrhage. Note the hematocrit level* ➔. ***(Right)*** *Axial T1WI C+ FS MR demonstrates a faint peripheral linear enhancement of the fibrous capsule* →*, but no significant enhancement of the lesion internally. Note the hematocrit level* ➔.

PORTAL BILIOPATHY

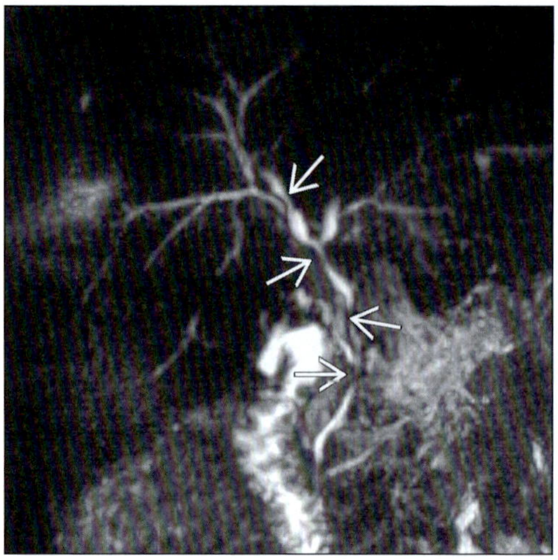

MRCP MIP image shows multiple focal areas of smooth indentation ➡ of the hepatic and bile ducts, resulting in focal areas of dilatation of the uninvolved segments.

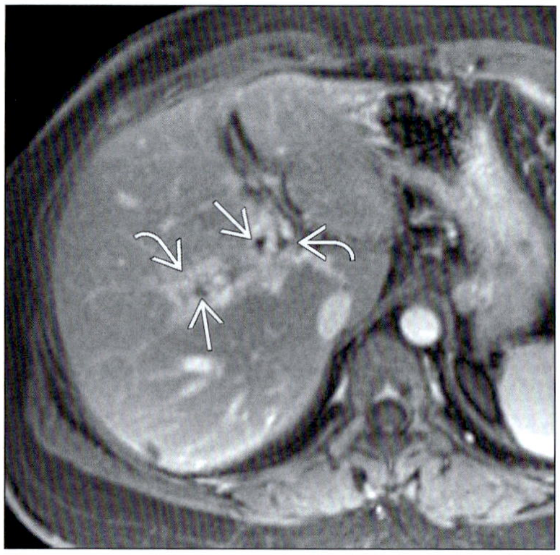

T1WI FS C+ MR in the same patient shows cavernous transformation of the portal vein ↪. The bile ducts ➡ appear as low signal intensity structures that can be mistaken for portal vein thrombus.

CLINICAL SCENARIO

History

- 58-year-old man with history of thrombocytosis

IMAGE INTERPRETATION

Pitfalls

- Apparent bile duct strictures can be mistaken for primary sclerosing cholangitis or cholangiocarcinoma
- Apparent filling defect within portal vein can be mistaken for portal vein thrombus

Actual Diagnosis

- Portal biliopathy due to cavernous transformation of portal vein surrounding hepatic and bile ducts

Clues to Correct Diagnosis

- Recognition of presence of cavernous transformation of portal vein
- Areas of narrowing are smooth, and degree of biliary dilatation is usually mild to moderate
- Filling defects caused by bile ducts can be traced into liver and are continuous with normal intrahepatic bile ducts

BACKGROUND

Epidemiology

- Rate of portal biliopathy in patients with extrahepatic portal venous obstruction is reported to be 70-100%
- Most commonly occurs in noncirrhotic patients with hypercoagulable states

Relevant Anatomy

- Common bile duct drains through
  - Epicholedochal plexus (Saint)
    - Fine reticular veins that are in contact with common bile duct
  - Paracholedochal venous plexus (Petren)
    - Runs parallel to common bile duct and drains into gastric, pancreatoduodenal, or portal veins

Relevant Pathology

- Portal biliopathy is believed to be due to
  - Extrinsic compression of collaterals on biliary tree
  - Fibrotic changes caused by ischemic injury
- Following portal obstruction, collaterals develop that bypass obstruction site
  - Cause mural irregularities and compression of biliary tree

IMAGING FEATURES

General

- Enlarged blood vessels surrounding bile ducts on US, CT, and MR
- Gallbladder varices
- Luminal narrowing of common bile duct as well as upstream biliary duct dilatation

MRCP

- Single or multiple biliary stenosis
- Wavy appearance of bile ducts
- Angulation of common bile duct
- Upstream dilatation of bile ducts with beaded appearance

RELATED REFERENCES

1. Aguirre DA et al: Portal biliopathy: imaging manifestations on multidetector computed tomography and magnetic resonance imaging. Clin Imaging. 36(2):126-34, 2012
2. Besa C et al: Portal biliopathy: a multitechnique imaging approach. Abdom Imaging. 37(1):83-90, 2012
3. Ozkavukcu E et al: Imaging features of portal biliopathy: frequency of involvement patterns with emphasis on MRCP. Eur J Radiol. 71(1):129-34, 2009

BALL ON THE WALL

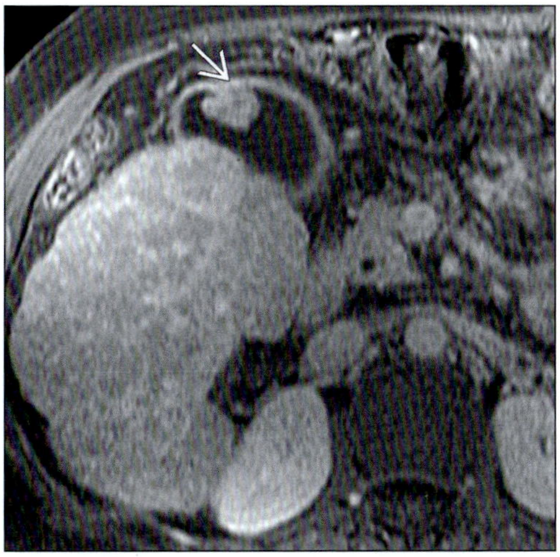

Axial T1WI C+ MR demonstrates a homogeneously enhancing polyp at the gallbladder fundus ➡ that has a sessile base and measures 2.3 x 1.5 cm.

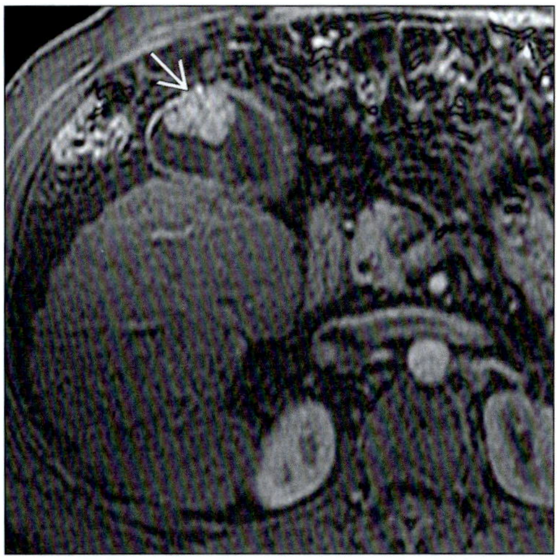

Axial T1WI C+ MR (at 6-month follow-up) demonstrates a homogeneously enhancing polyp at the gallbladder fundus ➡ with interval increase in size, measuring 2.9 x 2.3 cm.

CLINICAL SCENARIO

History
- 57-year-old man with abdominal pain

IMAGE INTERPRETATION

Pitfalls
- Gallbladder polyps should not be dismissed as insignificant findings
- Management should be based on morphology, size, patient age, and symptoms

Actual Diagnosis
- Surgically proven gallbladder adenocarcinoma

Clues to Correct Diagnosis
- Size > 1 cm and sessile base

Differential Diagnosis
- Cholesterol, inflammatory, adenoma, GB carcinoma, and metastasis
- Mimic of polyp: Focal adenomyomatosis and adherent stone/sludge

BACKGROUND

General
- Most gallbladder polyps are benign
- Most cases of benign polyps are asymptomatic
- Gallbladder cancer can present with right upper quadrant pain, jaundice, weight loss, and vomiting

Epidemiology
- Prevalence of gallbladder polypoid lesions is 2-12%
- Gallbladder polyps more common in men

Predictors of Malignancy
- Size > 1 cm, age > 50-60, solitary and sessile polyp
- History of primary sclerosing cholangitis (PSC)

Management
- < 5 mm: No follow-up needed
- 6-10 mm: Follow-up US (every 6 months for a year, then annually)
- > 10 mm: Cholecystectomy

IMAGING FEATURES

US
- Initial modality of choice: Low cost, good sensitivity and specificity
- Doppler: Increased vascularity greater with carcinoma
- Mucosal irregularity, sessile base, and thickening are ancillary findings suggestive of cancer

CT
- Polyps may not be well visualized on CT
- Modality of choice to evaluate extraluminal extension and staging of carcinoma

MR
- Most benign polyps are
  - T1WI: Isointense or hypointense
  - T2WI: Isointense or hyperintense
    - Malignant polyps may be heterogeneous and demonstrate hyperintense signal on T2WI
    - Gallstones appear hypointense
  - T1WI C+: Enhance homogeneously
- DWI: Gallbladder cancer shows restricted diffusion

PET/CT
- High FDG avidity in gallbladder cancer (FDG avidity in polyp > 1 cm is a risk factor for malignancy)

RELATED REFERENCES

1. Sebastian S et al: Managing incidental findings on abdominal and pelvic CT and MRI, Part 4: white paper of the ACR Incidental Findings Committee II on gallbladder and biliary findings. J Am Coll Radiol. 10(12):953-6, 2013
2. Andrén-Sandberg A: Diagnosis and management of gallbladder polyps. N Am J Med Sci. 4(5):203-11, 2012
3. Irie H et al: High b-value diffusion-weighted MRI in differentiation between benign and malignant polypoid gallbladder lesions. Acta Radiol. 52(3):236-40, 2011

RIGLER TRIAD

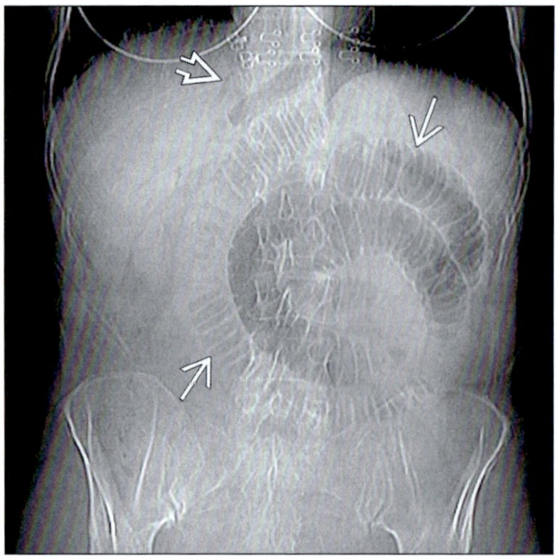

Frontal CT localizer shows dilated small bowel loops and air attenuation tubular structure projecting over the left lobe of the liver.

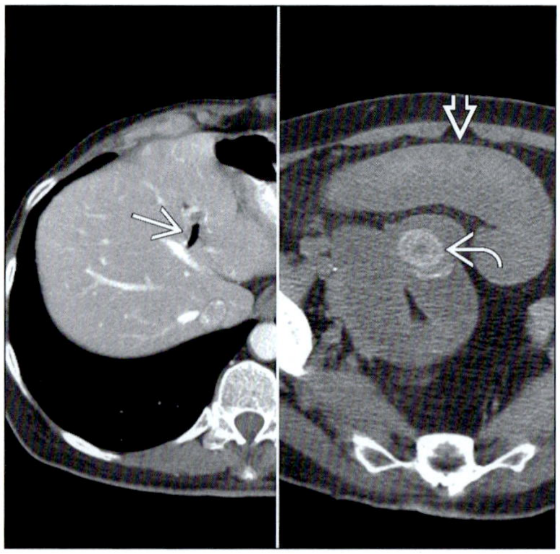

Composite CECT image shows pneumobilia, small bowel dilatation, and a calcified obstructing small bowel structure representing a gallstone.

IMAGING FEATURES

Appearance

- Rigler triad consists of
  - Biliary gas (pneumobilia)
    - Gas may be seen within gallbladder or intrahepatic bile ducts
  - Intestinal obstruction
  - Aberrantly located gallstone
    - May change position on serial radiographs

BACKGROUND

Clinical Significance

- Classic radiologic sign of gallstone ileus
- Rigler triad is best seen on abdominal CT
  - Sensitivity, specificity, and accuracy of CT in diagnosing gallstone ileus is 93%, 100%, and 99%, respectively
  - Other findings that may be seen include
    - Thickening and irregularity of gallbladder wall
    - Thickening of duodenal wall
- Can be easily missed on plain radiographs because most gallstones are radiolucent
  - Only 15% of cases show all 3 elements of Rigler triad

Epidemiology

- Gallstone ileus is complication in 0.3-0.5% of all cases of cholelithiasis
- Gallstone ileus causes ~ 0.1% of intestine obstruction
  - Almost 25% in patients are > 65 years old
- 70% of patients are > 65 years old
- Predominantly occurs in women
  - F:M = 3.5:1
- High mortality rate (12-27%)

Clinical Features

- Patients usually present with intermittent intestinal obstruction
- Most patients have preceding history of right upper quadrant pain

Relevant Pathology

- Gallstone ileus occurs in patients with subacute or chronic cholecystitis
  - Adhesions form between inflamed gallbladder and adjacent part of gastrointestinal tract
- Large stones within gallbladder → pressure necrosis with gallstone eroding into gastrointestinal tract → development of fistulous tract between gallbladder and bowel
  - Most fistulas involve duodenum
    - Fistulas to stomach and colon have been described
  - Gallstone ileus in absence of fistula may rarely occur
    - Due to passage of large stone into bowel through common bile duct following endoscopic sphincterotomy or cholecystectomy
- Terminal ileum is narrowest segment of small bowel and is thus, most likely site of obstruction
  - Bouveret syndrome describes gastric outlet obstruction secondary to impacted gallstone in duodenum or pylorus
- Most obstructive gallstones are ≥ 2.5 cm in diameter

RELATED REFERENCES

1. Halabi WJ et al: Surgery for gallstone ileus: a nationwide comparison of trends and outcomes. Ann Surg. 259(2):329-35, 2014
2. Patel NB et al: Multidetector CT of emergent biliary pathologic conditions. Radiographics. 33(7):1867-88, 2013
3. Lassandro F et al: Role of helical CT in diagnosis of gallstone ileus and related conditions. AJR Am J Roentgenol. 185(5):1159-65, 2005
4. Yu CY et al: Value of CT in the diagnosis and management of gallstone ileus. World J Gastroenterol. 11(14):2142-7, 2005

CALCIFIED GALLBLADDER WALL

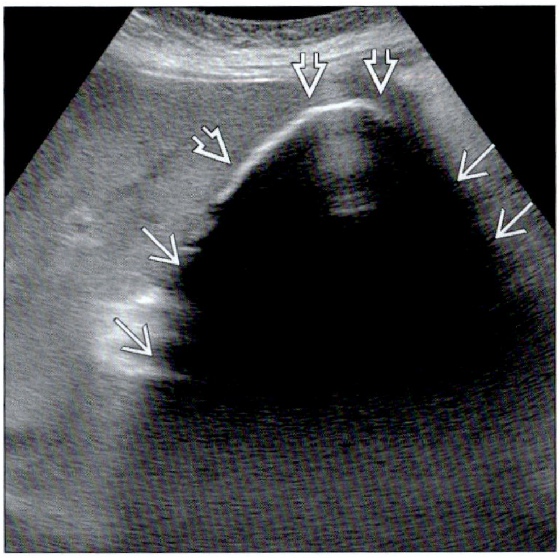

Grayscale ultrasound examination of the right upper quadrant demonstrates a curvilinear echogenic structure ➪ with posterior acoustic shadowing ➔.

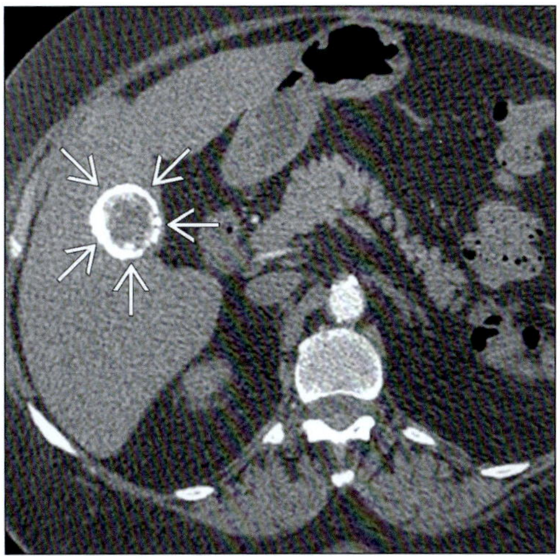

Axial CECT demonstrates densely calcified wall of the gallbladder ➔, consistent with porcelain gallbladder.

CLINICAL SCENARIO

History

- 55-year-old woman with right upper quadrant pain

IMAGE INTERPRETATION

Pitfall

- Extensive calcification of gallbladder wall is referred to as porcelain gallbladder

BACKGROUND

General

- Form of chronic cholecystitis
- Results from calcium deposits in gallbladder wall
- Usually asymptomatic and incidentally found on imaging

Epidemiology

- Prevalence in cholecystectomy specimens range from 0.06-0.8%
- F:M = 5:1
- Mean age: 54 years (range: 38–70 years)

Relevant Pathology

- Gross
  - "Porcelain" refers to gross appearance of blue discoloration of gallbladder found at surgery
- Microscopic
  - Extent of calcification can range from small focal mucosal plaques to full thickness intramural involvement with calcified fibrosis
- Most porcelain gallbladders (90%) are associated with gallstones
- May result from cystic duct obstruction leading to mucosal precipitation of calcium carbonate salts
- May also result from chronic irritation of wall by stone or low-grade inflammatory process
- May predispose to gallbladder adenocarcinoma
- Cholecystectomy should be considered

IMAGING FEATURES

Plain Radiography

- Curvilinear calcification can be seen projected over right upper quadrant

US

- Curvilinear hyperechoic gallbladder wall with posterior acoustic shadowing
- Should be differentiated from contracted gallbladder packed with stones in which wall of gallbladder appears external to echogenic curvilinear shadow representing stones

CT

- Most sensitive modality
- Curvilinear dense calcification of gallbladder wall

MR

- T1WI: Signal voids within gallbladder wall
- T2WI: Signal voids within gallbladder wall
- T1WI C+: No abnormal enhancement

HIDA

- Nonfunctioning gallbladder

RELATED REFERENCES

1. Revzin MV et al: The gallbladder: uncommon gallbladder conditions and unusual presentations of the common gallbladder pathological processes. Abdom Imaging. Epub ahead of print, 2014
2. Schnelldorfer T: Porcelain gallbladder: a benign process or concern for malignancy? J Gastrointest Surg. 17(6):1161-8, 2013
3. Gupta S et al: Rare presentation of malignant porcelain gallbladder with intrahepatic ductal calcification and surgical obstructive jaundice. Indian J Surg Oncol. 3(1):44-6, 2012
4. Ash-Miles J et al: More than just stones: a pictorial review of common and less common gallbladder pathologies. Curr Probl Diagn Radiol. 37(5):189-202, 2008

BRANCHING INTRAHEPATIC GAS

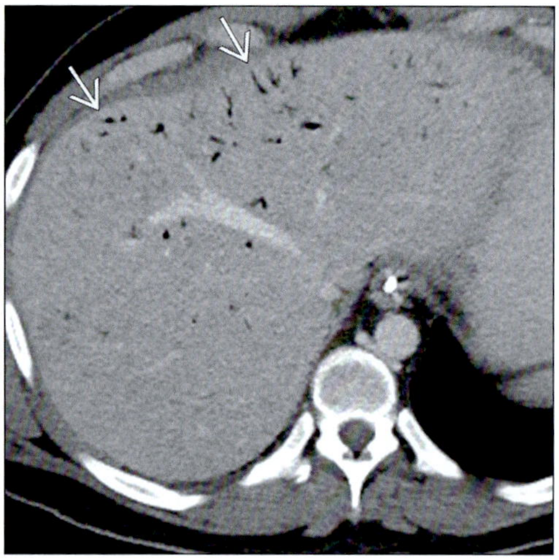

Axial CECT shows numerous small branching tubular structures of air attenuation ➔ in the periphery of the liver (within 2 cm of the liver capsule), due to the presence of gas in the intrahepatic portal veins.

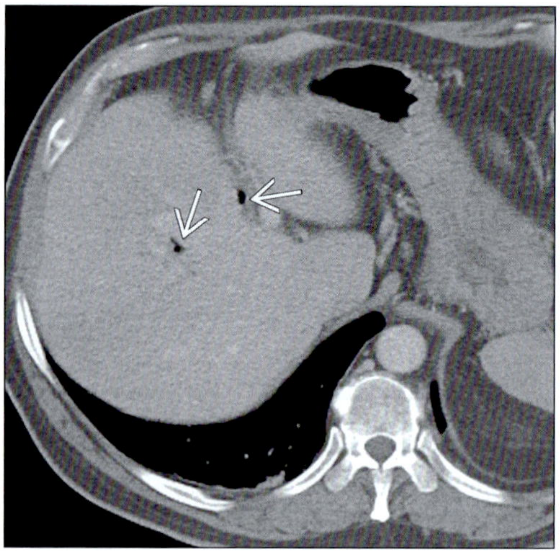

Axial CECT shows tubular areas of air attenuation ➔ centrally within the liver, not extending to within 2 cm of the liver capsule, due to pneumobilia.

IMAGING FEATURES

Clinical Scenario

- Both portal venous gas and pneumobilia present as intrahepatic branching air attenuation structures
  - Can be distinguished by pattern and distribution of gas within liver
    - Knowledge of patient clinical history and careful search for associated findings can also help to determine location of hepatic gas

Differential Diagnosis

- Portal venous gas
  - More peripherally located
    - Carried by centrifugal blood flow to hepatic periphery
  - Small and numerous branching gas attenuation on CT extending to within 2 cm of liver capsule
  - Predominantly in left lobe
  - ± mesenteric venous gas
  - May be able to demonstrate fluid-attenuation bile duct adjacent to gas-filled portal vein at CECT
  - Can be seen on ultrasound as small echogenic particles moving towards periphery of liver
- Pneumobilia
  - More centrally located
    - Carried by centripetal distribution related to direction of bile flow towards hilum of liver
  - Does not extend to within 2 cm of liver capsule
  - ± gas within common bile duct
  - May be able to demonstrate contrast-opacified portal vein adjacent to gas-filled bile duct at CECT
  - Can be seen on ultrasound as highly reflective linear echoes casting dirty shadow

BACKGROUND

Etiology

- Portal venous gas
  - Bowel ischemia
    - Accounts for ~ 50% of cases of portal venous gas
    - Presence of portal venous gas is not diagnostic sign of transmural necrosis in patients with bowel ischemia
  - Bowel dilatation (iatrogenic or noniatrogenic)
    - Following gastrointestinal endoscopic procedures such as colonoscopy
  - Gastrointestinal tract inflammation, trauma, ulcerations, and cancer
  - Intraabdominal sepsis (diverticulitis, pelvic abscess, etc.)
  - Idiopathic
  - Transplantation, corticosteroid therapy, and chronic obstructive pulmonary disease (COPD)
- Pneumobilia
  - Biliary instrumentation (ERCP, biliary stent, etc.)
  - Incompetent sphincter of Oddi
    - Sphincterotomy
    - Following passage of stone
    - Scarring as in chronic pancreatitis
  - Biliary enteric anastomosis
    - Surgically created
    - Spontaneous: Gallstone ileus, duodenal ulcer
  - Biliary infections and emphysematous cholecystitis

RELATED REFERENCES

1. Milone M et al: Computed tomography findings of pneumatosis and portomesenteric venous gas in acute bowel ischemia. World J Gastroenterol. 19(39):6579-84, 2013
2. Shah PA et al: Hepatic gas: widening spectrum of causes detected at CT and US in the interventional era. Radiographics. 31(5):1403-13, 2011
3. Sebastià C et al: Portomesenteric vein gas: pathologic mechanisms, CT findings, and prognosis. Radiographics. 20(5):1213-24; discussion 1224-6, 2000

GAS WITHIN GALLBLADDER WALL

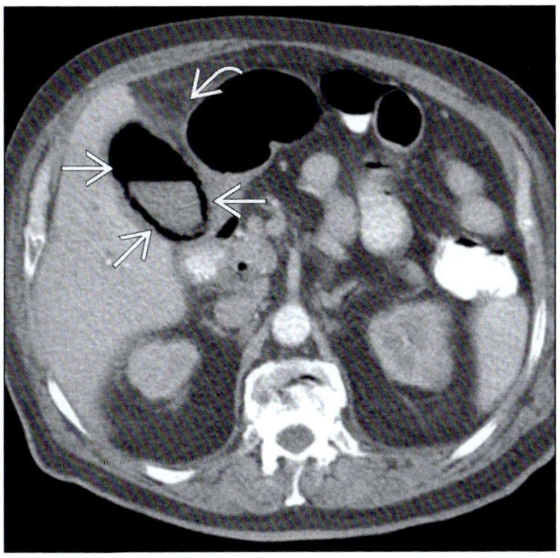

Axial CECT demonstrates linear gas attenuation ➔ within the gallbladder wall and lumen. Pericholecystic inflammatory changes ➔ are also noted.

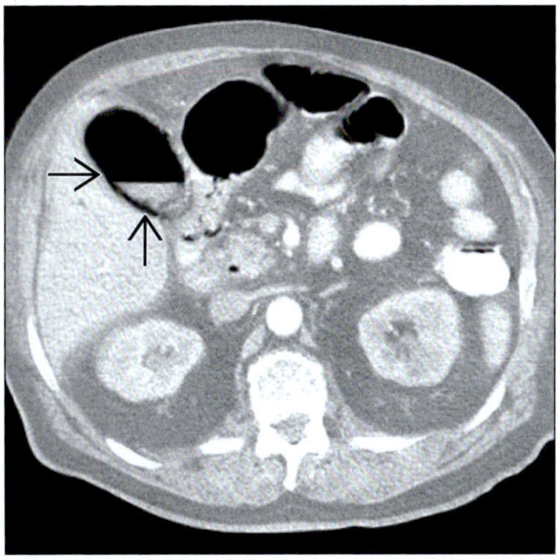

Axial CECT (in bone window) through the liver and gallbladder demonstrates linear gas attenuation ➔ within the gallbladder wall and gallbladder lumen.

CLINICAL SCENARIO

History

- 68-year-old man with right upper quadrant (RUQ) pain

IMAGE INTERPRETATION

Classic Sign

- Gas within gallbladder (GB) wall with pericholecystic inflammation is classic for emphysematous cholecystitis

BACKGROUND

General

- Gas-forming infection of GB
- Commonest organisms: *Clostridium Perfringens* and *Escherichia coli*
- Insidious onset with rapid clinical progression
- Patients may lack RUQ pain/tenderness
- Emergent condition typically treated with cholecystectomy and intravenous antibiotics
- Rare side effect of molecular targeted therapies

Epidemiology

- M > F
- Age: 50-70 years
- Typically seen in patients with diabetes mellitus &/or underlying peripheral vascular disease

Relevant Physiology

- Cystic artery ischemia and occlusion is important contributing factor

Relevant Pathology

- Gross: Gangrenous and necrotic GB
- Microscopic
  - Edema, hemorrhage, and necrosis of GB mucosa and wall
  - Mural abscesses may be seen
  - Microorganisms may be seen on Gram stains

IMAGING FEATURES

US

- Echogenic reflectors within GB wall &/or lumen with posterior ring down artifacts
- Champagne sign: Small echogenic foci, reflecting gas bubbles, floating to nondependent portions of GB
- Emphysematous cholecystitis may be mistaken for loop of bowel
- Sonographic Murphy sign may be negative, either due to denervation/neuropathy in setting of diabetes mellitus or from GB wall necrosis

CT

- Most sensitive for emphysematous cholecystitis
- Gas within GB lumen &/or wall
- Pericholecystic inflammatory change

Nuclear Imaging

- Hepatobiliary nuclear imaging may demonstrate nonvisualization of GB
- Increased tracer activity near GB fossa may be seen (a.k.a. rim sign), reflective of relative hyperemia due to inflammation; not specific to emphysematous cholecystitis

MR

- Signal voids within GB lumen &/or wall
- Signal voids accumulate in nondependent portions of GB, distinguishing them from gallstones, which appear as low signal intensity dependent foci

RELATED REFERENCES

1. Smith EA et al: Cross-sectional imaging of acute and chronic gallbladder inflammatory disease. AJR Am J Roentgenol. 192(1):188-96, 2009
2. Grand D et al: CT of the gallbladder: spectrum of disease. AJR Am J Roentgenol. 2004 Jul;183(1):163-70. Erratum in: AJR Am J Roentgenol. 183(20:543, 2004
3. Grayson DE et al: Emphysematous infections of the abdomen and pelvis: a pictorial review. Radiographics. 22(3):543-61, 2002

PEARL NECKLACE SIGN

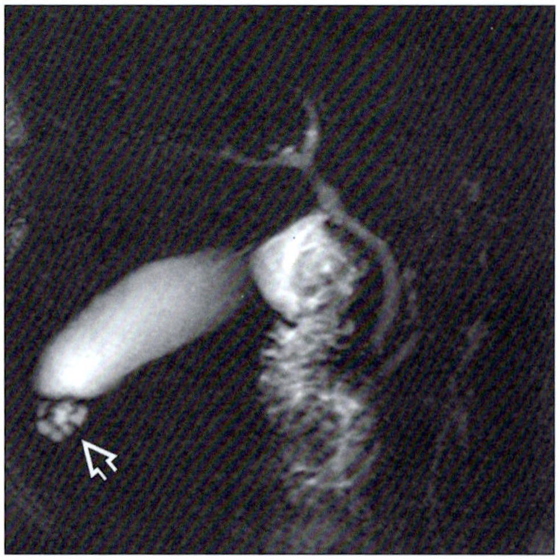

MRCP MIP image shows a collection of multiple small cystic structures ➡ in the region of the gallbladder fundus, demonstrating high signal intensity similar to that of intraluminal bile.

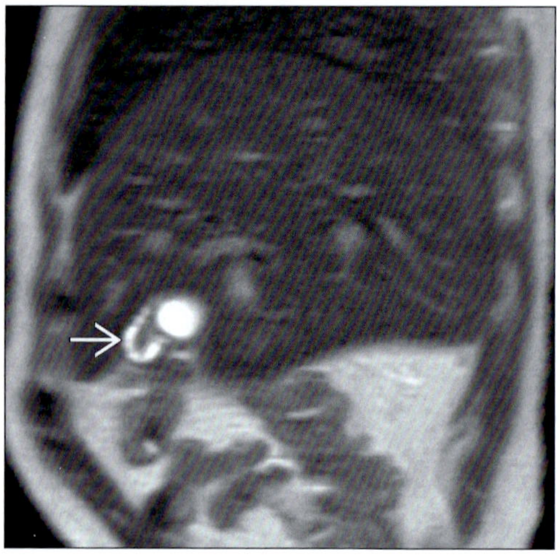

Sagittal T2WI MR in the same patient shows a curvilineal arrangement of small cystic structures ➡ within an area of gallbladder wall thickening, resembling a pearl necklace.

IMAGING FEATURES

Appearance

- Pearl necklace sign, also referred to as string of beads sign, describes curvilinear arrangement of multiple small foci of high signal intensity (similar to signal intensity of intraluminal bile) in gallbladder wall on MRCP or T2WI
  - May also be observed on CECT as small, hypoattenuating structures within focal area of gallbladder wall thickening

Significance

- Focal or segmental gallbladder adenomyomatosis can appear almost identical to mass and may be difficult to distinguish from benign and malignant gallbladder focal lesions
- Highly specific (92-100%) in diagnosing gallbladder adenomyomatosis vs. gallbladder cancer
- MR is superior to CECT in differentiating gallbladder adenomyomatosis from gallbladder malignancy

Limitation

- Low sensitivity (only 62%), as it may be absent in cases of
  - Small sinuses (> 3 mm)
  - Sinuses filled with inspissated proteinaceous bile or small calculi
    - May be better seen on ultrasound as echogenic foci with comet tail artifact &/or color Doppler twinkling artifact
- Gallbladder carcinoma in adenomyomatosis of gallbladder with pearl necklace sign has been described

BACKGROUND

Explanation

- Foci of high T2 signal intensity within gallbladder wall correspond to bile-filled Rokitansky-Aschoff sinuses
- Rokitansky-Aschoff sinuses are intramural diverticula lined by mucosal epithelium, frequently communicating with gallbladder lumen

Epidemiology

- Reported in 5-8.7% of cholecystectomy specimens
- More frequently seen in women than men
- 90% of cases are associated with gallstones

Relevant Pathology

- Adenomyomatosis is a benign hyperplastic cholesterolosis
  - Noninflammatory benign condition
  - Excessive proliferation of surface epithelium with deep and branching invaginations (Rokitansky-Aschoff sinuses) into thickened gallbladder wall
- Adenomyomatosis of gallbladder may manifest as diffuse, segmental, or focal disease
  - Diffuse adenomyomatosis
    - Diffuse mural thickening and luminal narrowing
  - Segmental adenomyomatosis
    - Circumferential thickening in midportion "waist" of gallbladder, producing hourglass configuration
  - Localized adenomyomatosis
    - Nodular, semilunar or crescentic, solid mass, usually in gallbladder fundus

RELATED REFERENCES

1. Bang SH et al: Differentiating between adenomyomatosis and gallbladder cancer: revisiting a comparative study of high-resolution ultrasound, multidetector CT, and MR imaging. Korean J Radiol. 15(2):226-34, 2014
2. Imai H et al: Gallbladder adenocarcinoma with extended intramural spread in adenomyomatosis of the gallbladder with the pearl necklace sign. Am Surg. 77(3):E57-8, 2011
3. Catalano OA et al: MR imaging of the gallbladder: a pictorial essay. Radiographics. 28(1):135-55; quiz 324, 2008
4. Haradome H et al: The pearl necklace sign: an imaging sign of adenomyomatosis of the gallbladder at MR cholangiopancreatography. Radiology. 227(1):80-8, 2003

ARCIFORM PATTERN OF ENHANCEMENT OF SPLEEN

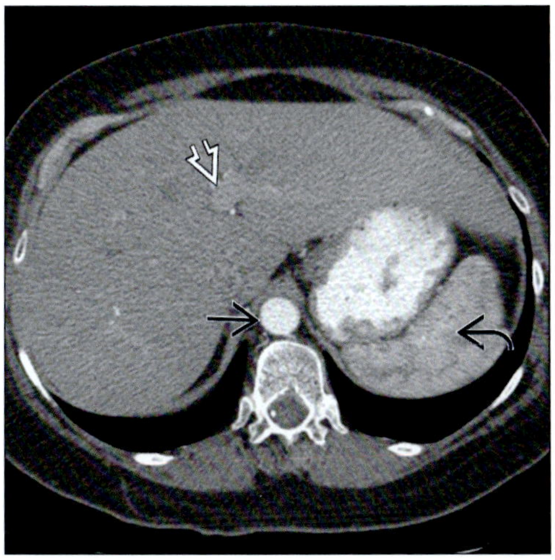
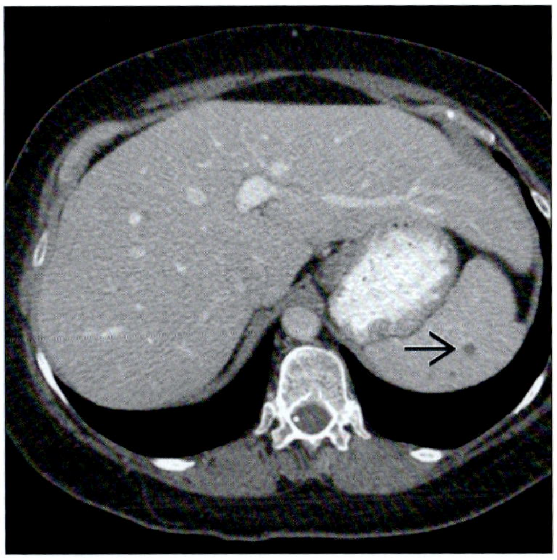

*(**Left**) Axial CT in the late arterial phase shows dense enhancement in the aorta → and hepatic artery branches and faint enhancement in the portal vein branch →. There are curvilinear hypoattenuating bands throughout the spleen, representing arciform enhancement →. No focal splenic lesion is seen. (**Right**) Axial CT in the portovenous phase in the same patient shows homogeneous enhancement of the spleen. Small focal hypodense lesions → are now apparent.*

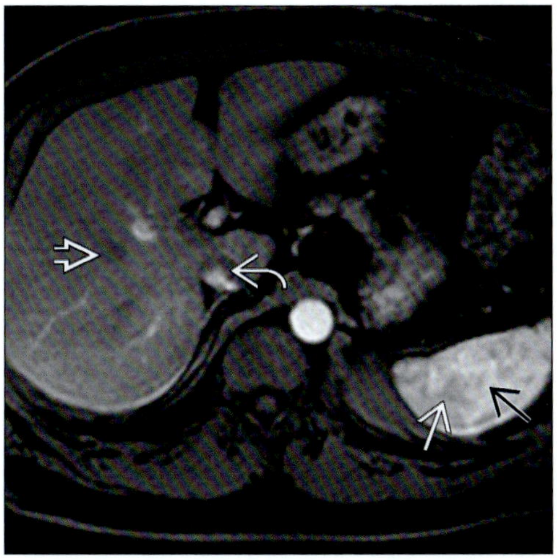
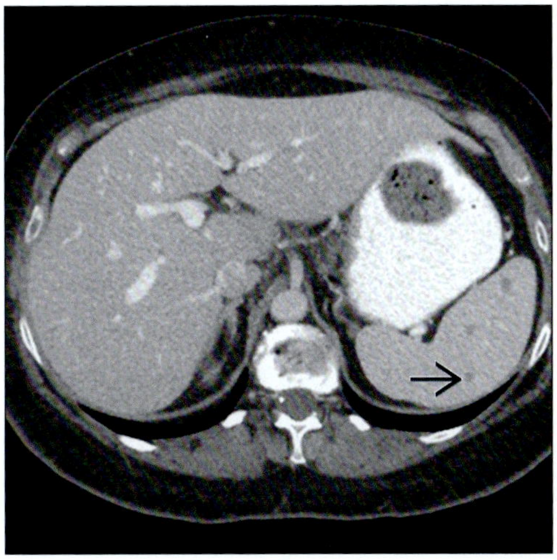

*(**Left**) T1WI MR (same patient) shows curvilinear alternating bands of high → & low → signal intensities compatible with arciform enhancement. Note dense enhancement in the aorta & hepatic artery branches. The hepatic veins are not opacified →. Note partial contrast enhancement in the IVC → from renal return. An accessory spleen is present. (**Right**) Axial CT in the portovenous phase (same patient) shows higher density enhancement in the portal vein branches & homogeneous enhancement of spleen. Small focal hypodense lesions → are now apparent.*

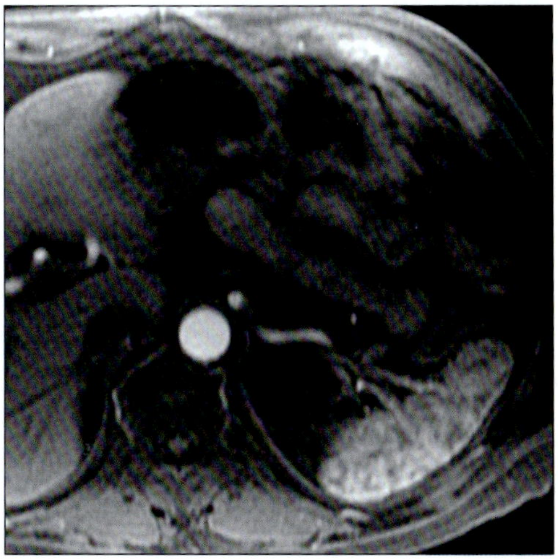
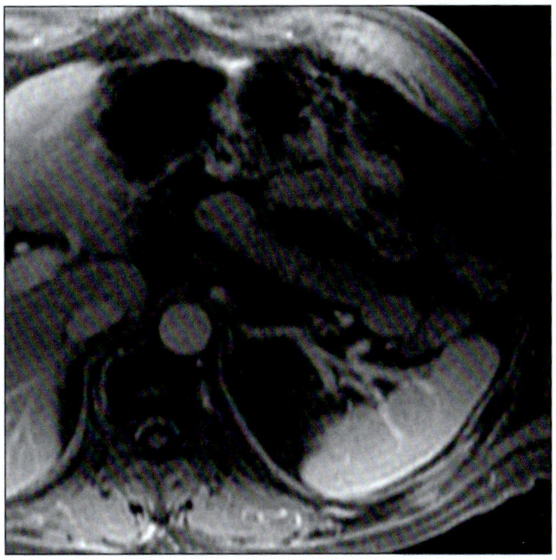

*(**Left**) Axial T1WI C+ in the arterial phase in a different patient demonstrates heterogeneous enhancement of the spleen (which can be misinterpreted as multiple focal lesions). (**Right**) Axial T1WI C+ in the venous phase demonstrates homogeneous enhancement of the spleen without evidence of focal lesions.*

EXTRAMEDULLARY HEMATOPOIESIS

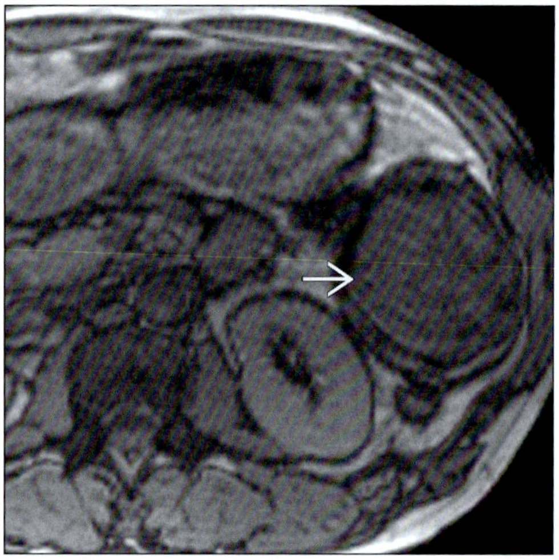

Axial out-of-phase T1WI MR demonstrates a large, well-circumscribed splenic mass lesion ➔ that appears slightly hypointense relative to the skeletal muscles.

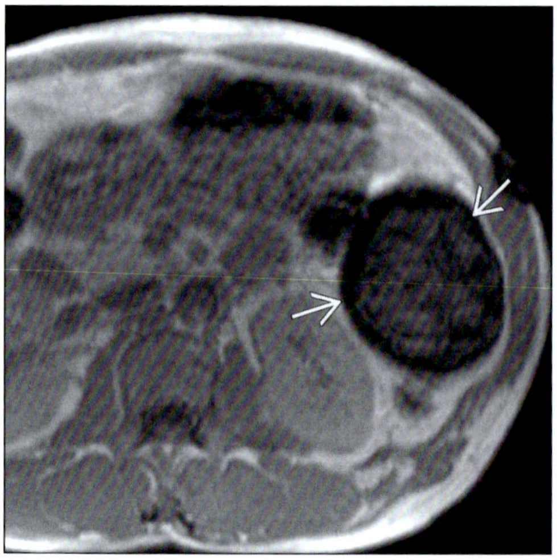

Axial in-phase MR shows a well-circumscribed splenic mass ➔ exhibiting lower signal intensity compared to out-of-phase, secondary to iron present in hemosiderin (magnetic susceptibility in longer TE).

CLINICAL SCENARIO

History

- 79-year-old man with lymphoma treated by chemotherapy

IMAGE INTERPRETATION

Pitfalls

- May be mistaken for splenic lymphoma, metastasis, hamartoma, pseudotumor, or granulomatous disease

Actual Diagnosis

- Extramedullary hematopoiesis (EMH)

Clues to Correct Diagnosis

- History of hematologic disorder/myelodysplasia
- Evidence of extramedullary hematopoiesis elsewhere, such as liver or paraspinal regions

BACKGROUND

Epidemiology

- Mass-like EMH in spleen is quite rare
- Spleen is most common site of EMH in myelodysplasia

Relevant Physiology

- Occurs in congenital hemolytic processes, marrow replacement; myelodysplastic syndromes, idiopathic, post-chemotherapy or post-radiation therapy
- Compensatory response to abnormal/insufficient medullary hematopoiesis
- Pluripotential stem cells develop in spleen, a site of hematopoiesis during fetal development

Relevant Pathology

- Gross: Encapsulated mass with fibrous capsule
- Active lesion
    - Hematopoietic elements with mature & immature granulocytic precursors, blast cells, erythroblasts, & megakaryocytes
    - Extracellular hemosiderin
- Inactive lesions: Fat and hemosiderin

IMAGING FEATURES

US

- Well-circumscribed, hyperechoic mass

CT

- Well-circumscribed, slightly heterogeneous mass
- Slightly hyperattenuating to spleen on NECT
- Mild gradual contrast enhancement (but hypoenhancing compared to spleen)

MR

- Depends upon evolution of hematopoiesis
    - Active hematopoietic lesions contain immature or mature erythroid and myeloid cells
        - T1WI: Intermediate signal intensity (SI)
        - T2WI: High signal intensity (SI)
    - Older inactive hematopoietic lesions
        - Low signal intensity on T1 and T2WI (secondary to iron deposition in hemosiderin) or high signal intensity (secondary to fat content)
        - Iron → decreased SI on pulse sequences having longer echo times (in 1.5 testa, in-phase compared to out-of-phase & T2WI compared to T1WI)

PET/CT

- FDG avid

Nuclear Medicine

- ↑ uptake on Tc-99m sulfur-colloid liver-spleen scan, unlike other lesions that are usually photopenic

RELATED REFERENCES

1. Wang CW et al: Focal extramedullary haematopoiesis of the spleen: unusual MR appearance with pathological correlation. Br J Radiol. 81(968):e211-4, 2008
2. Singer A et al: Extramedullary hematopoiesis presenting as a focal splenic mass: a case report. Abdom Imaging. 29(6):710-2, 2004

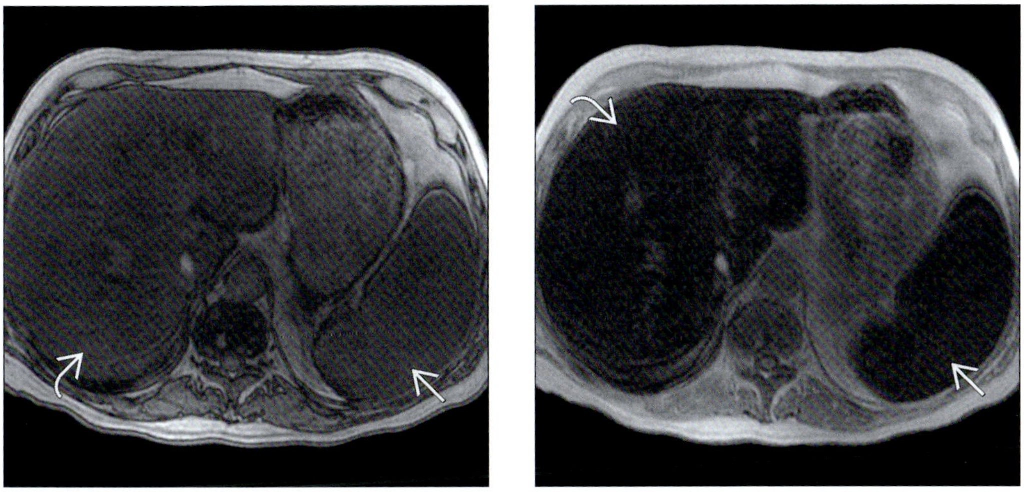

(Left) *Axial out-of-phase MR at the level of the liver and spleen demonstrates no definite evidence of significant abnormality.* ***(Right)*** *Axial in-phase (longer TE) MR in the same patient demonstrates diffuse loss of signal within the liver and spleen, consistent with iron deposition, secondary to repeated blood transfusions.*

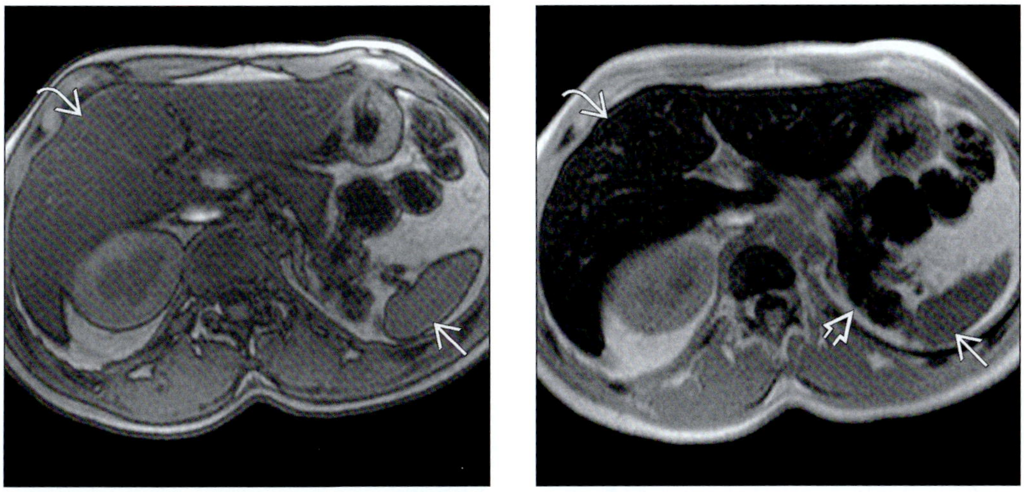

(Left) *Axial out-of-phase T1WI MR in a 45-year-old man at the level of the liver and spleen demonstrates homogeneous signal intensity, which is nearly isointense to the skeletal muscles.* ***(Right)*** *Axial in-phase (longer TE) MR in the same patient shows diffuse loss of signal within the liver and pancreas, consistent with iron deposition. The spleen shows no evidence for iron deposition, suggesting primary hemochromatosis.*

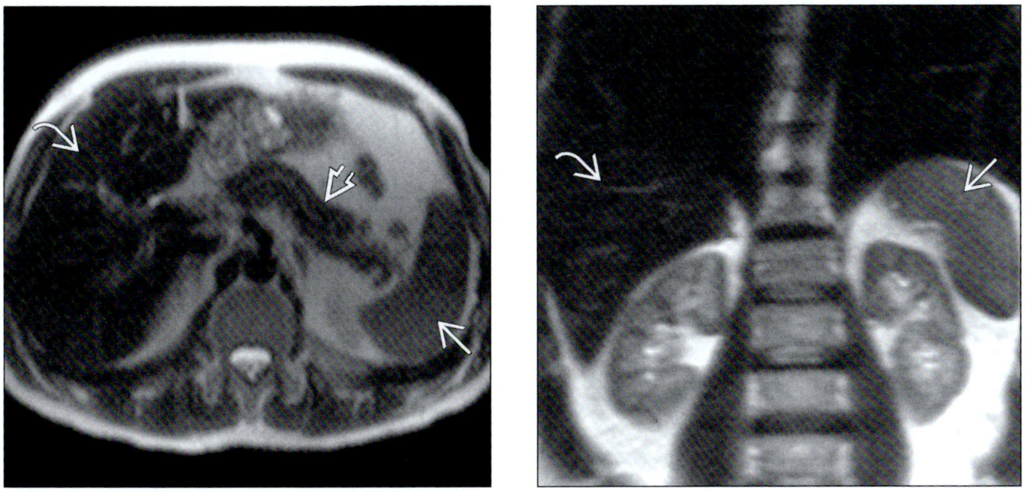

(Left) *Axial T2WI MR in the same patient demonstrates diffuse loss of signal within the liver and pancreas, consistent with iron deposition. Involvement of the liver and pancreas and sparing of the spleen is consistent with primary hemochromatosis.* ***(Right)*** *Coronal T2WI MR in the same patient demonstrates diffuse loss of signal within the liver, consistent with iron deposition. The spleen shows no evidence for iron deposition, suggesting primary hemochromatosis.*

SENTINEL CLOT SIGN: SPLENIC RUPTURE

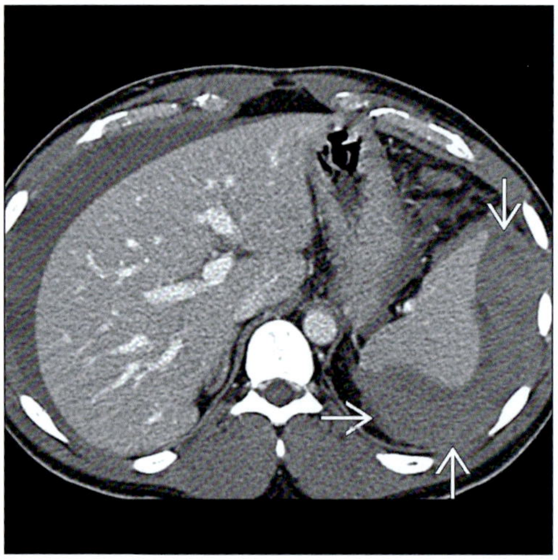

Axial CECT shows high-attenuation intraperitoneal fluid (hemoperitoneum) with the highest attenuation fluid noted adjacent to the spleen compatible with a sentinel clot ➡.

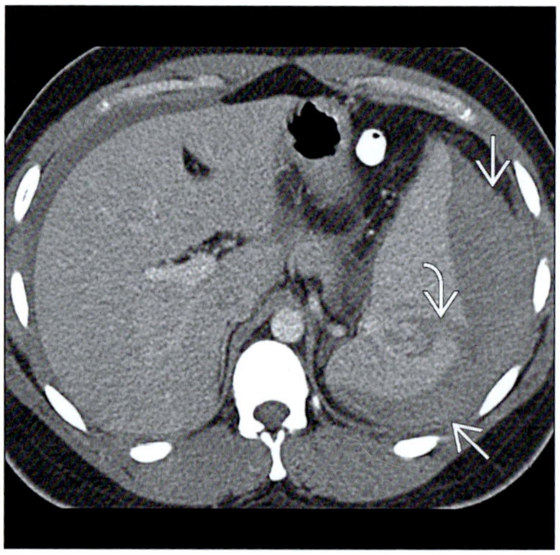

Axial CECT in a different patient demonstrates a sentinel clot ➡, adjacent to the spleen, which has an irregular hypoattenuating laceration ➡ extending to the splenic surface.

CLINICAL SCENARIO

History

- 35-year-old man with no prior medical problems presents with abdominal pain after motor vehicle accident

IMAGE INTERPRETATION

Classic Sign

- In absence of visible laceration in spleen, presence of adjacent sentinel clot is highly suggestive of underlying splenic injury (known as sentinel clot sign)

Description

- CT is fairly sensitive (86%) in detecting visceral injury, which causes hemoperitoneum in abdominal trauma patients
- In about 14% of cases, CT is not able to visualize parenchymal injury itself
  - In such cases, sentinel clot sign may be only clue that organ adjacent to it is injured

BACKGROUND

General

- Hemoperitoneum is frequently present in patients with significant visceral abdominal injuries after trauma
- Sentinel clot sign may be even more valuable in mesenteric injuries as only finding of mesenteric injury can be nonspecific, such as bowel wall thickening
- Sentinel clot sign is not that helpful for liver trauma as most liver lacerations are easily visualized on CT

Relevant Pathology

- At time of extravasation, extravasated blood is isoattenuating to circulating blood
- Shortly after extravasation, extravasated blood starts to clot and increases in attenuation
- Blood that is closest to the injury has more time to clot and become hyperattenuating

IMAGING FEATURES

NECT

- Most hyperattenuating localized region of a hemoperitoneum is known as a sentinel clot, which is suggestive of adjacent visceral injury
- CT should be performed in patients with abdominal trauma for detection of extent of injury

CECT

- Important to detect any underlying vascular involvement and active extravasation

Ultrasound

- Hemoperitoneum and sentinel clot appear as complex heterogeneous fluid

MR

- Hemoperitoneum and sentinel clot follow signal intensity of blood degradation products

Key Teaching Points

- In abdominal trauma patients with hemoperitoneum without direct signs of visceral injury, such as laceration or contrast extravasation, sentinel clot can help localize injured organ

RELATED REFERENCES

1. Lubner M et al: Blood in the belly: CT findings of hemoperitoneum. Radiographics. 27(1):109-25, 2007
2. Orwig D et al: Localized clotted blood as evidence of visceral trauma on CT: the sentinel clot sign. AJR Am J Roentgenol. 153(4):747-9, 1989
3. Federle MP et al: Hemoperitoneum studied by computed tomography. Radiology. 148(1):187-92, 1983

SPLENIC CLEFT MIMICKING LACERATION

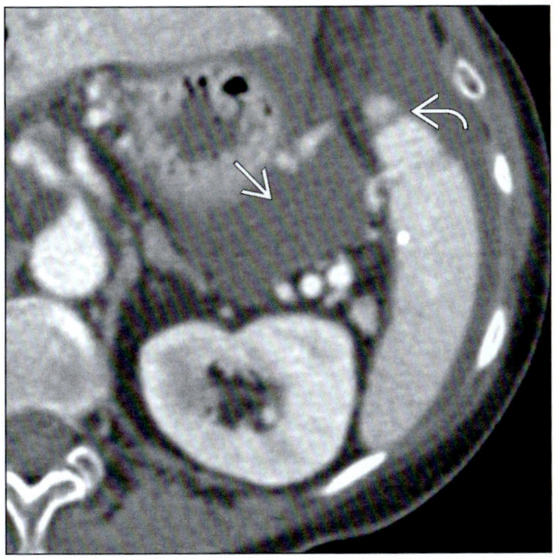

Axial CECT demonstrates perisplenic fluid ➡ and a well-defined linear hypoattenuation ➡ traversing through the anterior pole of the spleen.

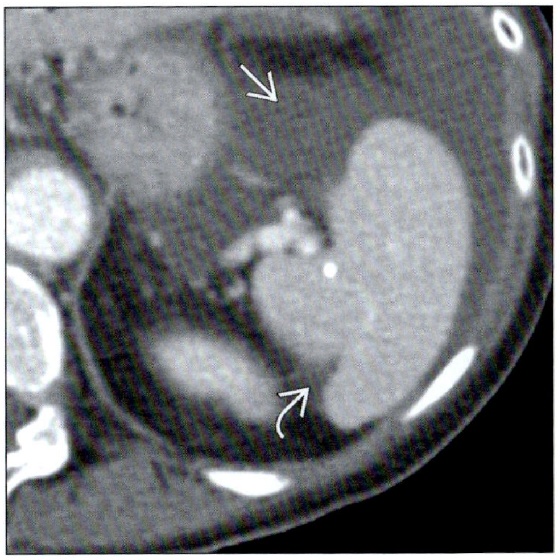

Axial CECT shows perisplenic fluid ➡ and a well-defined linear hypoattenuation ➡ at the posteromedial surface of the spleen.

CLINICAL SCENARIO

History

- 33-year-old man with trauma

IMAGE INTERPRETATION

Pitfalls

- Can be mistaken for splenic tear

Actual Diagnosis

- Congenital splenic cleft

Clues to Correct Diagnosis

- Splenic clefts have smooth or rounded margin
- Usually found along medial splenic surface, whereas lacerations mostly originate from lateral surface
- On delayed imaging, cleft remains hypoattenuating because it contains fat, while lacerations can be hyperattenuating (blood)
- Other associated findings such as subcapsular hematoma can support diagnosis of splenic tear

BACKGROUND

General

- Fetal spleen is normally lobulated
- Notches or clefts on adult spleen are remnants of grooves that originally separated fetal lobules

Epidemiology of Splenic Trauma

- Spleen is most commonly injured organ following trauma (motor vehicle accident being most common cause), followed by direct blows and falls
    - Splenomegaly is more susceptible to trauma

IMAGING FEATURES

General

- Splenic cleft is seen as smooth indentation of splenic surface, while laceration is usually associated with abnormal bleeding

US

- Can be useful for screening of splenic injury, especially in hemodynamically unstable patient
- Lacerations and hematomas may appear echogenic but both fresh and chronic hemorrhage can appear hypoechoic

CT

- Primary imaging technique for screening of splenic injury
- Portal venous phase is needed in addition to arterial phase to evaluate splenic parenchymal injury because normally heterogeneous enhancement during early arterial phase may mimic injury

MR

- Splenic hematoma can be seen as high signal intensity on both T1WI and T2WI
- Plays little role in patients with splenic trauma because of time factor, especially in hemodynamically unstable patients

Nuclear Medicine

- Tc-99m sulfur colloid scan has been shown to be sensitive but nonspecific

Angiography

- Useful in therapeutic embolization of splenic vessels

RELATED REFERENCES

1. Kamaya A et al: Multiple lesions of the spleen: differential diagnosis of cystic and solid lesions. Semin Ultrasound CT MR. 27(5):389-403, 2006
2. Madoff DC et al: Splenic arterial interventions: anatomy, indications, technical considerations, and potential complications. Radiographics. 25 Suppl 1:S191-211, 2005

AUTOSPLENECTOMY IN SICKLE CELL ANEMIA

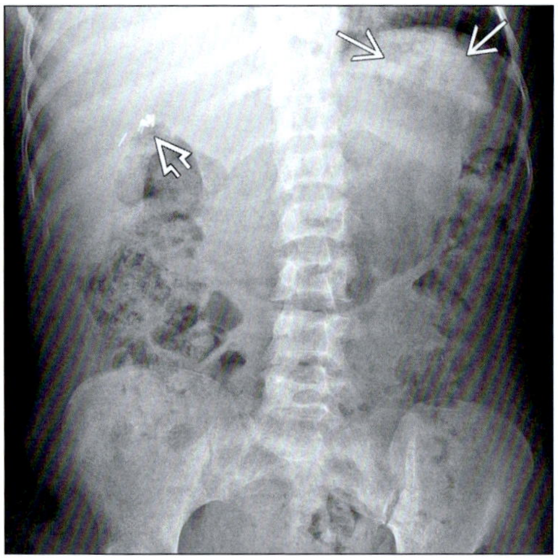

Frontal supine radiograph shows a crescent-shaped dense left upper quadrant structure →. Note also right upper quadrant surgical clips ⇨ due to prior cholecystectomy.

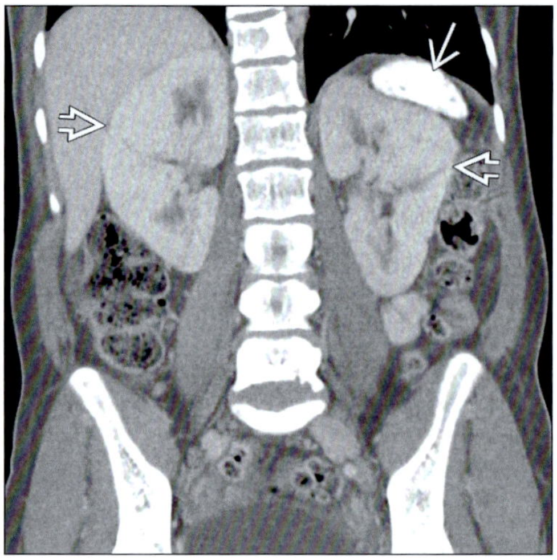

Coronal CECT shows a small, densely calcified spleen → and enlargement of both kidneys ⇨. No hepatic or lymph nodal calcifications are present.

CLINICAL SCENARIO

History

- 29-year-old woman with history of sickle cell anemia (SCA)

Imaging Findings

- Small, densely calcified spleen on plain radiography and CT

Differential Diagnosis

- Thorium dioxide exposure
  - Can result in areas of splenic increased attenuation
    - Clinical history of exposure to agent
    - Liver and lymph nodal increased attenuation are also frequently seen

Other Abdominal Manifestations of SCA

- Pigmented gallstones
  - Most common gastrointestinal manifestation of SCA
  - Seen in around 50% of patients
- Intrahepatic biliary duct stones and cholestasis
- Enlarged kidneys
  - Seen in up to 50% of patients
  - If renal failure develops, kidneys become small

BACKGROUND

General

- SCA is common in Afro-descendent population
- Prevalence of 0.2% (homozygous form) and 8-10% (heterozygous form)

Relevant Pathology

- Slow, tortuous microcirculation of spleen makes it susceptible to repeated episodes of focal venoocclusive disease
  - Results in splenic infarction, which progresses over time to functional autosplenectomy
  - Infarcted spleen is replaced by fibrous tissue, with deposition of hemosiderin and calcium
  - Loss of splenic function makes SCA patients prone to infection
    - Particularly *Streptococcus pneumoniae*, *Haemophilus influenzae* type B, and *Salmonella*, *Klebsiella*, and other encapsulated bacteria

IMAGING FEATURES

Plain Radiography

- Small calcified spleen is visible on plain radiographs as crescent-shaped left upper quadrant dense structure

US

- Small highly echogenic spleen with dense shadowing
  - ± small islands of preserved splenic tissue with echogenicity similar to that of normal spleen

CT

- Small spleen of very high attenuation
  - ± small islands of preserved splenic tissue with attenuation similar to that of normal spleen

MR

- Low signal intensity on all MR pulse sequences, secondary to ferrocalcinosis
  - ± small islands of preserved splenic tissue with signal intensity similar to that of normal spleen

Tc-99m Sulfur Colloid

- Uptake of Tc-99m sulfur colloid may totally disappear
  - Islands of preserved splenic tissue or regrowth of splenic tissue occasionally may be present in older children and adults with SCA

RELATED REFERENCES

1. Lonergan GJ et al: Sickle cell anemia. Radiographics. 21(4):971-94, 2001
2. Adler DD et al: MRI of the spleen: normal appearance and findings in sickle-cell anemia. AJR Am J Roentgenol. 147(4):843-5, 1986

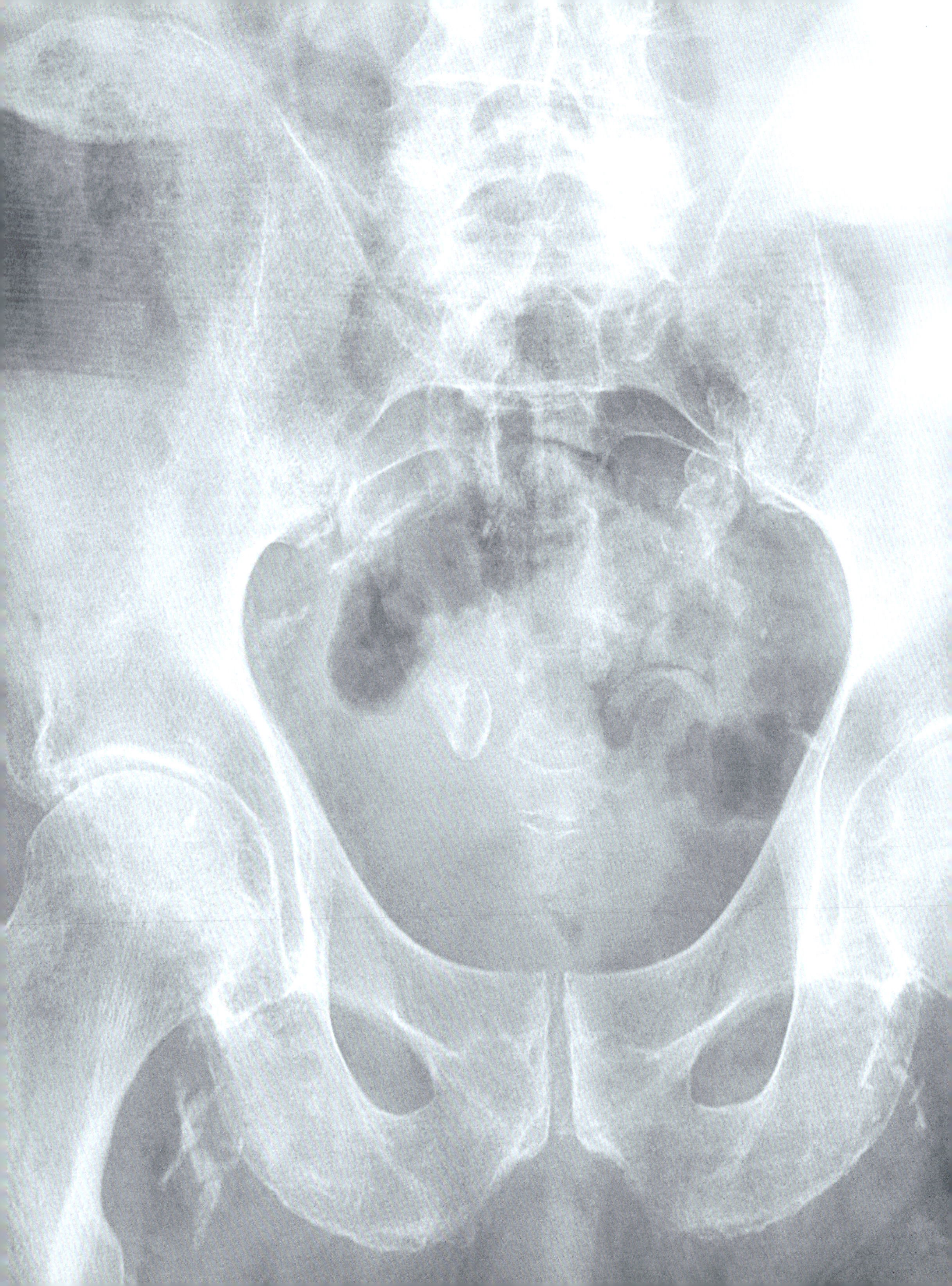

SECTION 5
Abdominal Wall, Peritoneum, Retroperitoneum, and Diaphragm

Benign Conditions Simulating Malignancy

Treatment-Related Conditions Simulating Diseases

Classic Signs and Appearances

PRESACRAL MYELOLIPOMA

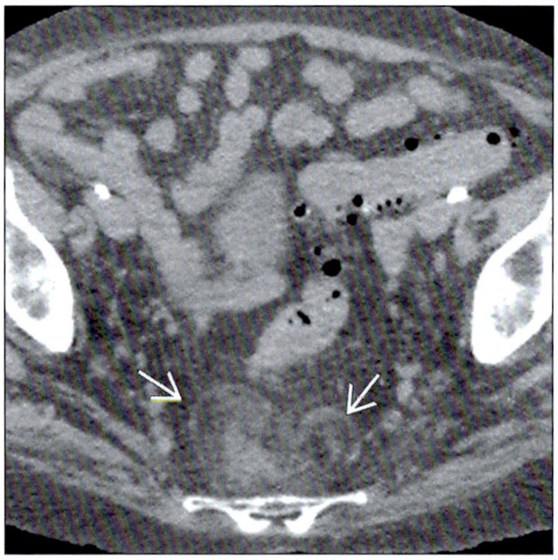

Axial CECT in a 79-year-old woman shows a lobulated presacral mass → composed of low-attenuation fatty elements intermixed with areas of soft tissue attenuation.

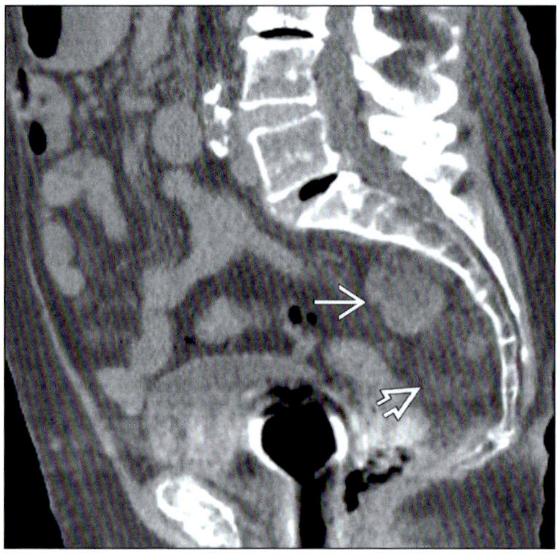

Coronal CECT in the same patient shows 2 lobulated presacral masses. The superior lesion → is predominantly soft tissue density while the inferior lesion ⇨ is more fatty intermixed with soft tissue attenuation.

CLINICAL SCENARIO

History

- 79-year-old woman with incidental imaging finding

IMAGE INTERPRETATION

Pitfalls

- Presacral fat-containing lesion can be mistaken for liposarcoma

Actual Diagnosis

- Presacral myelolipoma

Clues to Correct Diagnosis

- Characteristic location in presacral space and characteristic patient population (older patients) should suggest diagnosis
- No characteristic CT, MR, or US findings to differentiate from liposarcoma
- Absence of aggressive features such as bone destruction
- Tc-99m sulfur colloid scan

BACKGROUND

General

- Benign tumors consisting of myeloid elements (hematopoietic tissue) and mature fat
- Almost always occur in adrenal glands
- Presacral region is most common extraadrenal location
- Other reported locations include retroperitoneum, mediastinum, kidney, stomach, and liver
- Multifocal disease has been reported

Etiology

- Unknown; possible mechanisms include
  - Metaplasia of uncommitted adrenal cortical mesenchymal cells
  - Reactivation of connective tissue hematopoiesis (normally seen in embryonic life)

Epidemiology

- Mostly in older patients
- F:M = 2:1
- ↑ incidence with Cushing syndrome, 21-hydroxylase deficiency, nonhyperfunctioning adrenal adenoma, and multiple endocrine neoplasia, type 2 (MEN2A) syndrome

IMAGING FEATURES

US

- Hyperechoic mass if predominately fatty, or mostly hypoechoic if tumor is predominately myeloid

CT

- Encapsulated mass with macroscopic fatty tissue intermixed with areas of soft tissue
- Variable amount of fat
- Soft tissue elements may enhance

MR

- T1WI
  - Fat elements demonstrate high signal intensity (SI) with loss of signal on fat-suppression sequences
  - Hematopoietic elements demonstrate lower SI
- T2WI
  - Heterogeneous with fatty elements demonstrating high SI
- T1WI C+ FS
  - Hematopoietic soft tissue elements may enhance

Tc-99m Sulfur Colloid Imaging

- ↑ uptake due to presence of reticuloendothelial components

RELATED REFERENCES

1. Itani M et al: Radiologic-pathologic correlation in extra-adrenal myelolipoma. Abdom Imaging. 39(2):394-7, 2014
2. Baker KS et al: Presacral myelolipoma: a case report and review of imaging findings. J Radiol Case Rep. 6(6):1-9, 2012

GOSSYPIBOMA

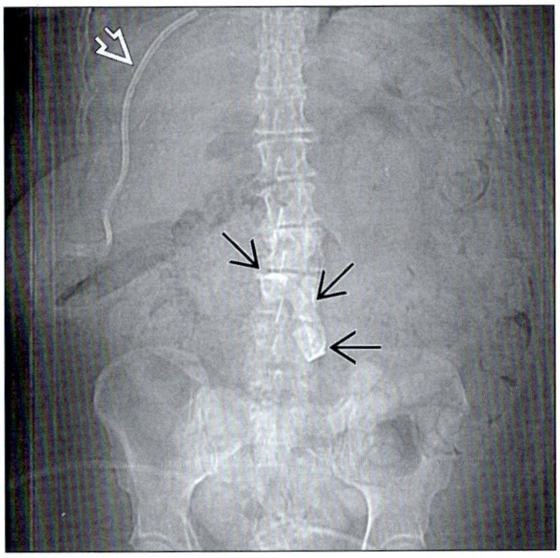

Plain radiographic examination demonstrates a radiopaque, metallic marker → seen within the lower abdomen. A surgical drainage tube ➡ is noted along the right upper quadrant.

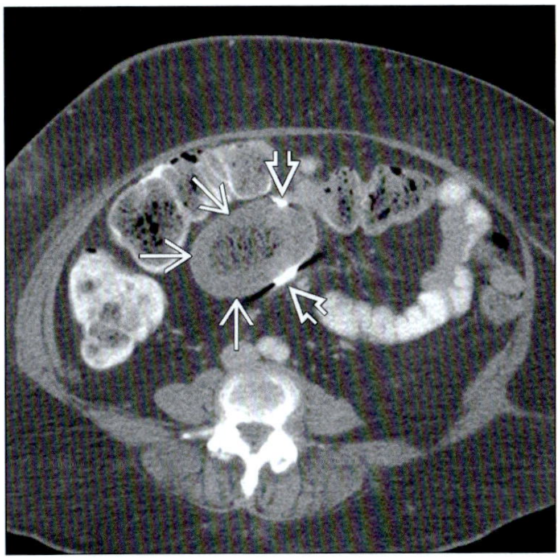

Axial CECT demonstrates a well-circumscribed, mass-like structure ➡ containing multiple mottled gas foci in the lower abdomen with a metallic marker noted at the periphery ➡.

CLINICAL SCENARIO

History

- Recent segmental hepatectomy and cholecystectomy
- Postoperative wound dehiscence with abdominal pain

IMAGE INTERPRETATION

Pitfalls

- Can be misinterpreted as abscess when gas is present
- Misinterpreted as solid tumor in absence of gas

Actual Diagnosis

- Gossypiboma: Retained sponge

Clues to Correct Diagnosis

- Presence of radiopaque marker & gas within sponge
- Recent abdominal surgery

BACKGROUND

General

- Definition: Retained surgical towel
  - Synonym: Textiloma
  - Latin: Gossypium = cotton
  - Surgical material of cotton matrix left behind in body cavity during surgical operation

Epidemiology

- Cotton pads, towels, gauzes, or sponges used for primary homeostasis can result in gossypibomas
  - Surgical sponge is most common type
- Mean age: 49 years (range: 6-92 years)
- Locations: Abdomen (56%), pelvis (18%), thorax (11%)
  - Detection method: CT (61%), radiography (35%)

Pathology

- Foreign bodies lead to 2 types of reactions
  - Exudative tissue reaction → abscess formation
  - Aseptic fibrous tissue reactions → adhesions → encapsulation and formation of granulomas

Clinical Presentation

- Most patients are asymptomatic during this process
  - However, patient may present with abdominal pain, nausea, vomiting, anemia, abdominal mass, diarrhea, malnutrition, weight loss, or intestinal obstruction
  - Symptoms can develop 1 day to years postoperatively
  - May be spontaneously expelled through rectum, bladder, or surgical wound

IMAGING FEATURES

Plain Radiograph

- Radiopaque marker can be seen if present
- May not be diagnostic if no opaque marker
- Sponge seen as multiple mottled, small, gas lucencies

US

- Well-circumscribed mass with hypoechoic and echogenic areas with posterior acoustic shadowing

CT

- Most sensitive and specific modality
- Thin, metallic, radiopaque marker strip
- Thick, calcified, reticulate rind sign: Seen many years after surgery, thought to result from gradual calcium deposition along fiber network of surgical gauze
- Sponge-like with gas bubbles is most characteristic
- Occasionally enhanced peripheral capsule

PET/CT

- Low central uptake
- ↑ uptake of periphery secondary to fibroblastic capsule

RELATED REFERENCES

1. Gümüş M et al: A serious medicolegal problem after surgery: gossypiboma. Am J Forensic Med Pathol. 33(1):54-7, 2012
2. Manzella A et al: Imaging of gossypibomas: pictorial review. AJR Am J Roentgenol. 193(6 Suppl):S94-101, 2009
3. Wan W et al: Improving safety in the operating room: a systematic literature review of retained surgical sponges. Curr Opin Anaesthesiol. 22(2):207-14, 2009

DEPENDENT VISCERA SIGN

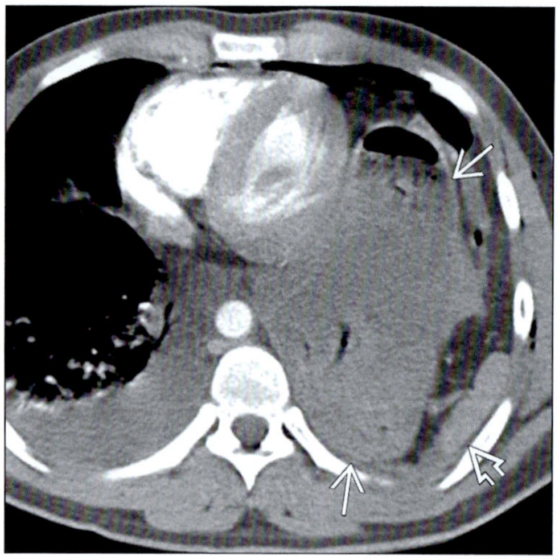

Axial CECT shows the presence of the stomach and spleen within the left hemithorax, abutting the posterior ribs without intervening lung due to obliteration of the posterior costophrenic recess.

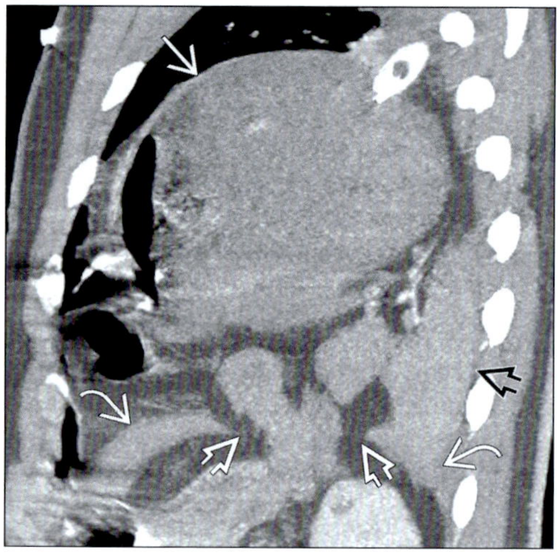

Sagittal CECT shows herniation of the stomach and spleen into the chest. Note thickening of the visualized diaphragm and the large diaphragmatic defect.

IMAGING FEATURES

Appearance

- Dependent viscera sign is seen at supine CT in thoracoabdominal area
- Viscera (i.e., bowel or solid organs) are positioned against posterior ribs, with obliteration of posterior costophrenic recess
  - On right side, liver or bowel abuts posterior ribs
  - On left side, stomach, bowel, or spleen abuts posterior ribs, or stomach or bowel lies posterior to spleen

Significance

- Dependent viscera sign is seen with diaphragmatic rupture
  - 100% sensitivity for diagnosing diaphragmatic rupture
- Dependent viscera sign is not a reliable indicator of diaphragmatic injury in penetrating trauma
  - Owing to small size and variable position of defect

Other Imaging Findings

- Diaphragmatic discontinuity
  - Observed in 95.7% of patients
  - 71-80% sensitive for diaphragmatic rupture
  - In ~ 6% of general population, discontinuity is a normal variant
    - Seen more commonly in older patients, women, and those with emphysema
- Collar sign
  - Diaphragm constricts herniated bowel or solid organs in a waist-like manner
  - 67% sensitive for left-sided rupture and 50% sensitive for right-sided rupture
- Thickening of visualized diaphragm
  - Observed in 69.6% of patients
- Dangling diaphragm sign
  - Free edge of torn hemidiaphragm curls medially from its normal course parallel to body wall
  - Sensitivity: 54%; specificity: 98%
- Intrathoracic herniation of abdominal contents
  - 32-64% sensitive for diaphragmatic rupture
  - Late feature of this condition

BACKGROUND

Explanation

- Loss of diaphragmatic support after rupture may cause abdominal organs to fall into a dependent position against posterior thoracic wall when patient is supine

Incidence

- Diaphragmatic injuries occur in 0.8-8% of patients with blunt abdominal trauma
- Blunt diaphragmatic rupture remains undiagnosed at initial presentation in 7-66% of cases

Pathophysiology

- Spontaneous healing of diaphragmatic ruptures has never been reported
  - Normally negative pleuroperitoneal pressure gradient (7-22 cm H_20), along with continuous diaphragmatic motion, prevent diaphragmatic healing
- Abdominal structures generally herniate into thorax
  - Because of negative intrapleural pressure
- Herniation may be delayed for days or years (from 1 day to 48 years)
  - Herniation occurs within 3 years in 80% of cases

RELATED REFERENCES

1. Panda A et al: Traumatic diaphragmatic injury: a review of CT signs and the difference between blunt and penetrating injury. Diagn Interv Radiol. 20(2):121-8, 2014
2. Desir A et al: CT of blunt diaphragmatic rupture. Radiographics. 32(2):477-98, 2012

DEPENDENT VISCERA SIGN

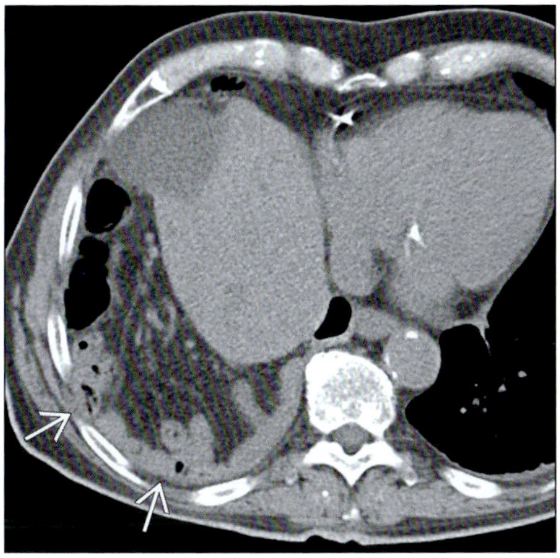

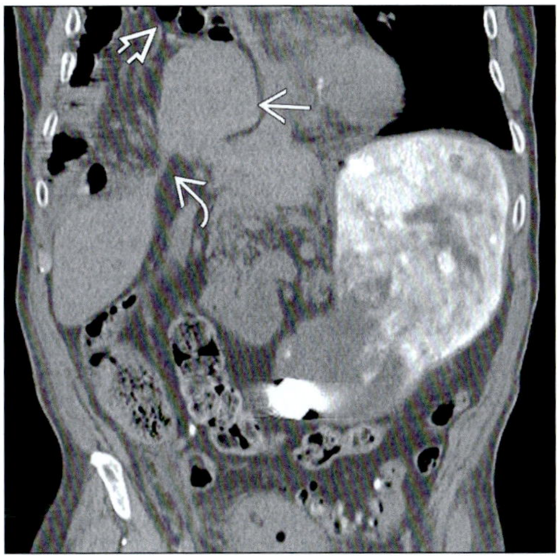

(Left) *Axial NECT shows dependent viscera sign on the right side where the small bowel loops abut the posterior ribs →.* ***(Right)*** *Coronal NECT in the same patient shows herniation of the liver → and small bowel → into the chest. Note also the constriction of the liver → at the site of diaphragmatic defect in a waist-like manner (collar sign).*

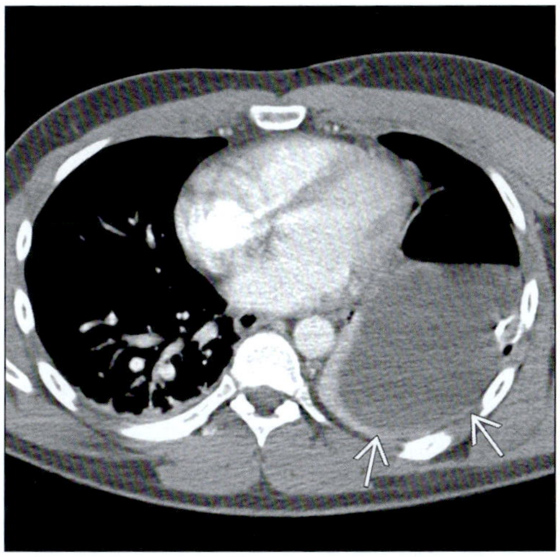

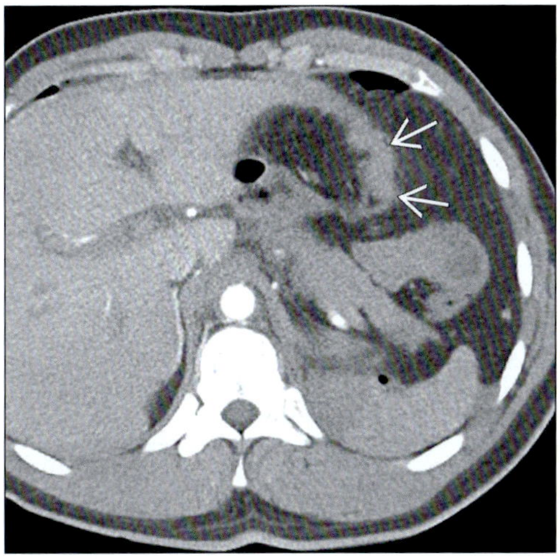

(Left) *Axial CECT shows dependent viscera sign on the left side where the stomach abuts the posterior ribs →.* ***(Right)*** *Axial CECT in the same patient shows a curvilinear flap → extending away from the chest wall toward the center of the abdomen (dangling diaphragm sign), a finding that represents the torn-free edge of the left hemidiaphragm, the distal part of which is thickened (thickening of the diaphragm sign).*

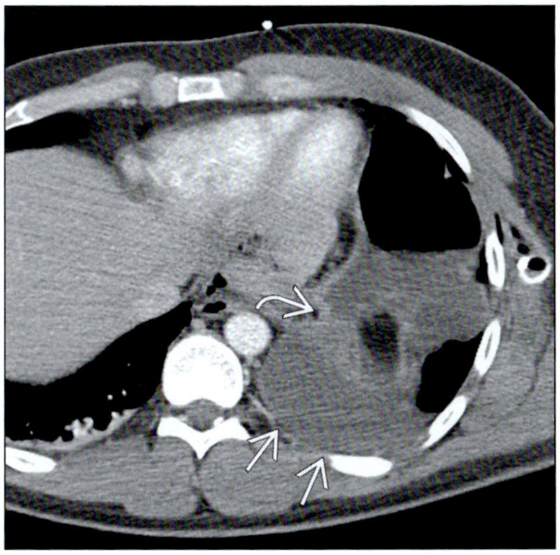

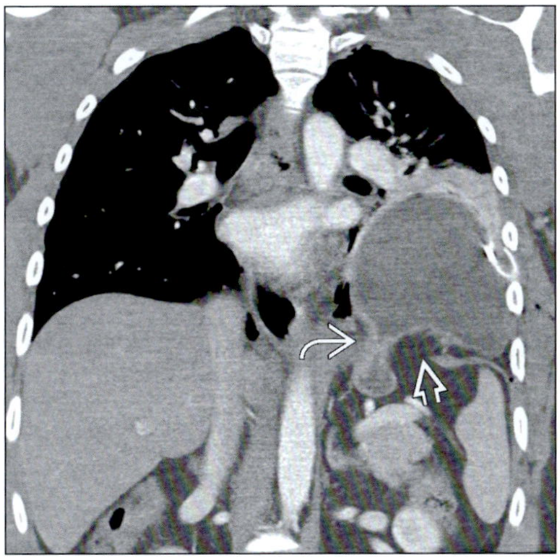

(Left) *Axial CECT shows dependent viscera sign on the left side where the stomach abuts the posterior ribs →. Note also the constriction of the stomach → at the site of diaphragmatic defect in a waist-like manner (collar sign).* ***(Right)*** *Coronal CECT shows constriction of the stomach → at the site of diaphragmatic defect in a waist-like manner (collar sign). Also note diaphragmatic discontinuity →.*

PERITONEAL LOOSE BODY (PERITONEAL MOUSE)

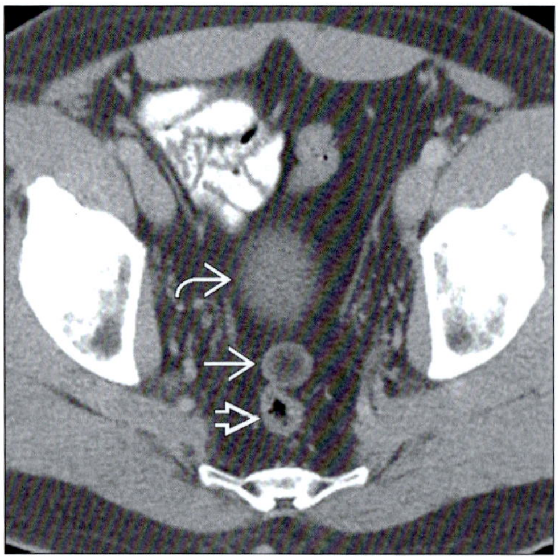

Axial CECT shows a round pelvic mass ➔ anterior to the rectum ➔ and posterosuperior to the urinary bladder ➔ that is composed of a central area of fat attenuation and a peripheral rim of soft tissue attenuation.

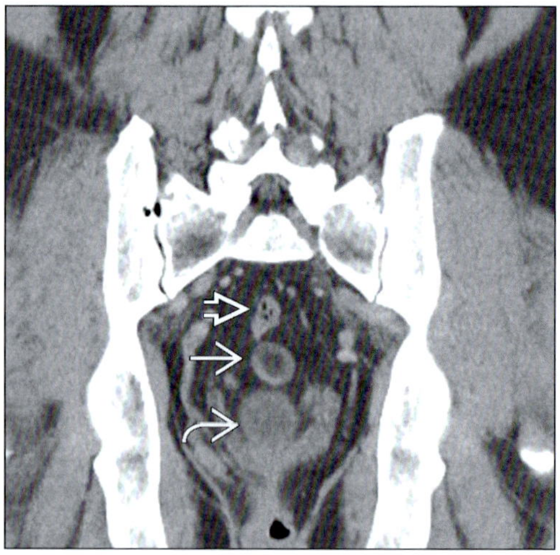

Coronal CECT in the same patient shows a round pelvic mass ➔ composed of a central area of fat attenuation and a peripheral rim of soft tissue attenuation between the rectum ➔ and urinary bladder ➔.

CLINICAL SCENARIO

History

- 75-year-old man with history of prostatic carcinoma

IMAGE INTERPRETATION

Pitfalls

- Can be mistaken for primary malignant neoplasm or metastatic disease

Actual Diagnosis

- Peritoneal loose body (peritoneal mouse)

Clues to Correct Diagnosis

- Intraperitoneal location of a round mass with central fat attenuation or calcifications
- Pelvic location
- Change in position on serial examinations

BACKGROUND

Relevant Anatomy

- Presumably a result of evolution of infarcted epiploic appendage
  - Infarcted appendage undergoes necrosis → fibrotic or calcified mass
  - Becomes detached from wall of colon → loose body within peritoneal cavity
- Mostly pelvic in location
  - Gravitate to most dependent part of abdominal cavity
- Usually small (0.5-2.5 cm in diameter) and asymptomatic
- Larger lesions may reach diameter of 5-10 cm (giant peritoneal mice)
  - Rarely cause acute urinary retention and small bowel obstruction due to extrinsic compression

Relevant Pathology

- Core of necrotic, calcified fat laminated by layers of acellular hyalinized fibrous tissue

IMAGING FEATURES

Plain Radiography

- Different calcification patterns have been described
  - Dense nodular
  - Small ring-shaped
  - Peripheral shell

CT

- Round or oval-shaped, well-defined soft tissue attenuation mass
  - No enhancement of soft tissue component
- Central fat attenuation, central dense calcification, or ring-shaped calcification around a core of fat attenuation
- Peripheral shell of calcification may be seen

MR

- Well-circumscribed, low-intensity mass on both T1- and T2WI
  - MR signal is similar to that of muscle
- Central high-intensity area may be seen on T1WI with suppression on fat suppressed sequences
  - Due to fat content
- Mass does not exhibit any enhancement

PET/CT

- No metabolic activity

RELATED REFERENCES

1. Allam T et al: Peritoneal mouse as detected on (18)F-FDG PET-CT. Front Oncol. 3:83, 2013
2. Jang JT et al: Giant peritoneal loose body in the pelvic cavity. J Korean Soc Coloproctol. 28(2):108-10, 2012
3. Gayer G et al: CT diagnosis of a large peritoneal loose body: a case report and review of the literature. Br J Radiol. 84(1000):e83-5, 2011

PERITONEAL LOOSE BODY (PERITONEAL MOUSE)

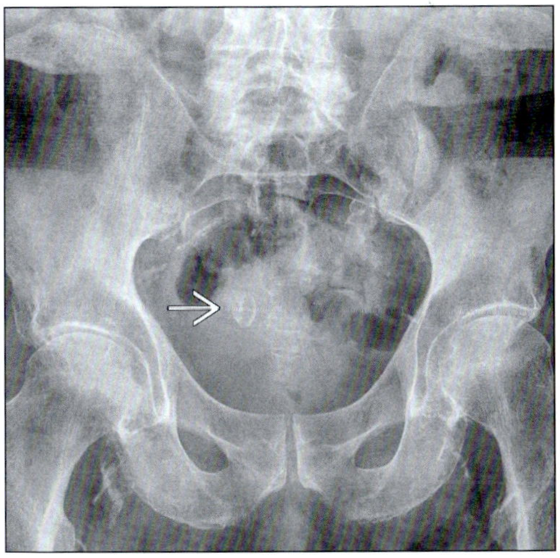

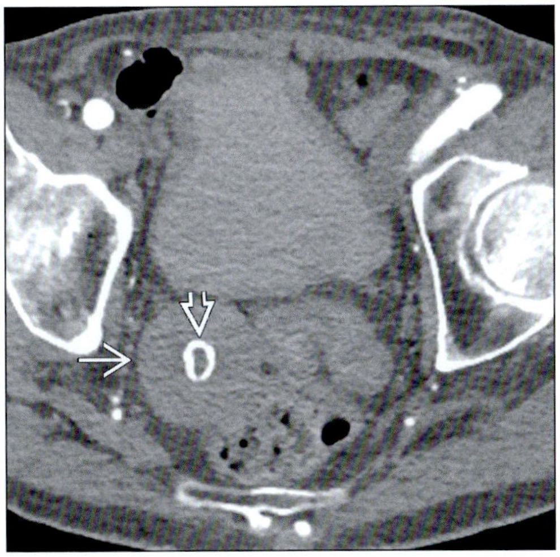

(Left) *Plain radiograph of the pelvis shows an abnormal calcific attenuation* ➔ *in the right side of the pelvis.* ***(Right)*** *Axial CECT in the same patient shows a rounded right pelvic lesion* ➔ *of soft tissue attenuation with a central ring-shaped area of calcification* ⇨.

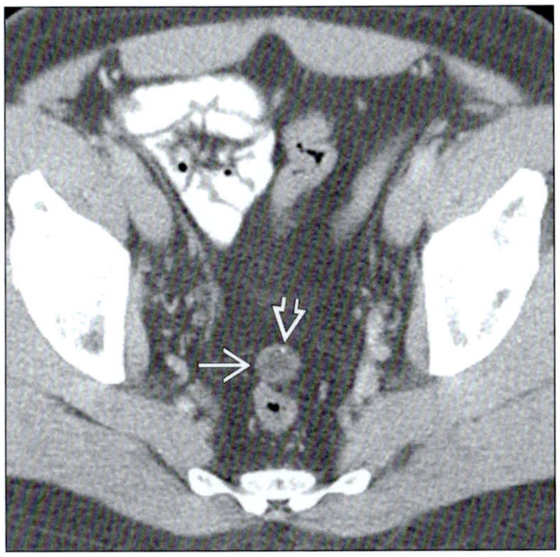

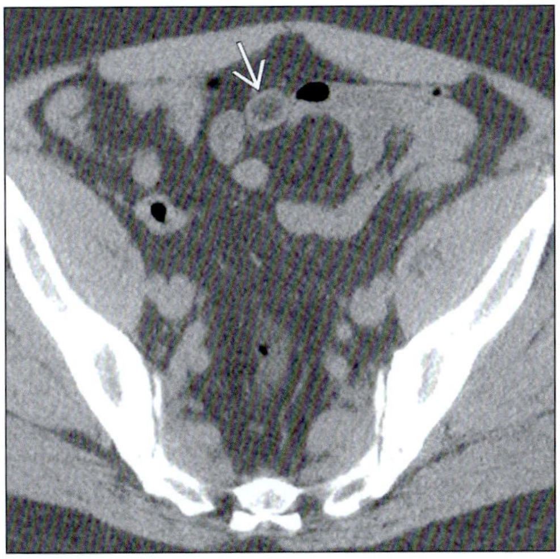

(Left) *Axial CECT in a 75-year-old man with a history of prostate cancer shows a round pelvic mass* ➔ *composed of a central area of fat attenuation and a peripheral rim of soft tissue attenuation. Tiny calcific attenuation is present in the wall* ⇨. ***(Right)*** *Axial NECT in the same patient obtained as part of PET/CT shows change in the position of the previously seen pelvic mass* ➔*, which is now located between small bowel loops.*

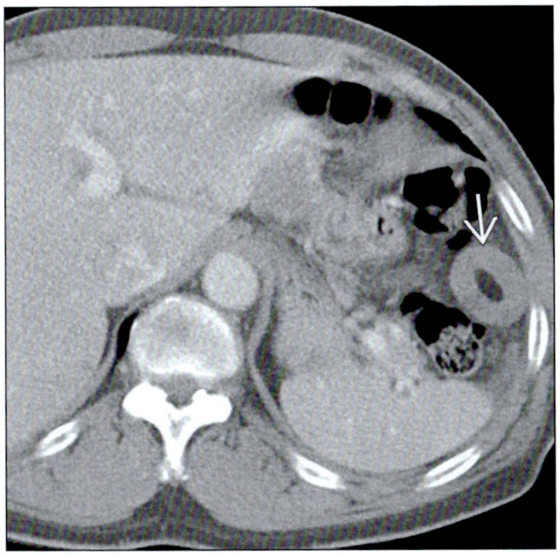

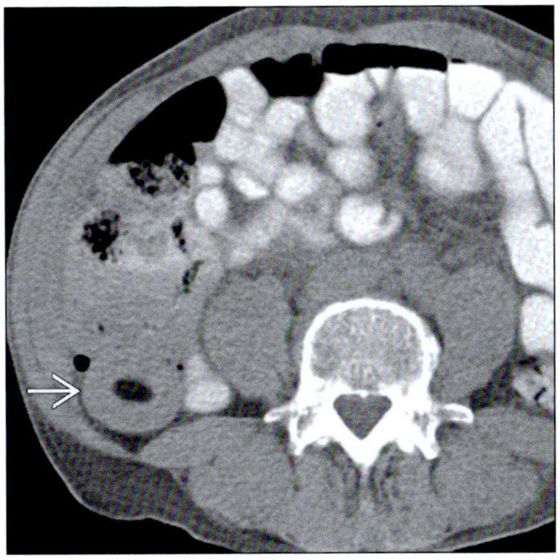

(Left) *Axial CECT in a 78-year-old man with a history of prostate cancer shows a round left upper quadrant mass* ➔ *composed of a central area of fat attenuation and a peripheral rim of soft tissue attenuation.* ***(Right)*** *Axial CECT in the same patient shows interval migration of the mobile mass* ➔*, which is now located along the right paracolic gutter.*

JELLY BELLY

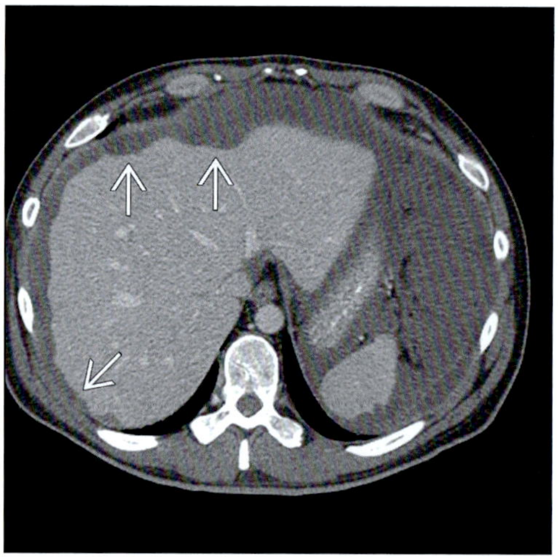

Axial CECT demonstrates a moderate to large amount of intraperitoneal fluid with indentation/scalloping of the underlying liver surface ➡, indicating increased cellularity.

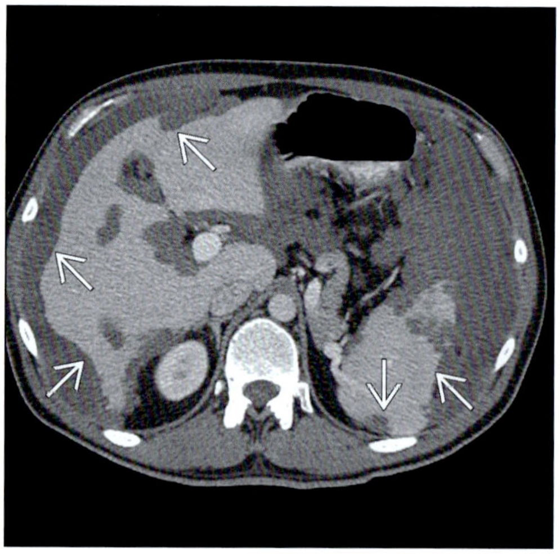

Axial CECT demonstrates large amounts of intraperitoneal fluid with scalloping of the underlying liver and spleen surfaces ➡, giving a jelly belly appearance.

CLINICAL SCENARIO

History

- 49-year-old woman with progressive abdominal pain, increased abdominal girth, and weight loss

IMAGE INTERPRETATION

Classic Sign

- Low-attenuation ascites, which causes mass effect (scalloping) on solid organs, is classic for pseudomyxoma peritonei (PMP)

BACKGROUND

General

- Rupture of appendiceal mucinous tumor → copious amounts of mucinous ascites in peritoneal cavity
  - Ovaries can be secondarily involved (likely by transcoelomic spread)

Relevant Pathology

- PMP can be classified pathologically into
  - Low-grade process: Diffuse peritoneal adenomucinosis (DPAM): Mucin-secreting cells without cellular atypia
    - 2° to rupture of mucinous cystadenoma
    - Good prognosis: 5-year overall survival was 75%
  - High-grade process: Peritoneal mucinous carcinoma (PMCA)
    - 2° to rupture of mucinous cystadenocarcinoma
    - Poor prognosis: 5-year overall survival was14%
  - Intermediate/discordant subtype (PMCA-I/D)
    - Intermediate prognosis: 5-year overall survival was 50%

Treatment

- Usually by debulking cytoreductive surgery and heated intraperitoneal chemotherapy

IMAGING FEATURES

Plain Radiography

- Massive ascites, increased opacity of abdomen with obliteration of psoas muscle border, and medial displacement of bowel
- Curvilinear calcifications may be present

US

- Echogenic ascitic fluid and echogenic debris
  - Unlike proteinaceous ascites, echoes are not mobile
- Centrally displaced bowel
- Scalloping of hepatic and splenic margins

CT

- Low-attenuation ascites with scalloping of liver and spleen with medial displacement of bowel
- Scalloping of organs differentiates from simple ascites
- Coarse calcifications are not uncommon
- In most cases, primary appendiceal tumors could not be detected

MR

- PMCA can demonstrate deep invasion of the peritoneal surfaces
- On T1WI, T2WI, & immediate T1WI C+: Ascites, mucin, & solid tumors are indistinct & difficult to distinguish
- Solid masses in PMCA demonstrate enhancement in delayed T1WI C+
  - Higher grade pathological subtype is associated with more intense enhancement

RELATED REFERENCES

1. Nakakura EK. Pseudomyxoma peritonei: more questions than answers. J Clin Oncol. 10;30(20):2429-30, 2012
2. Levy AD et al: Secondary tumors and tumorlike lesions of the peritoneal cavity: imaging features with pathologic correlation. Radiographics. 29(2):347-73, 2009

MUSHROOM SIGN

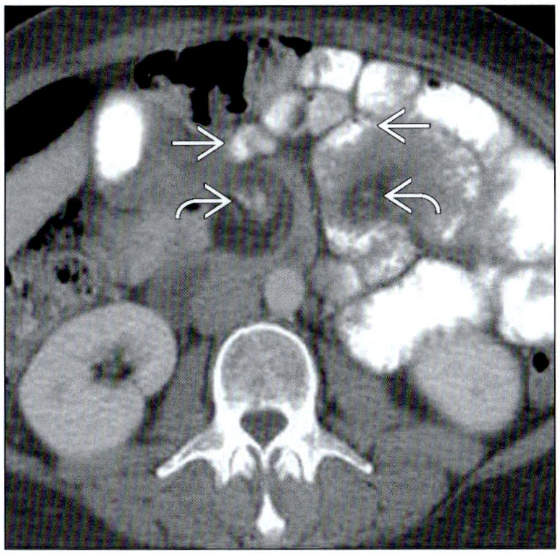

Axial CECT shows mushroom sign ➡ of the internal hernia as bowel passes through a narrow opening between mesenteric vessels ➡ at the root of the mesentery.

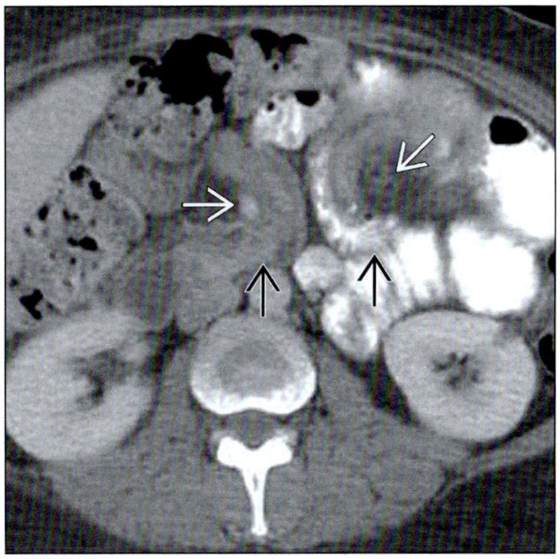

Axial CECT shows the mesenteric fat and bowel ➡ passing through a narrow defect between mesenteric vessels ➡ at the root of the mesentery, demonstrating the mushroom sign.

IMAGE INTERPRETATION

Appearance & Explanation

- Mushroom shape occurs when root of mesentery passes through a narrow opening between mesenteric vessels
- Seen with internal hernias where bowel herniates through peritoneal or mesenteric defect

BACKGROUND

Clinical Presentation

- Most common presentation: Acute intestinal obstruction
- Other symptoms: Postprandial pain, nausea, and emesis
- Internal hernias can be incidentally found on imaging

Relevant Anatomy

- Locations: Foramen of Winslow, paraduodenal, transmesenteric, transomental, pericecal, sigmoid mesocolon, and supravesical and pelvic hernias

Relevant Pathology

- Herniation of bowel into abnormal space due to defect of mesentery and visceral peritoneum caused by congenital mechanisms, surgery, trauma, and inflammation
- Excessive weight loss may precipitate internal hernia because of loss of protective space-occupying effect of mesenteric fat
- Laparoscopic Roux-en-Y gastric bypass is more prone to internal hernia than open operation

IMAGING FEATURES

Enteroclysis

- Contraindicated with closed loop obstruction and in suspected hernial strangulation
- May show small bowel to be bunched up or clustered
- Colon may be deviated by internal hernia sac
- Bowel proximal to hernia may be dilated

US

- In small bowel obstruction, dilated small bowel loops can be seen showing active peristalsis

CT

- Aids in evaluation of small intestine and surrounding structures
- More active role in identification of site, level, and cause of small bowel obstruction, including internal hernias
- Several signs that may indicate internal hernia include
  - Swirled appearance of mesenteric fat or vessels at root of mesentery is best indicator of internal hernia
  - Small bowel obstruction
  - Clustered loops of small bowel
  - Mushroom shape of herniated mesenteric root with crowding and stretching of mesenteric vessels
  - Small bowel other than duodenum passing posterior to superior mesenteric artery

RELATED REFERENCES

1. Lockhart ME et al: Internal hernia after gastric bypass: sensitivity and specificity of seven CT signs with surgical correlation and controls. AJR Am J Roentgenol. 188(3):745-50, 2007
2. Vijayaraghavan SB: Sonographic features of internal hernia. J Ultrasound Med. 25(1):105-10, 2006
3. Takeyama N et al: CT of internal hernias. Radiographics. 25(4):997-1015, 2005

OMENTAL CAKE SIGN

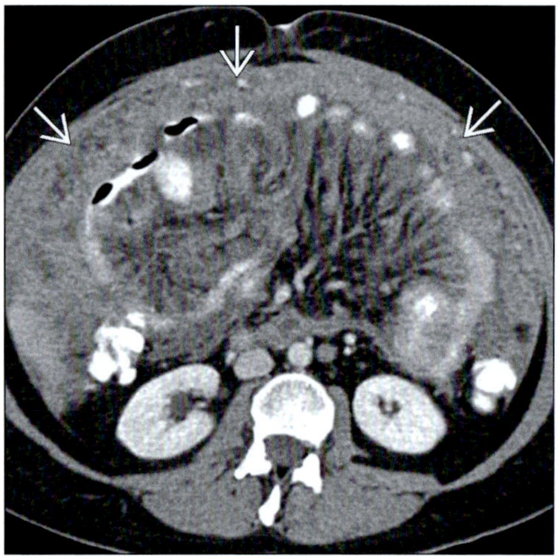

Axial CECT demonstrates significant omental thickening with multiple coalescent masses forming thick omental cake ➔ in the anterior abdomen.

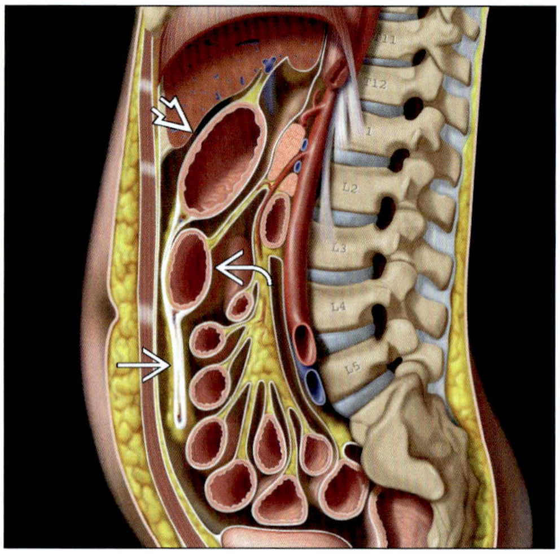

Graphic demonstrates the anatomy of the greater omentum ➔, the largest peritoneal fold. It extends from the greater gastric curvature ➔ to the free border of the transverse colon ➔.

IMAGE INTERPRETATION

Appearance and Explanation

- Omental cake refers to infiltration of omental fat by coalescent soft tissue attenuation masses

Differential Diagnosis and Epidemiology

- Ranges from inflammation, to infection, to malignancy
- Malignancy can be either primary tumor of peritoneum or spread from adjacent or remote areas
- Most common causes are metastases from ovary, stomach, pancreas, or colon
- Tuberculous peritonitis may also give this appearance
- More common in adult population
- Uncommon in children, though reported in cases of rhabdomyosarcoma and lymphoma
  - Best clue in lymphoma is significant multicompartmental lymphadenopathy

BACKGROUND

Clinical Presentation

- Abdominal fullness and pain

Pathology

- Different patterns of omental involvement include seedlings, localized or diffuse infiltration of omental fat by soft tissue attenuation, and coalescent masses resulting in what is called omental cake
- Caking is indicator of advanced stage of disease

IMAGING FEATURES

US

- May have variable echogenicity with respect to bowel loops and may appear hypoechoic, isoechoic, or slightly hyperechoic, and may be homogeneous or heterogeneous
- Degree of vascularity may be demonstrated using color or power Doppler ultrasound

CT

- Sensitive in cases of omental pathologies
- Normal omentum looks like bands of fatty tissue with fine blood vessels
- Omental pathology may appear as diffuse haziness, soft tissue nodules; omental cake arises when these nodules coalesce to form diffusely thickened mass
- Ascites may be accompanying feature
- Associated intraabdominal findings such as hepatic metastases and lymphadenopathy may be only clues to origin of omental disease if diagnosis is unknown

US- or CT-Guided Biopsy

- Biopsy is performed if no abdominal or pelvic primary lesion is noted on imaging

MR

- May be utilized in patients with contraindications to CT (contrast allergy, pregnancy) or for problem solving with inconclusive CT
- Imaging features included omental stranding, nodules, cake, and occasional ascites
- Delayed enhancement improves detection of peritoneal metastases

PET/CT

- FDG PET/CT demonstrates increased activity of omental cake
- Sensitive in identifying active lesions, defining extent of disease, and monitoring therapeutic response

RELATED REFERENCES

1. Mamlouk MD et al: Omental cakes: unusual aetiologies and CT appearances. Insights Imaging. 2(4):399-408, 2011
2. Zamir N et al: Omental cake: a radiological diagnostic sign. APSP J Case Rep. 2(3):27, 2011
3. Toma P et al: Multimodality imaging of Hodgkin disease and non-Hodgkin lymphomas in children. Radiographics. 27(5):1335-54, 2007

MOLAR TOOTH EXTRAPERITONEAL RUPTURE

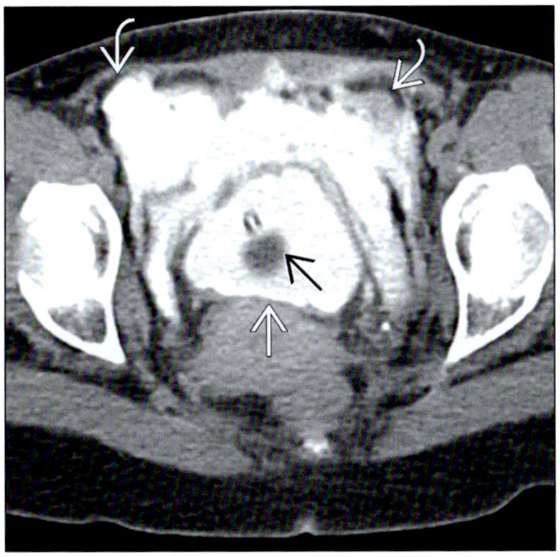

Axial CT cystography shows distension of the urinary bladder with dense contrast injected through Foley catheter with extraluminal contrast to prevesical space, giving the molar tooth appearance.

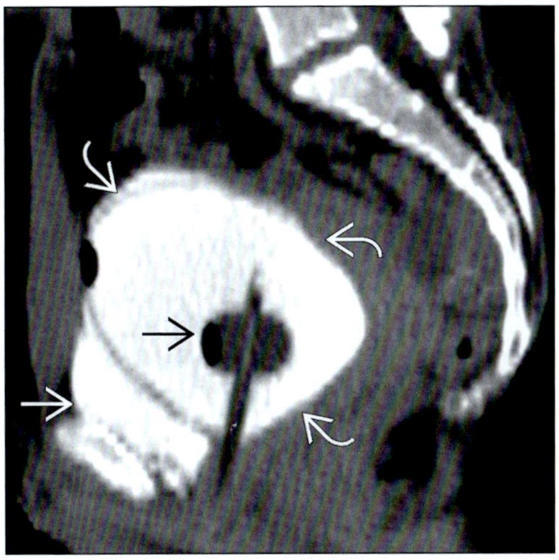

Sagittal reconstructed CT cystography demonstrates localization of extraluminal contrast to prevesical space anterior to the distended urinary bladder. An intravesical Foley catheter is seen.

CLINICAL SCENARIO

History

- 34-year-old man with history of motor vehicle accident

IMAGE INTERPRETATION

Classic Sign

- Accumulation of extraluminal contrast in prevesical space giving a molar tooth configuration is consistent with extraperitoneal urinary bladder (UB) rupture in context of trauma

BACKGROUND

Epidemiology

- Extraperitoneal rupture is most common type of UB injury (> 2/3 of cases)

Relevant Anatomy

- Molar tooth sign results from accumulation of contrast in prevesical extraperitoneal space
- "Crown" portion lies anterior to UB between umbilicovesical fascia and transversalis fascia of anterior abdominal wall and displaces UB posteriorly
- "Root" portion extends posteriorly on either side of UB between fascia and either peritoneum superiorly or parietal pelvic fascia inferiorly

Relevant Pathology

- Bladder injury should be suspected in patient who has sustained pelvic trauma has gross hematuria or fails to void
- Extraperitoneal bladder ruptures are generally managed with bladder catheter drainage alone
- Etiology
  - Usually caused by penetrating trauma
    - Trauma from knife or gunshot wounds
  - In blunt trauma
    - Most commonly 2° to motor vehicle accident
    - Due to direct laceration of bladder by bone fragments from pelvic fracture
  - Possibility of UB rupture is increased when it is fully distended at time of injury
- Extraperitoneal bladder ruptures are generally managed with bladder catheter drainage alone

IMAGING FEATURES

Conventional Cystography

- Used to be diagnostic test of choice
- Extraperitoneal UB rupture: Flame-shaped extraluminal contrast into perivesical soft tissues
- Pelvic bony fractures may be seen

US

- May demonstrate soft tissue hematomas
- Demonstration of fluid outside urinary bladder
- May not distinguish intraperitoneal from extraperitoneal UB rupture

CT

- Delayed phase or CT cystogram technique are most sensitive
- Molar tooth sign is characteristic of extraperitoneal rupture
- Fractures of pelvic bones are commonly seen

MR

- Time-consuming examination; not practical in setting of trauma

RELATED REFERENCES

1. Titton RL et al: Urine leaks and urinomas: diagnosis and imaging-guided intervention. Radiographics. 23(5):1133-47, 2003
2. Vaccaro JP et al: CT cystography in the evaluation of major bladder trauma. Radiographics. 20(5):1373-81, 2000

SANDWICH SIGN

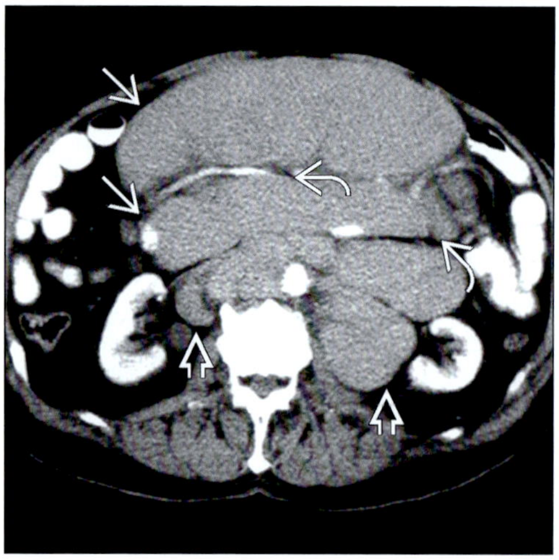

Axial CECT demonstrates significant mesenteric lymphadenopathy ➔ sandwiching mesenteric vessels and fat ↪. Extensive retroperitoneal adenopathy is also noted ⇨.

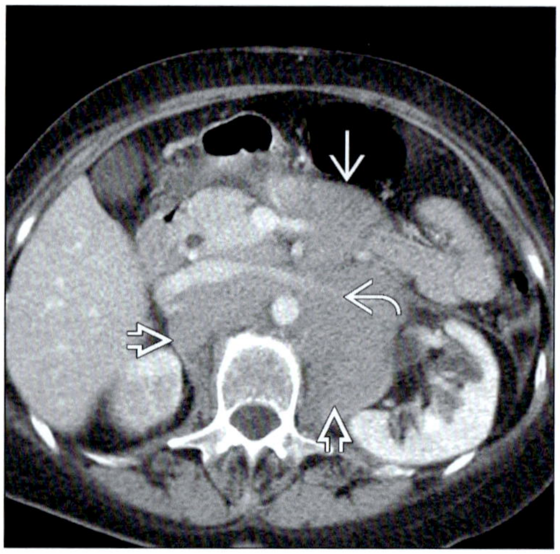

Axial CECT in a patient with non-Hodgkin lymphoma shows a sandwich sign made by mesenteric lymphadenopathy ➔ sandwiching mesenteric vessels ↪. Retroperitoneal lymphadenopathy is also seen ⇨.

CLINICAL SCENARIO

History

- 58-year-old man with AIDS, abdominal pain, and abdominal mass on palpation

IMAGE INTERPRETATION

Sandwich Sign

- Mesenteric fat and vessels resemble sandwich filling
- Soft tissue adenopathy represents the bun
- With IV and oral contrast administration, mesenteric tubular structures enhance → enhancing appearance of layers within sandwich filling
- As adenopathy enlarges, mesenteric vessels compress, which partially obstructs venous return, leading to engorgement and more prominent mesenteric veins

Classic Sign

- Classic for mesenteric lymphomas
- Other causes of mesenteric adenopathy (e.g., carcinomas, sarcomas, carcinoid, and lymphadenopathy syndrome associated with AIDS as well as infectious and inflammatory bowel diseases) do not produce large bulky adenopathy that results in sandwich sign

BACKGROUND

General

- Most mesenteric lymphomas are non-Hodgkin lymphoma (NHL)
- Immunocompromised individuals such as AIDS and post-transplantation patients are particularly susceptible
- Post-transplantation patients develop post-transplantation lymphoproliferative disorder (PTLD)
  - Although morphologically indistinguishable from aggressive NHL, considered unique lymphoproliferative disease due to its substantially different pathogenesis and management

Epidemiology

- Traditionally seen in immunocompromised patients, particularly those with AIDS
- Concomitant increase of PTLD with increasing number of people receiving solid organ and bone marrow transplants

Relevant Pathology

- Mesenteric lymphomas are unique because they can grow to a large size and can envelop fat, bowel, and vessels without causing clinical symptoms
- PTLD is an Epstein-Barr virus-driven B-cell lymphoproliferation in immunosuppressed who have undergone transplantation

IMAGING FEATURES

US

- 2 layers of plaque-like sonolucent masses surrounding a central, linear, hyperechoic area
  - Hyperechoic area represents fat with leaves of mesentery

CECT

- Enlarged mesenteric lymph nodes sandwiching mesenteric vessels and fat
- Extensive retroperitoneal lymphadenopathy is commonly seen
- With administration of intravenous and oral contrast material, mesenteric tubular structures enhance relative to fat

RELATED REFERENCES

1. Hardy SM: The sandwich sign. Radiology. 226(3):651-2, 2003
2. Mueller PR et al: Appearance of lymphomatous involvement of the mesentery by ultrasonography and body computed tomography: the "sandwich sign". Radiology. 134(2):467-73, 1980

HYDROCELE OF THE CANAL OF NUCK

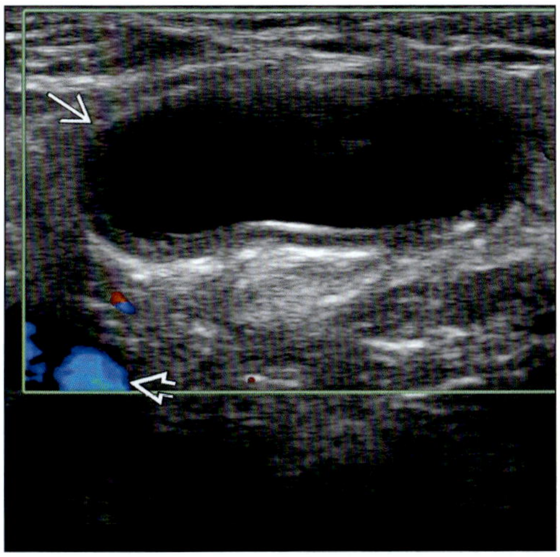

Axial color Doppler ultrasound of the right inguinal region shows an anechoic cystic structure ➔ lying medial and superficial to the femoral vein ➲. The cystic structure has a thin uniform wall.

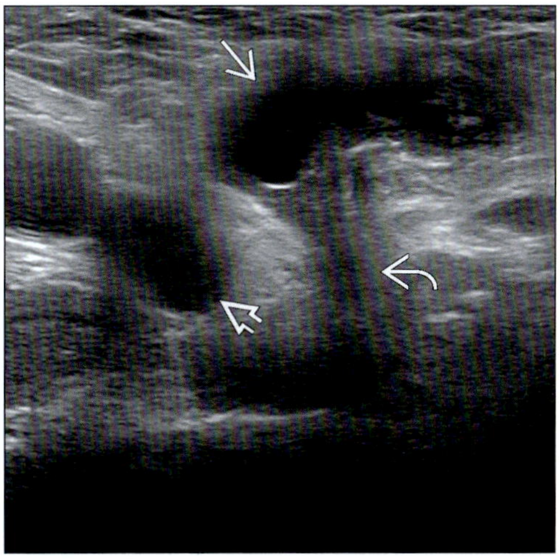

Axial ultrasound of the right inguinal region in the same patient shows the anechoic cystic structure ➔ with a hypoechoic tail ➲ extending medial to the femoral vein ➲ toward the abdomen.

CLINICAL SCENARIO

History

- 28-year-old woman with palpable right inguinal mass

IMAGE INTERPRETATION

Pitfalls

- Can be misdiagnosed as inguinal hernia and even cystic neoplasms

Actual Diagnosis

- Hydrocele of canal of Nuck

Clues to Correct Diagnosis

- Classic location of simple-appearing cystic structure with thin or imperceptible wall
- Valsalva maneuver or coughing during real-time US can differentiate a hydrocele of canal of Nuck from inguinal hernia
  - No change in shape or size in case of hydrocele of canal of Nuck
- Tail directed toward inguinal canal may be seen

BACKGROUND

Relevant Anatomy

- In women, small pouch of patent peritoneal fold extending along round ligament into inguinal canal through inguinal ring during development is called canal of Nuck
  - Canal of Nuck is homologous to processus vaginalis in men
  - During 1st year of life, it undergoes complete obliteration
    - It becomes obliterated in a superior to inferior direction
- Incomplete obliteration → fluid entrapment in peritoneal remnant

Relevant Pathology

- Complications of hydrocele of canal of Nuck are infection, hemorrhage, or large cyst with retroperitoneal extension

IMAGING FEATURES

General Features

- Variable appearances have been described
  - Well-defined, thin-walled, tubular or sausage-shaped structure along round ligament
  - Comma-shaped lesion with tail directed toward inguinal canal
  - Cyst within cyst
  - Multicystic

US

- Cyst contains simple anechoic fluid
- No change in appearance on Valsalva or during coughing

CT

- Thin-walled cystic structure in inguinal region, appearing as fluid attenuation

MR

- Thin-walled cystic structure in inguinal region, appearing as fluid signal intensity (low signal intensity at T1WI and high signal intensity at T2WI)
- Wall of hydrocele may show mild enhancement on gadolinium-enhanced studies

RELATED REFERENCES

1. Hosseinzadeh K et al: Imaging of the female perineum in adults. Radiographics. 32(4):E129-68, 2012
2. Safak AA et al: Hydrocele of the canal of Nuck: sonographic and MRI appearances. J Clin Ultrasound. 35(9):531-2, 2007

CISTERNA CHYLI

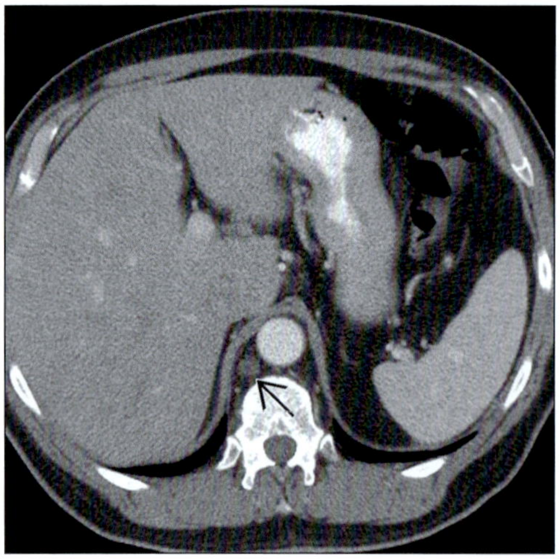

Axial CECT shows a small, oval-shaped, relatively low-attenuation structure ⇒ in the right retrocrural region.

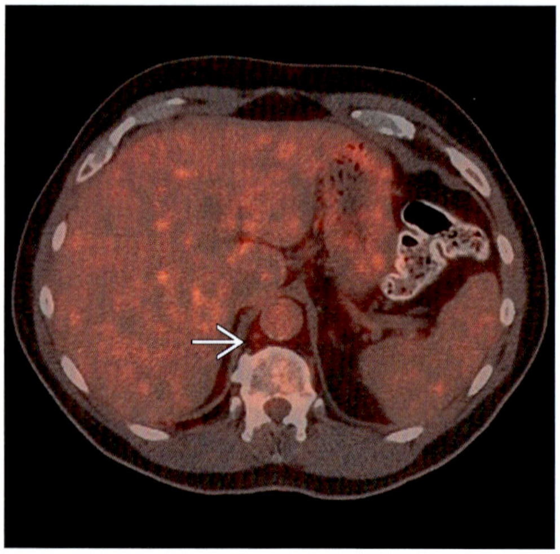

Axial fused image of PET/CT demonstrates no definite evidence of abnormal FDG uptake of the retrocrural structure ➡.

CLINICAL SCENARIO

History

- 61-year-old man with history of follicular lymphoma

IMAGE INTERPRETATION

Pitfalls

- Could be misdiagnosed as enlarged retrocrural lymph node

Actual Diagnosis

- Prominent cisterna chyli (normal anatomical structure in right retrocrural region)

Clues to Correct Diagnosis

- Characteristic location in right retrocrural region at level of L1-2 vertebrae
- Classic tubular shape
- Typical fluid attenuation on CT
- Low SUV on PET scan

BACKGROUND

Epidemiology

- Seen in 50% of lymphangiographic studies and 20% of autopsies

Relevant Anatomy

- Cisterna chyli is a dilated lymphatic sac typically located in paravertebral space usually in right retrocrural location
- Most commonly at L1-L2 vertebral level
- Extends 5-7 cm in caudocephalic direction
- Cisterna chyli is origin of thoracic lymphatic duct
- Classically, cisterna chyli receives lymph from 3 lymphatic vessels
  - 2 lumbar lymphatic trunks from lower extremities
  - Intestinal trunk drains fatty lymph from intestines
- From cisterna chyli, lymph continues superiorly into thoracic duct, draining into left internal jugular vein (or junction of left internal jugular and subclavian veins)

IMAGING FEATURES

Lymphangiography

- Variable appearances: Inverted letter Y or V, string of pearls, or comma-like configuration

US

- Unusually large cisterna chyli may mimic other pathologic conditions of retroperitoneum
- Typically seen as anechoic oval retrocrural structure

CT

- NECT: Fluid attenuation oval structure in characteristic location
- CECT: No significant post-contrast enhancement

MR

- T1WI: Low signal intensity similar to cerebrospinal fluid (CSF)
- T2WI: High signal intensity similar to CSF
- T1WI C+: No significant enhancement
- DWI: No diffusion restriction

PET/CT

- Low FDG uptake (↓ metabolic activity and ↓ SUV)

RELATED REFERENCES

1. Tamsel S et al: Unusually large cisterna chyli: US and MRI findings. Abdom Imaging. 31(6):719-21, 2006
2. Pinto PS et al: Cisterna chyli at routine abdominal MR imaging: a normal anatomic structure in the retrocrural space. Radiographics. 24(3):809-17, 2004
3. Smith TR et al: The cisterna chyli: incidence and characteristics on CT. Clin Imaging. 26(1):18-22, 2002
4. Gollub MJ et al: The cisterna chyli: a potential mimic of retrocrural lymphadenopathy on CT scans. Radiology. 199(2):477-80, 1996

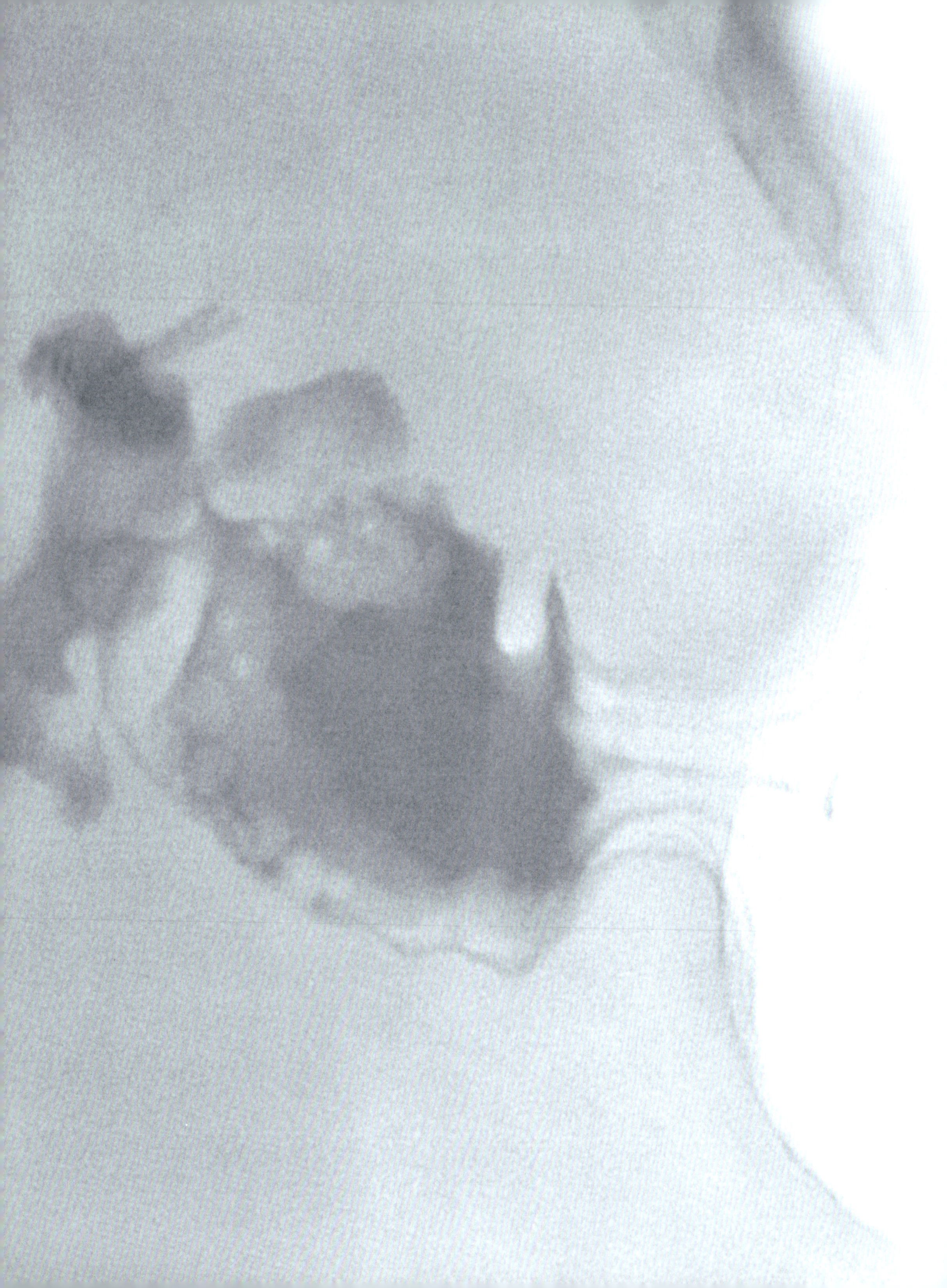

SECTION 6
Gastrointestinal Tract

Benign Conditions Simulating Malignancy

Malignant Lesions Mimicking Benign Conditions

Classic Signs and Appearances

FUNDAL PSEUDOTUMOR

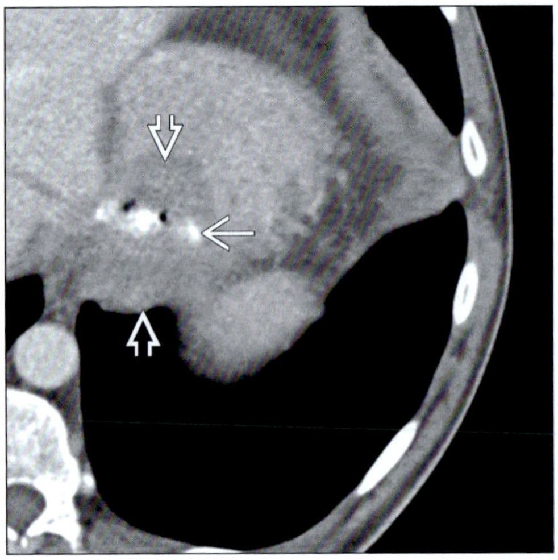

Axial CECT through the diaphragmatic hiatus demonstrates circumferential soft tissue thickening ➔ at the gastric fundus with the esophageal lumen seen centrally ➔.

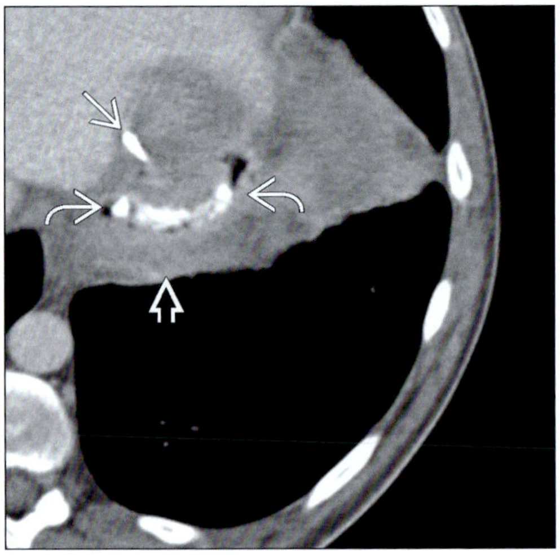

Axial CECT shows a pseudotumor representing a Nissen fundoplication defect. A suture ➔ is seen near the esophageal hiatus. Fundoplication is seen as soft tissue ➔ surrounding the lower esophagus ➔.

CLINICAL SCENARIO

History

- 50 year old with history of surgery for gastroesophageal reflux disease (GERD) presents for evaluation of abdominal pain

IMAGE INTERPRETATION

Pitfalls

- Can be misinterpreted as soft tissue mass at gastric fundus

Actual Diagnosis

- Normal appearance of Nissen fundoplication defect

Clues to Correct Diagnosis

- Knowledge of surgical procedure and its details
- Symmetrical, smoothly marginated soft tissue attenuation surrounding distal esophagus
- Surgical sutures surrounding cardia

BACKGROUND

General

- Laparoscopic Nissen fundoplication is considered standard surgical approach for severe GERD
- Recent literature suggests long-term outcome from antireflux surgery may be superior to medical treatment
- Failure of medical management, complications of GERD, and need for long-term medical therapy are most frequent indications for Nissen fundoplication
- First-line treatment for paraesophageal hernia

Epidemiology

- Gastroesophageal reflux affects approximately 20% of USA population

Relevant Pathophysiology

- Reflux due to mechanical dysfunction centered around lower esophageal sphincter
- Loss of sphincter function leads to symptoms of reflux
- Most fundoplications are performed laparoscopically
- Fundoplication: Gastric fundus is wrapped and sutured around lower esophagus to create intraabdominal esophagus
  - Reinforces closing function of lower esophageal sphincter
  - Esophageal hiatus narrowed down by sutures

IMAGING FEATURES

Fluoroscopy

- Prominent smooth filling defect of gastroesophageal junction
- Symmetric on both sides of esophagus
- Esophagus seen in center of wrap
- Distal esophagus may be dilated in elderly with impaired primary peristalsis

CT

- Circumferential soft tissue attenuation around distal esophagus
- Pseudomass defect on gastric fundus
- "Mass" is smoothly marginated
- Clips may be seen at site of fundoplication

Key Teaching Points

- Fundoplication defect can be pitfall for fundal tumor
- Defect appears as smoothly marginated mass surrounding distal esophagus

RELATED REFERENCES

1. Hamdy E et al: Response of atypical symptoms of GERD to antireflux surgery. Hepatogastroenterology. 56(90):403-6, 2009
2. Salminen P: The laparoscopic Nissen fundoplication--a better operation? Surgeon. 7(4):224-7, 2009
3. Canon CL et al: Surgical approach to gastroesophageal reflux disease: what the radiologist needs to know. Radiographics. 25(6):1485-99, 2005

APPENDICEAL CARCINOMA

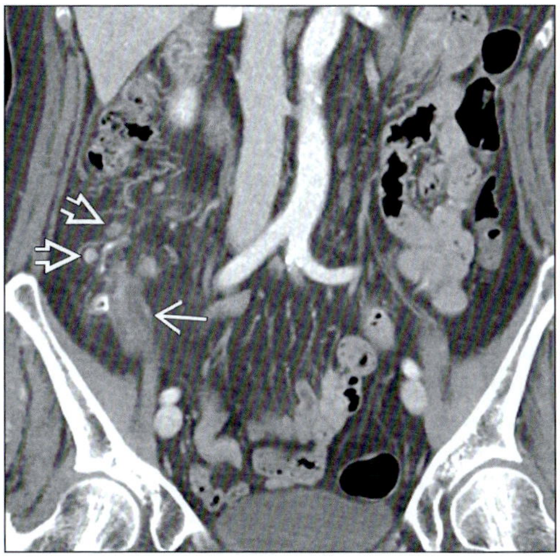
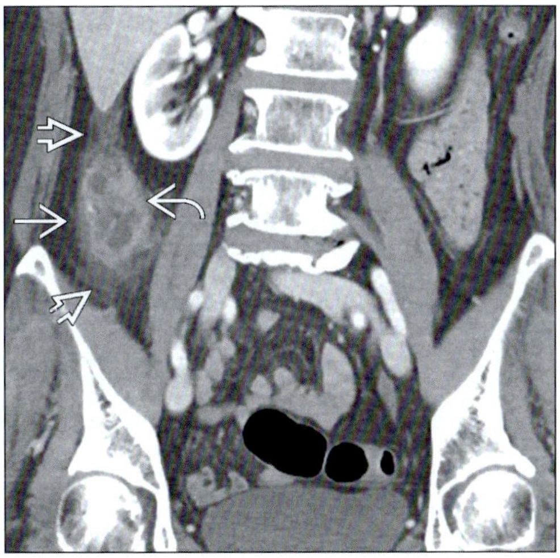

(Left) *Coronal CECT in a 77-year-old woman who presented with a 1-month history of right lower quadrant abdominal pain shows an enlarged appendix ➔ with multiple, rounded, slightly prominent, regional lymph nodes ➔.* ***(Right)*** *Coronal CECT in the same patient shows cystic dilatation of the appendiceal tip ➔ with mild periappendiceal stranding ➔ and a thick irregular and enhancing appendiceal wall ➔. Pathology revealed perforated appendiceal carcinoma.*

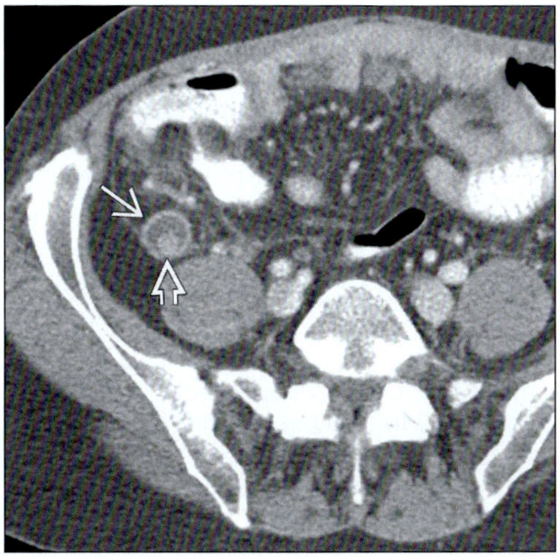
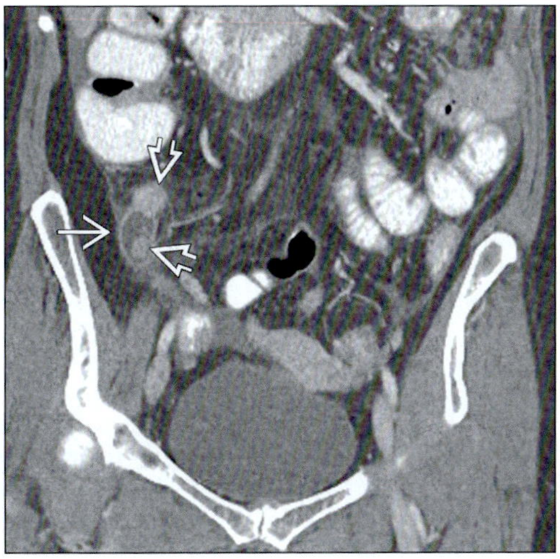

(Left) *Axial CECT in a 66-year-old man who presented with right lower quadrant pain, fever, and elevated white blood cell count shows cystic dilatation of the appendix (mucocele) ➔ with an enhancing mural nodule ➔.* ***(Right)*** *Coronal CECT in the same patient shows appendiceal mucocele ➔ with soft tissue enhancing nodules ➔. Pathology revealed mucocele with appendiceal mucinous carcinoma.*

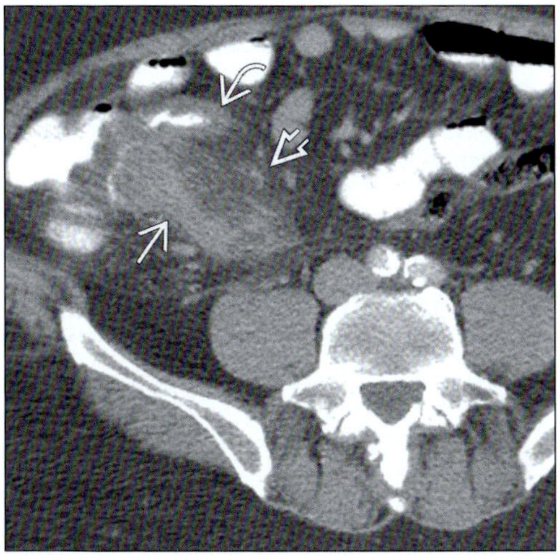
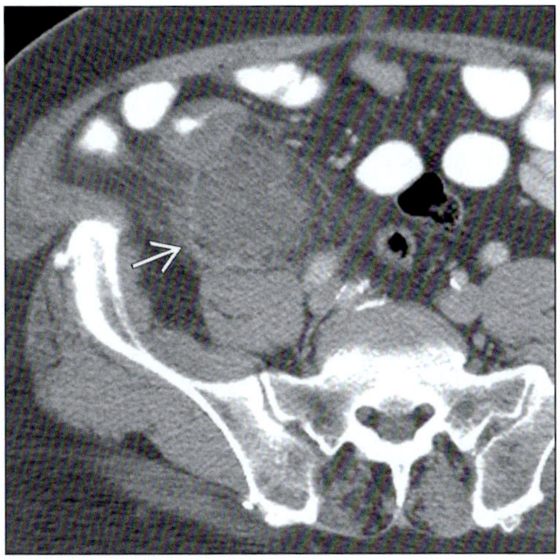

(Left) *Axial CECT in a 65-year-old man who presented with clinical features of acute appendicitis shows an enlarged appendix measuring 16 mm in diameter ➔ with periappendiceal stranding ➔ and thickening of the wall of the terminal ileum ➔.* ***(Right)*** *Axial CECT in the same patient shows phlegmonous changes ➔ with surrounding inflammatory stranding. Pathology revealed perforated appendicitis with abscess due to low-grade appendiceal carcinoma.*

BOWEL TARGET SIGN

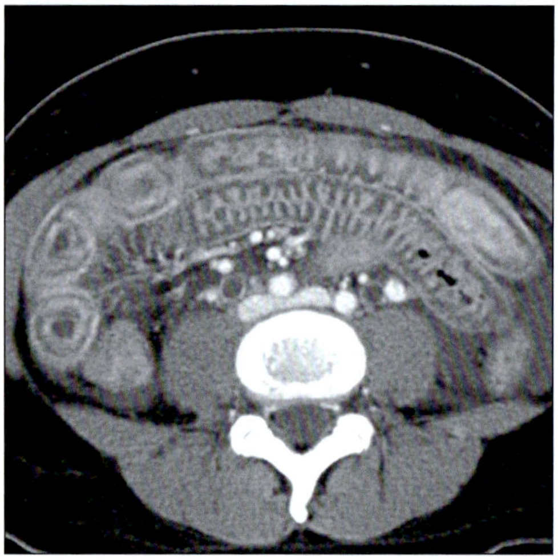

Axial CECT in a patient with systemic lupus erythematosus shows diffuse thickening of small bowel wall with enhancing inner, outer layers & hypoattenuating middle layer, giving the target appearance.

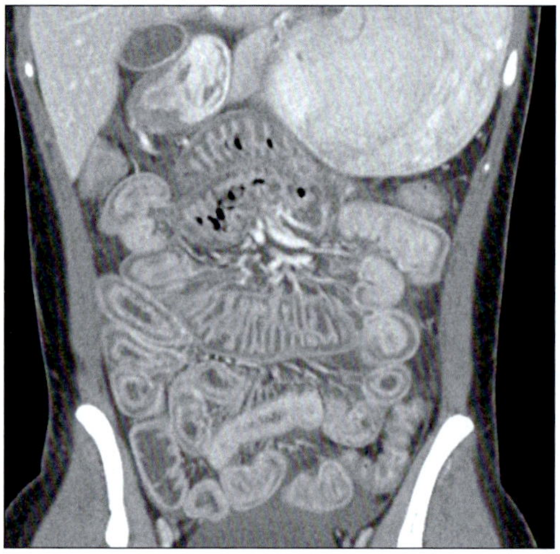

Coronal CECT in the same patient shows diffuse thickening of the small bowel wall with enhancing inner and outer layers and hypoattenuating middle layer, giving the target appearance.

IMAGING FEATURES

Appearance

- Bowel wall thickening with mural stratification into hypoattenuating middle layer between enhancing inner and outer layers
- Seen on contrast-enhanced CT of abdomen

Differential Diagnosis

- Target sign is seen with various diseases of bowel in which submucosal edema, inflammation, or both are present
  - Inflammatory bowel diseases (Crohn disease and ulcerative colitis)
    - During acute phase of Crohn disease
  - Ischemic bowel disease
  - Intramural intestinal hemorrhage
    - Anticoagulation therapy or underlying bleeding diathesis
  - Vascular disorders (Henoch-Schönlein purpura)
  - Other vasculitis (systemic lupus erythematosus [SLE])
  - Angioedema (hereditary and due to ACE inhibitor therapy)
  - Infectious diseases (infectious colitis and pseudomembranous colitis)
  - Radiation (enteritis and radiation colitis)
  - Bowel edema associated with portal hypertension

Clinical Significance

- Although target sign does not allow specific diagnosis, its presence virtually excludes malignancy as cause of bowel thickening
  - Notable exception is occurrence of target sign in cases of infiltrating rectal scirrhous carcinoma

BACKGROUND

Explanation

- Inner and outer layers of target sign represent mucosa and muscularis propria &/or serosa, respectively
  - High attenuation is result of contrast enhancement due to hyperemia
- Lower attenuation of middle layer results from edema and is assumed to be within submucosa

Imaging Technique

- Best appreciated during late arterial and early portal venous phases of contrast enhancement
- Best demonstrated when bowel is distended with neutral oral contrast material

IMAGING FEATURES

Fluoroscopy

- Corresponds to stack of coins appearance
  - Uniformly thickened folds with relatively parallel configuration
  - Fold thickening is defined as folds > 3 mm in thickness in jejunum and 2 mm in ileum

CT

- Associated findings may include ascites and mesenteric engorgement and edema

RELATED REFERENCES

1. Levine MS et al: Pattern approach for diseases of mesenteric small bowel on barium studies. Radiology. 249(2):445-60, 2008
2. Ahualli J: The target sign: bowel wall. Radiology. 234(2):549-50, 2005
3. Harisinghani MG et al: Halo sign: useful CT sign for differentiating benign from malignant colonic disease. Clin Radiol. 58(4):306-10, 2003
4. Wittenberg J et al: Algorithmic approach to CT diagnosis of the abnormal bowel wall. Radiographics. 22(5):1093-107; discussion 1107-9, 2002

COMB SIGN

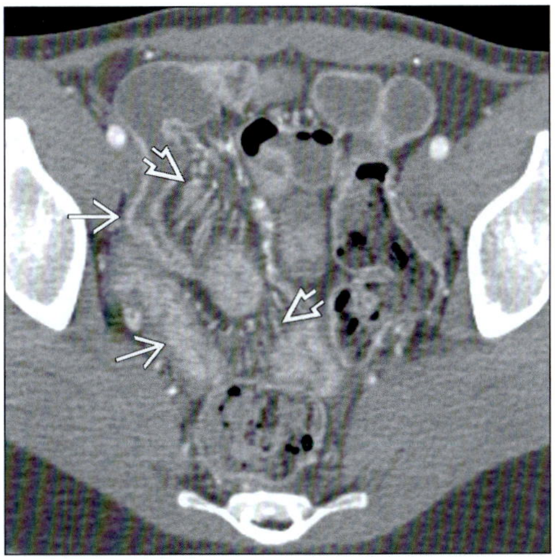

Axial CECT shows engorgement of the vasa recta, giving the characteristic comb sign. Note also mucosal enhancement of the small bowel.

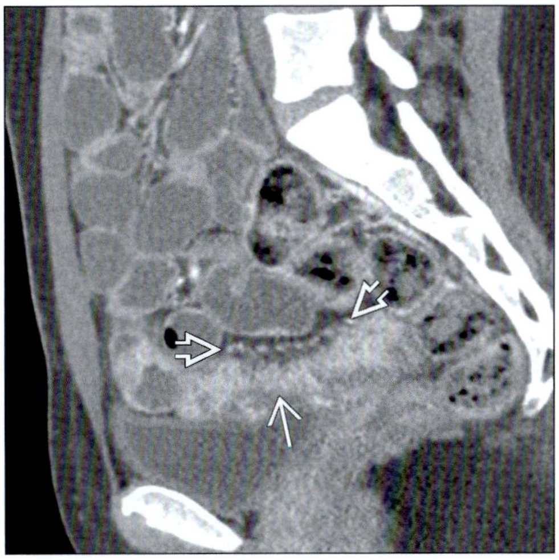

Sagittal CECT shows engorgement of the vasa recta and mucosal enhancement of involved segment of small bowel.

COMB SIGN

Appearance

- Seen on CECT scans as multiple fine tubular, tortuous structures on mesenteric side of ileum, which are aligned as teeth of a comb

Explanation

- Hypervascularity of mesentery with vascular dilatation, tortuosity, and wide spacing of vasa recta
  - Attributed to increased flow and fibrofatty proliferation in mesentery of involved bowel

Significance

- Presence of comb sign should suggest an acute exacerbation in patients with known Crohn disease

BACKGROUND

Anatomy

- Arteries that supply small bowel branch off within mesentery as series of intestinal arteries interconnected by arcades
- Vasa recta, or terminal branches, are taller and more widely spaced in jejunum compared to ileum

Relevant Pathology

- Crohn disease is a chronic granulomatous process characterized by transmural inflammation of bowel wall
- Any portion of alimentary tract may be involved
  - Most commonly involves terminal ileum and proximal colon

Differential Diagnosis

- Comb sign is not pathognomonic for Crohn disease and has been described in other conditions including
  - Vasculitis (such as lupus, polyarteritis nodosa, Henoch-Schönlein syndrome, microscopic polyangiitis, Behçet syndrome)
  - Mesenteric thromboembolism
  - Strangulated bowel obstruction
  - Ulcerative colitis
- These conditions can be differentiated on the basis of clinical history, bowel segments involved, and associated findings
- Absence of comb sign may be useful in differential diagnosis of lymphoma and metastases, which are usually hypovascular lesions

Other Imaging Findings of Crohn Disease

- Bowel-related findings
  - Aphthoid ulcerations at double-contrast barium studies
  - Bowel wall thickening
    - Occurs in up to 82% of patients
    - Usually ranges between 5 and 10 mm but can reach 20 mm
    - Frequently observed in terminal ileum but can also affect other portions of gastrointestinal tract
    - Mucosal and serosal enhancement and submucosal edema → mural stratification → target appearance at CT, during acute phase of disease
    - Mural stratification is lost in longstanding disease
  - Mesenteric lymph nodes
  - Mesenteric fibrofatty proliferation "creeping fat"
  - Abscesses, fistulas, sinus tracts, and perianal disease
- Extra-bowel findings
  - Fatty infiltration of liver
  - Primary sclerosing cholangitis
  - Nephrolithiasis
  - Cholelithiasis
  - Sacroiliitis

RELATED REFERENCES

1. Lo Re G et al: CT enterography as a powerful tool for the evaluation of inflammatory activity in Crohn's disease: relationship of CT findings with CDAI and acute-phase reactants. Radiol Med. 119(9):658-66, 2014
2. Madureira AJ: The comb sign. Radiology. 230(3):783-4, 2004

RING SIGN: EPIPLOIC APPENDAGITIS

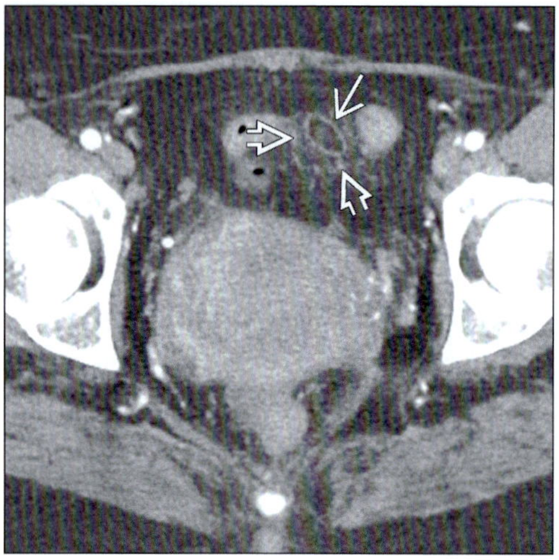

Axial CECT demonstrates a well-circumscribed fatty mass ➔ with a thin rim of soft tissue attenuation adjacent to the sigmoid colon. There is mild stranding of the surrounding fat ➔.

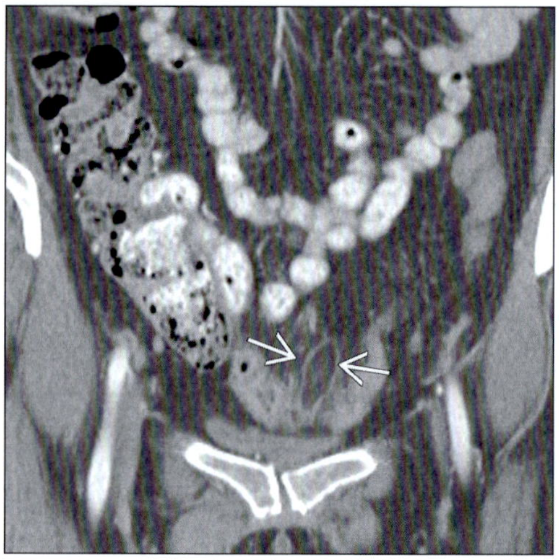

Coronal CECT in the same patient shows a well-circumscribed, elongated fatty mass ➔ with a thin rim of soft tissue attenuation adjacent to the sigmoid colon.

CLINICAL SCENARIO

History

- 49-year-old man with left lower quadrant pain

IMAGE INTERPRETATION

Classic Sign

- Ring-enhancing, fat-containing lesion adjacent to left colon is consistent with epiploic appendagitis

Differential Diagnosis

- Omental torsion is main differential diagnostic possibility but it is more common on right side

BACKGROUND

General

- Acute epiploic appendagitis is a self-limited inflammation of appendices epiploicae
- Acute onset of pain, commonly in left lower quadrant

Epidemiology

- Mean age at diagnosis: 40 years
- Most are treated conservatively

Relevant Anatomy

- Epiploic appendages are peritoneal pouches arising from serosal surface of colon attached by vascular stalk
- Composed of adipose tissue and blood vessels
- Size: 1-2 cm thick and 2-5 cm long
- Frequently associated with colonic diverticula
- Typically are most abundant near sigmoid colon
- May reach 100 in number
- Typically only seen on CT when inflamed &/or surrounded by fluid

Relevant Pathology

- Etiology: Torsion of epiploic appendages, resulting in venous occlusion, leading to ischemia and inflammation
- Can be associated with obesity, hernia, and strenuous exercise

IMAGING FEATURES

US

- Small, oval, hyperechoic, noncompressible mass, with occasional peripheral hypoechoic halo

CT

- Most sensitive modality
- Fatty-attenuation lesion contacting colon
- Surrounded by hyperattenuating peripheral rim, representing inflamed visceral peritoneal lining (ring sign)

MR

- T1WI: High signal intensity pedunculated paracolic small lesion
- T1WI FS: Low signal intensity due to fat suppression
- T1WI C+: Peripheral rim enhancement
- T2WI: Intermediate signal intensity of fat

Key Teaching Points

- Epiploic appendagitis is a pedunculated paracolic small fatty lesion
- Most common location near sigmoid colon
- Typically present with acute left lower quadrant pain
- Typically treated conservatively

RELATED REFERENCES

1. Schnedl WJ et al: Insights into epiploic appendagitis. Nat Rev Gastroenterol Hepatol. 8(1):45-9, 2011
2. Singh AK et al: Acute epiploic appendagitis and its mimics. Radiographics. 25(6):1521-34, 2005
3. Singh AK et al: CT appearance of acute appendagitis. AJR Am J Roentgenol. 183(5):1303-7, 2004
4. Mollà E et al: Primary epiploic appendagitis: US and CT findings. Eur Radiol. 8(3):435-8, 1998

BIRD'S BEAK SIGN

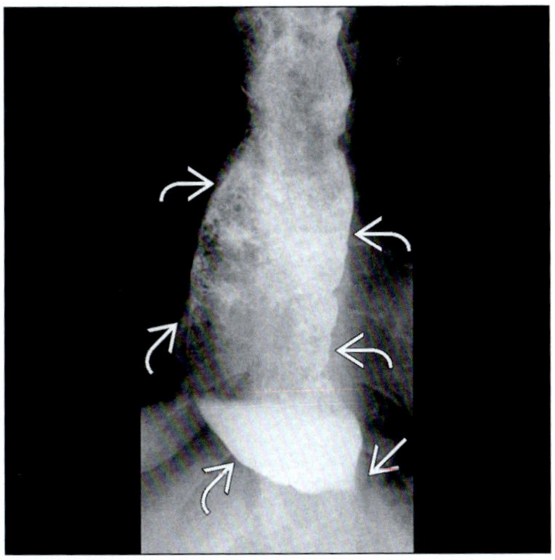

Frontal view of a barium swallow examination demonstrates significant dilatation of the proximal esophagus ➔ with distal tapering bird's beak ➔ sign, consistent with achalasia.

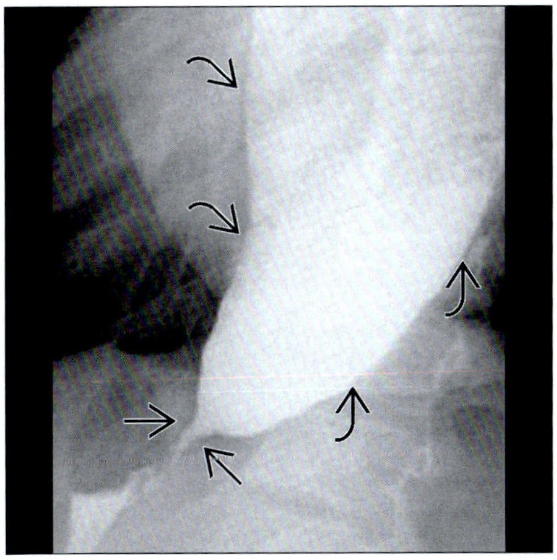

Oblique view of a barium swallow examination demonstrates significant distension of the proximal esophagus with barium ➔ and distal smooth narrowing bird's beak ➔ sign, consistent with achalasia.

CLINICAL SCENARIO

History

- 47-year-old man with several months history of dysphagia, intermittent chest pain, and regurgitation

IMAGE INTERPRETATION

Clues to Correct Diagnosis

- Bird's beak sign of esophagus is classic fluoroscopic finding seen in achalasia

BACKGROUND

General

- Bird's beak sign refers to dilation and smooth tapering of distal esophagus
- Achalasia is a primary esophageal motility disorder
- Incomplete relaxation of lower esophageal sphincter
- Symptoms: Dysphagia (solids & liquids), regurgitation (saliva & undigested food), chest pain, & weight loss
- Manometry: Loss of primary peristalsis and incomplete relaxation of lower esophageal sphincter (LES)
- Endoscopy: Dilated esophagus with retained saliva and undigested food particles
- Must rule out pseudoachalasia secondary to stricture, surgery (fundoplication, gastric banding), or tumor (esophageal, gastric cardia)
- May be sequela of Chagas disease
- Medical therapy: Botulinum toxin, nitrates, calcium channel blockers
- Surgical management: Myotomy or pneumatic dilation

Epidemiology

- Incidence of 1 in 100,000; prevalence of 10 in 100,000
- Often present at early adult age
- Occurs equally in men and women

Relevant Physiology

- Unclear etiology; likely inflammatory process due to autoimmune, viral, or neurodegenerative causes
- Results in loss of inhibitory neurotransmitters

Relevant Pathology

- Degeneration of ganglion cells in LES and esophageal myenteric plexus

IMAGING FEATURES

Fluoroscopy

- Imaging study of choice; must be used in conjunction with manometry to increase sensitivity
- Aperistalsis of esophagus
- Esophageal dilation with smooth, tapered narrowing of distal esophagus, giving bird's beak appearance
- Poor emptying due to incomplete relaxation of LES
- Advanced stage: Tortuosity, angulation, megaesophagus
- Differentiation from pseudoachalasia is difficult
  - Evaluate gastric cardia and fundus (may be difficult due to delayed emptying of barium)
  - May see eccentricity, nodularity, or shouldering of distal esophageal segment in pseudoachalasia
  - Larger esophageal diameter (> 4 cm) more suggestive of primary achalasia than pseudoachalasia

Plain Radiography

- Widened mediastinal contour
- Dilated esophagus (with air-fluid level) with anterior deviation of trachea

CT

- Not routinely ordered for evaluation of achalasia
- No wall thickening seen in achalasia
- May be useful to distinguish from pseudoachalasia
  - Tumor or esophagitis may → wall thickening or mass

RELATED REFERENCES

1. Ba-Ssalamah A et al: Dedicated multi-detector CT of the esophagus: spectrum of diseases. Abdom Imaging. 34(1):3-18, 2009

CORKSCREW ESOPHAGUS

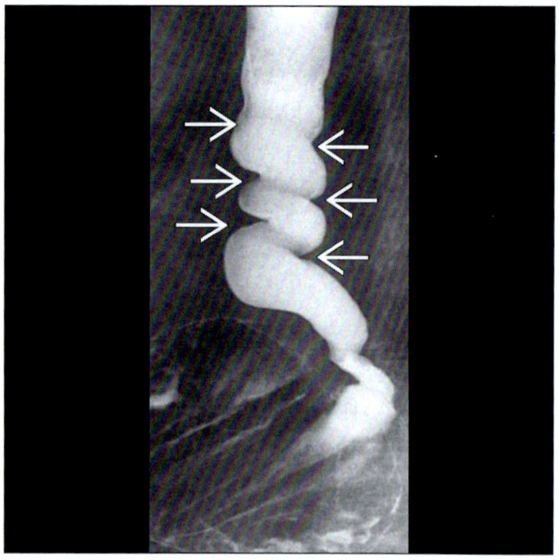

Oblique view fluoroscopy image during barium swallow show simultaneous, nonperistaltic contractions of the distal esophagus corkscrew ➔.

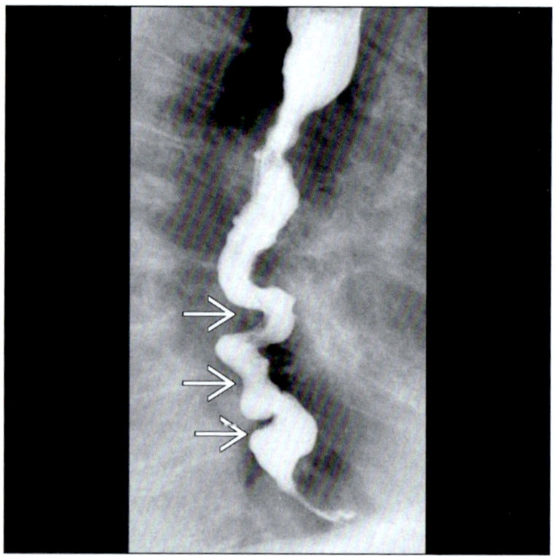

Lateral view fluoroscopy image during barium swallow confirms findings of a corkscrew appearance. These tertiary contractions ➔ are a classic fluoroscopic finding of diffuse esophageal spasm.

CLINICAL SCENARIO

History

- 65-year-old woman with several month history of intermittent dysphagia and chest pain

IMAGE INTERPRETATION

Classic Sign

- Corkscrew appearance of esophagus (seen on barium swallow) is the classic fluoroscopic finding of distal esophageal spasm (DES)

BACKGROUND

General

- Corkscrew appearance of esophagus, a.k.a. rosary bead appearance
- Due to multiple simultaneous, nonperistaltic, lumen-obliterating contractions (tertiary contractions)
- Seen in distal esophagus
- Corkscrew appearance may not be present during episodes of pain

Clinical Relevance

- Presents clinically as intermittent chest pain and dysphagia for seconds to minutes
- Reflux-related symptoms, such as heartburn, regurgitation, and cough, can be encountered
- Symptoms may or may not occur with ingestion of food
- Esophageal manometry has a central role in diagnosis, along with high-resolution esophageal pressure topography
- Frequently coexists with gastroesophageal reflux disease (GERD)
- Should be distinguished from other esophageal motility disorders such as achalasia
- May be treated medically with calcium channel blockers, nitrates, anticholinergic agents

Epidemiology

- Infrequently seen, accounts for 5-15% of esophageal motility disorders

Relevant Physiology

- Unclear etiology
- May be related to deficiency of nitric oxide, leading to abnormalities in neural inhibition
- Results in premature contractions of muscles of distal esophagus → increased intraluminal pressure
- Recent studies have shown that DES may progress to achalasia

Relevant Pathology

- Hypertrophy of muscularis propria may be present

IMAGING FEATURES

Fluoroscopy

- Normal primary peristalsis in upper esophagus
- Corkscrew or rosary bead appearance is classic finding in distal esophagus
  - Not frequently seen in patients with DES (as low as 4%) in a recent series
- Can also show abnormal primary and tertiary peristalsis without classic corkscrew appearance of esophagus (more frequently seen)
- Differentiated from achalasia by normal relaxation of lower esophageal sphincter (LES)
  - Achalasia has LES dysfunction

Other Imaging Modalities

- Have no role in diagnosis of DES

RELATED REFERENCES

1. Achem SR et al: Distal esophageal spasm: an update. Curr Gastroenterol Rep. 15(9):325, 2013
2. Roman S et al: Distal esophageal spasm. Dysphagia. 27(1):115-23, 2012
3. Adler DG et al: Primary esophageal motility disorders. Mayo Clin Proc. 76(2):195-200, 2001

SHAGGY ESOPHAGUS

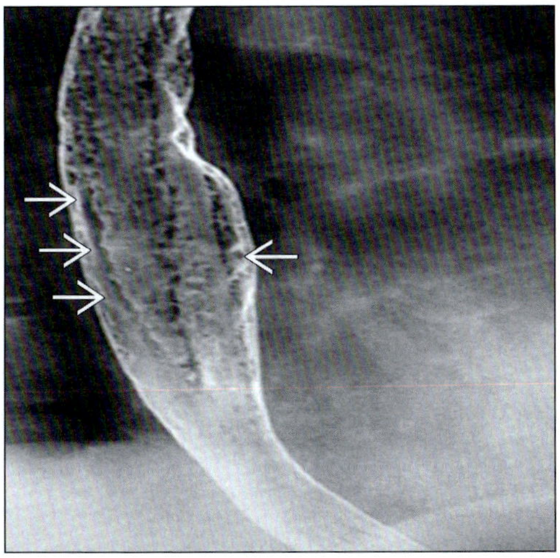

Double-contrast esophagram shows the shaggy appearance of the esophagus due to multiple ulcers and coalescent longitudinal plaques ➡.

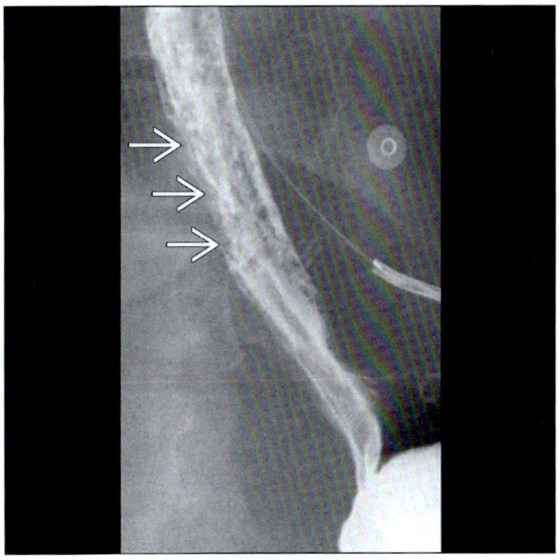

Oblique view of double-contrast esophagram demonstrates multiple ulcers and coalescent longitudinal plaques ➡, giving a shaggy appearance.

CLINICAL SCENARIO

History

- 53-year-old HIV-positive man with odynophagia

IMAGE INTERPRETATION

Classic Sign

- Multiple longitudinal ulcers and plaques on esophagogram that coalesce to give shaggy appearance of esophagus, with trapping of contrast between lesions
- Shaggy esophagus is classic for candidal esophagitis

BACKGROUND

General

- *Candida* infection of esophagus is seen mostly in
  - Immunocompromised patients (such as AIDS)
  - Patients with mechanical obstruction and local stasis
- Etiology
  - Infectious esophagitis is usually caused by fungi of *Candida* (typically *Candida albicans)*
- Clinical presentation
  - Patients usually present with odynophagia, commonly associated with oral thrush (50% of cases)
- Prognosis
  - Usually self-limited and responds rapidly to oral therapy
- May coexist with herpes or cytomegalovirus (CMV) esophagitis

Epidemiology

- Occurs in all ages
- Involves both genders equally
- Occurs in 15-20% of patients with AIDS

Relevant Pathology

- Downward spread of *C. albicans* from mouth to esophagus
- *Candida* surface-binding molecules adhere to mucosa
- Protease secretion → tissue breakdown
- Adenosine secretion → blockage of neutrophil oxygen radical production → resistance to phagocytosis
- May be associated with esophageal intramural pseudodiverticulosis, tiny outpouchings representing dilated excretory ducts of esophageal submucosal glands

IMAGING FEATURES

Fluoroscopic Findings (Double-Contrast Esophagram)

- Discrete plaques in mid to upper esophagus with longitudinal orientation
- Cobblestone or snakeskin appearance with confluent plaques
- Shaggy esophagus, usually in AIDS patients

CECT

- Uniform circumferential wall thickening (> 5 mm)
- Usually involves relatively long segment
- Target sign
  - Edematous wall that shows
    - Low-attenuation submucosa
    - Inflamed mucosa showing avid enhancement

RELATED REFERENCES

1. Manfredi R et al: Recurring Candida albicans esophagitis in a HIV-infected patient undergoing long-Term antiretroviral therapy, and with absent-negligible immunodeficiency. Braz J Infect Dis. 11(6):605-9, 2007
2. Levine MS et al: Diseases of the esophagus: diagnosis with esophagography. Radiology. 237(2):414-27, 2005
3. Luedtke P et al: Radiologic diagnosis of benign esophageal strictures: a pattern approach. Radiographics. 23(4):897-909, 2003
4. Berkovich GY et al: CT findings in patients with esophagitis. AJR Am J Roentgenol. 175(5):1431-4, 2000

FAT HALO SIGN

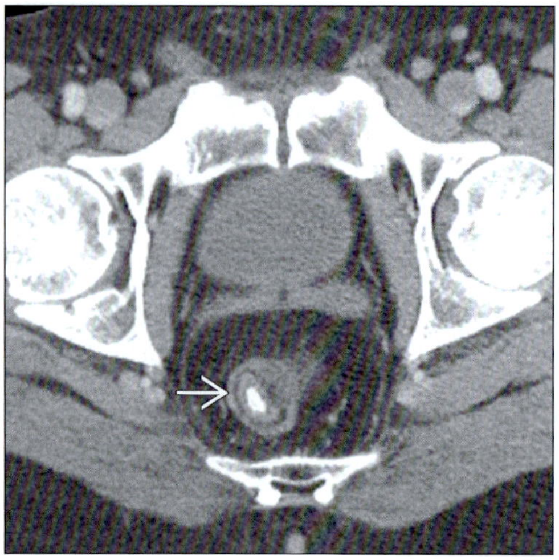

Axial CECT in a patient with chronic ulcerative colitis shows submucosal fat ➡, resulting in differentiation of the rectal wall into 3 layers (fat halo sign).

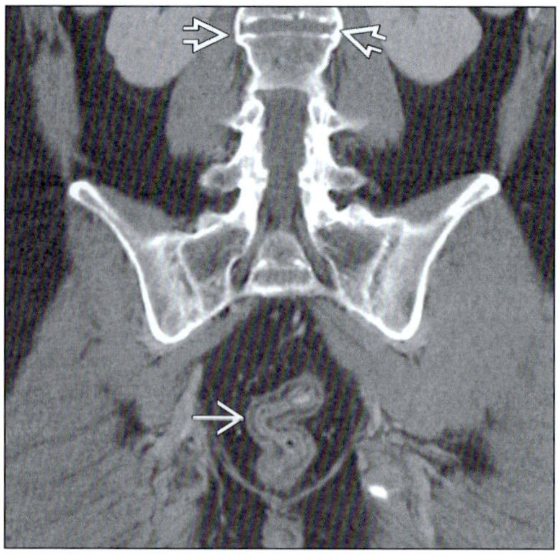

Coronal CECT in the same patient shows rectal submucosal fat ➡, resulting in the fat halo sign. Note also the spinal syndesmophytes ⇨, resulting in bamboo spine.

IMAGING FEATURES

Appearance

- Fat halo sign seen on CT of abdomen appears as thickened bowel wall demonstrating 3 layers: Inner and outer layer of soft tissue attenuation, which enclose 3rd layer of fatty attenuation
- Fat halo sign can be appreciated on both contrast-enhanced and nonenhanced CT

Differential Diagnosis

- Abnormal fatty infiltration of submucosa can be seen in different pathological conditions
  - Chronic inflammatory bowel disease (Crohn disease and ulcerative colitis)
  - Cytoreductive therapy
  - Graft-vs. -host disease
  - In absence of clinical or radiologic evidence of inflammatory bowel disease, presence of fat halo sign may represent a normal finding, possibly related to obesity
- Intramural fat may exist in both distal ileum and colon as a normal variant in patients without gastrointestinal symptoms or history of gastrointestinal disease
  - Normal intramural fat layer is generally very thin, usually thinner than the fat layer seen with inflammatory bowel disease
    - Noted in 21% of individuals with no history of inflammatory bowel disease
    - Most frequently seen in underdistended or poorly distended bowel loops

Pitfall

- Fat halo sign should be differentiated from target sign, where middle layer has fluid or soft tissue attenuation and results from submucosal edema or hemorrhage

BACKGROUND

Explanation

- Abnormal wall of small bowel or colon consists of 3 layers
  - Inner layer of soft tissue attenuation represents mucosa
  - Middle layer of low attenuation (-18 to -64 HU)
    - Results from widening and fatty infiltration of submucosa
  - Outer soft tissue attenuation layer represents muscularis propria and serosa

Distribution

- When fat halo sign is seen in both small and large bowel, it is considered evidence of Crohn disease
  - Typically terminal ileum and ascending colon
- When only colon is affected, degree and geographic distribution of bowel wall thickness are signs used to distinguish ulcerative colitis from Crohn disease
  - Ulcerative colitis
    - Symmetric and diffuse wall thickening
  - Crohn disease
    - Eccentric and discrete wall thickening, with affected segments alternating with spared areas (skip areas)

Incidence

- Fat halo sign has been reported in 61% of patients with ulcerative colitis and in 8-27% of patients with Crohn disease

RELATED REFERENCES

1. Ahualli J: The fat halo sign. Radiology. 242(3):945-6, 2007
2. Amitai MM et al: Fat halo sign in the bowel wall of patients with Crohn's disease. Clin Radiol. 62(10):994-7, 2007
3. Harisinghani MG et al: Bowel wall fat halo sign in patients without intestinal disease. AJR Am J Roentgenol. 181(3):781-4, 2003

SCLEROSING ENCAPSULATING PERITONITIS ABDOMINAL COCOON

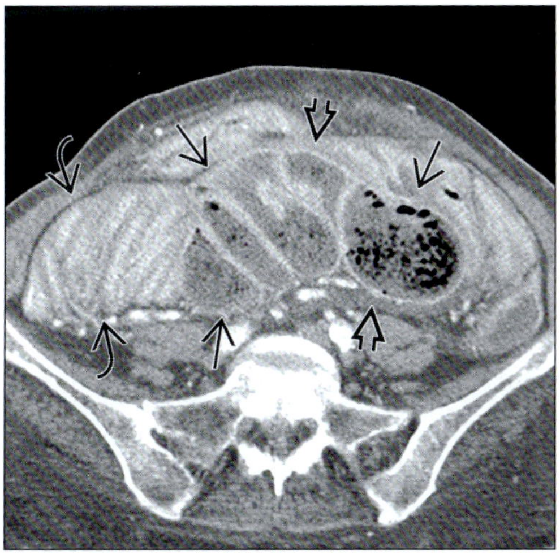

Axial CECT shows a collection of dilated small bowel loops → that are adherent together and surrounded by a thin rim of abnormal soft tissue density ⇨. Compressed loops ↗ also appear adherent together.

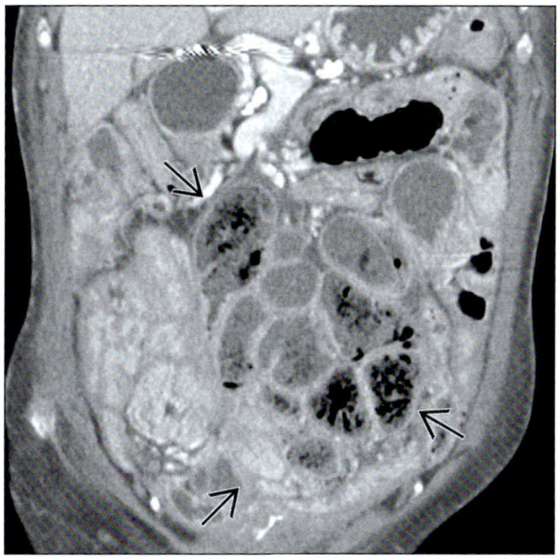

Coronal CECT shows a collection of dilated small bowel loops → in the middle of the abdomen with small bowel feces sign. Other decompressed bowel loops in the right abdomen also appear matted together.

IMAGING FEATURES

Appearance

- Abdominal cocoon or sclerosing encapsulating peritonitis (SEP) is a condition characterized by total or partial encasement of the small bowel by fibrocollagenous cocoon-like sac
- Clustered small bowel loops encased by thin membrane-like sac
  - Can be seen at radiography and barium studies
- Abnormally thickened, fibrotic peritoneum that encapsulates small bowel loops, resulting in obstruction

Differential Diagnosis

- Should be differentiated from other conditions involving peritoneum, such as peritoneal carcinomatosis and pseudomyxoma peritonei

Other Imaging Features

- Peritoneal thickening, calcification, and enhancement
  - Serosal bowel wall calcification
  - Calcification over liver capsule, spleen, posterior peritoneal wall
- Gross ascites and loculated fluid collections
- Tethering or matting of small bowel loops
- Thickening of bowel wall

BACKGROUND

General

- While exact etiology is unclear, chronic irritation of peritoneum has been postulated as cause
- Many risk factors exist for sclerosing encapsulating peritonitis
  - Long-term peritoneal dialysis and continuous ambulatory peritoneal dialysis (CAPD)
    - Prevalence of abdominal cocoon in patients undergoing CAPD ranges from 0.5-2.8%
    - Incidence increases with duration of peritoneal dialysis
    - Incidence and mortality of 2.1% and 8.3%, respectively, at 8 years
    - Incidence and mortality of 17.2% and 100%, respectively, after 15 years
  - Prior abdominal surgery
  - Practolol therapy
  - Sarcoidosis
  - Liver transplantation
  - Peritoneal tuberculosis
  - Ventriculoperitoneal shunts and peritoneovenous shunts
  - Idiopathic
    - Adolescent females
    - May result from retrograde menstruation that leads to subclinical peritoneal infection

Pathology

- Diffuse inflammatory process affecting peritoneum may involve small bowel along its antimesenteric wall, causing mural fibrosis and thickening
- Can lead to adhesions between adjoining bowel loops, narrowing of bowel lumen, and eventually small bowel obstruction
- Small bowel necrosis and perforation may also occur

Clinical Features

- Intestinal obstruction presenting with abdominal pain and vomiting
- History of similar episodes that resolved spontaneously
- Nontender soft mass on abdominal palpation

RELATED REFERENCES

1. Caldwell J et al: Sclerosing encapsulating peritonitis (cocoon bowel) presenting after laparotomy for splenic abscess. J Radiol Case Rep. 7(10):17-23, 2013
2. George V et al: Chronic fibrosing conditions in abdominal imaging. Radiographics. 33(4):1053-80, 2013
3. Serter A et al: Supposed to be rare cause of intestinal obstruction; abdominal cocoon: report of two cases. Clin Imaging. 37(3):586-9, 2013

RIBBON BOWEL: GRAFT-VS.-HOST DISEASE

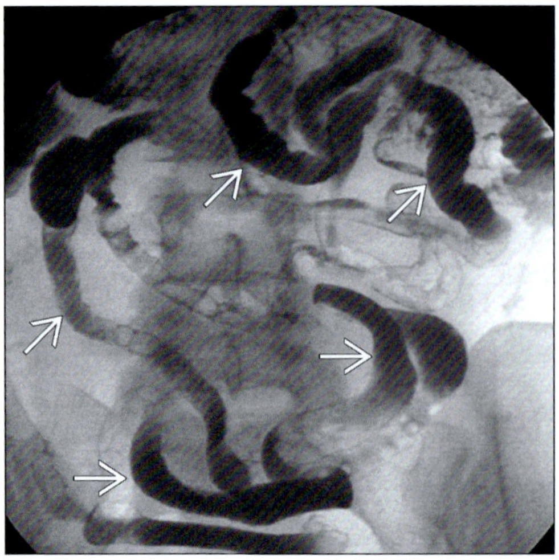

Small bowel follow-through image of the abdomen demonstrates normal-caliber small bowel ➔ with smooth appearance of the lumen.

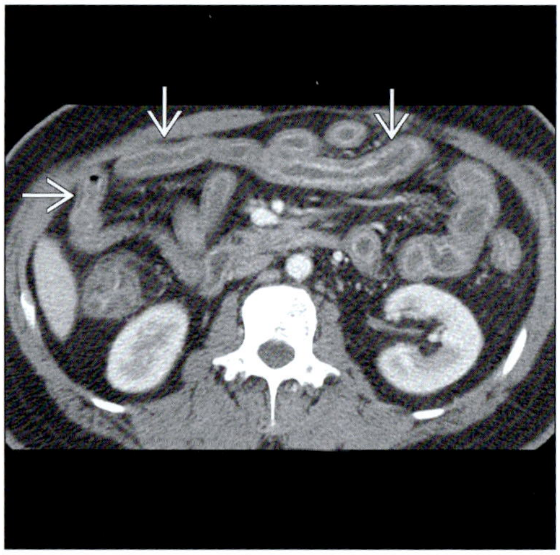

Axial CECT through the abdomen demonstrates significant wall thickening of small bowel loops ➔, which demonstrates mucosal hyperenhancement with associated mesenteric edema.

CLINICAL SCENARIO

History

- 33-year-old man with leukemia presents with nausea, skin rash, and diarrhea 8 weeks after allogeneic hematopoietic stem cell transplantation

IMAGE INTERPRETATION

Classic Sign

- Smooth, ribbon-like appearance of small bowel on contrast in patient with recent hematopoietic stem cell transplantation is classic for graft-vs.-host disease (GVHD)

BACKGROUND

General

- Seen in setting of allogeneic hematopoietic stem cell transplantation
- Results from donor T cells reacting to antigens of host
- 2 forms of GVHD exist: Acute and chronic
- Classically, acute form occurs within 100 days post transplantation
- 4 grades of GVHD exist, depending on degree of skin, gastrointestinal tract, and liver involvement
- Clinically: Rash, diarrhea, pain, ascites, and nausea
- Treated with immunosuppression, including corticosteroids

Epidemiology

- M = F
- GVHD with GI involvement occurs in 30-75% after allogeneic hematopoietic stem cell transplantation
- Risk of GVHD increases with increased age of donor or recipient
- Risk increases when gender of donor & recipient differ
- Risk decreases with increasing human antigen matching & genetic relation between donor & recipient

Relevant Physiology

- Donor T cells react to antigens on host tissues of immunocompromised recipient

Relevant Pathology

- Gross: Bowel wall edema
- Microscopic: Epithelial cell apoptosis, crypt cell necrosis, mucosal inflammation, and lymphocytic infiltration

IMAGING FEATURES

Plain Radiography

- May demonstrate nonspecific findings

Fluoroscopy

- Contrast may demonstrate small bowel wall thickening, featureless, ribbon-like loops

CT

- Gastrointestinal tract involvement often manifests as bowel wall thickening, which may be discontinuous
- Small bowel is involved in 75-100% of cases
- Mucosal enhancement in up to 54% of patients
- Serosal enhancement in up to 31% of patients
- Simultaneous mucosal and serosal enhancement has been described as halo sign
- Engorgement of vasa recta of affected bowel segments and mesenteric edema are common findings
- Ascites can be seen

US

- Findings may be nonspecific; bowel wall thickening and ascites could be seen

RELATED REFERENCES

1. del Campo L et al: Abdominal complications following hematopoietic stem cell transplantation. Radiographics. 34(2):396-412, 2014

NORTHERN EXPOSURE SIGN

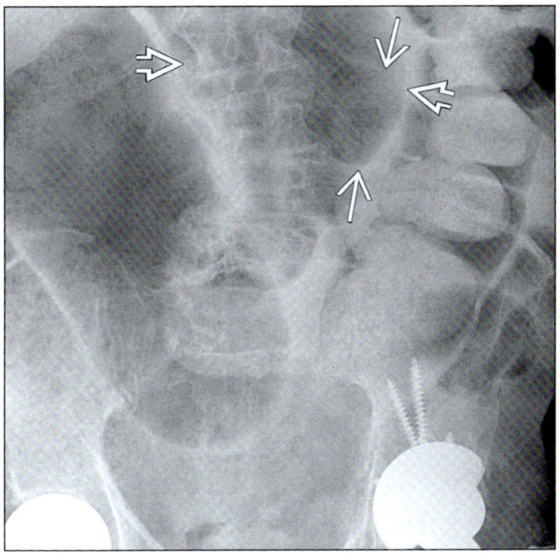

Abdominal supine radiograph shows nondilated, feces-filled transverse colon ➔ crosses shadow of markedly dilated, gas-filled sigmoid colon ➲ that ascends vertically to reach uppermost abdomen.

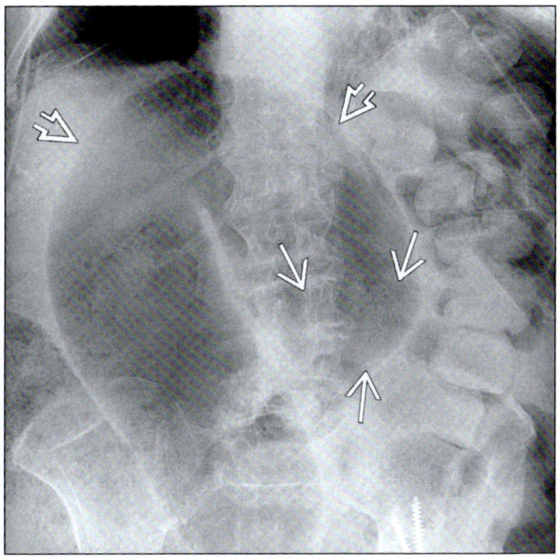

Abdominal radiograph obtained with the patient in the supine position shows nondilated, feces-filled transverse colon ➔ that crosses shadow of markedly dilated sigmoid colon ➲.

CLINICAL SCENARIO

History

- 73-year-old man with abdominal pain, vomiting, and obstipation

IMAGE INTERPRETATION

Classic Sign

- Northern exposure sign: Dilated, twisted, U-shaped sigmoid colon that projects above transverse colon on supine AP radiograph
  - White line in middle of inverted "U" represents opposed inner walls of sigmoid colon pointing toward pelvis
- Classic for sigmoid volvulus
  - Sign has sensitivity of 86% and specificity of 100% for differentiating sigmoid volvulus from other causes of distal colonic obstruction

BACKGROUND

General

- Twisting or torsion of sigmoid colon around its mesenteric axis
- Predisposing factors: Longstanding constipation and redundant colonic mesentery
- It could be midline, directed to right or left upper quadrants, or causing elevation of hemidiaphragm
- If sigmoid volvulus arises in midline, it could extend above 10th thoracic vertebral body
- Northern exposure sign has sensitivity of 86% and specificity of 100%

Epidemiology

- Associated abnormalities: Comorbid disease: 30% with psychiatric disease, 13% are institutionalized at time of diagnosis

Relevant Pathology

- Gross: Twisted segment with dilation of proximal bowel loops
- Microscopic: Localized thickening of mucosal folds with ischemic and necrotic changes

IMAGING FEATURES

Plain Radiography

- Supine images demonstrate northern exposure sign: Massively dilated sigmoid colon that extends superiorly above level of transverse colon

Contrast Enema (Using Water-Soluble Contrast Material)

- Bird's beak sign: Smooth tapering of contrast column

CT

- Bird's beak could also be demonstrated with progressive tapering of afferent and efferent limbs leading into twist
- Whirl sign: Tightly twisted mesentery and bowel
- Signs of ischemia (such as wall thickening, pneumatosis, and stranding) should be sought

RELATED REFERENCES

1. Tiah L et al: Sigmoid volvulus: diagnostic twists and turns. Eur J Emerg Med. 13(2):84-7, 2006
2. Matsumoto S et al: Computed tomographic imaging of abdominal volvulus: pictorial essay. Can Assoc Radiol J. 55(5):297-303, 2004
3. Javors BR et al: The northern exposure sign: a newly described finding in sigmoid volvulus. AJR Am J Roentgenol. 173(3):571-4, 1999

SHOCK BOWEL

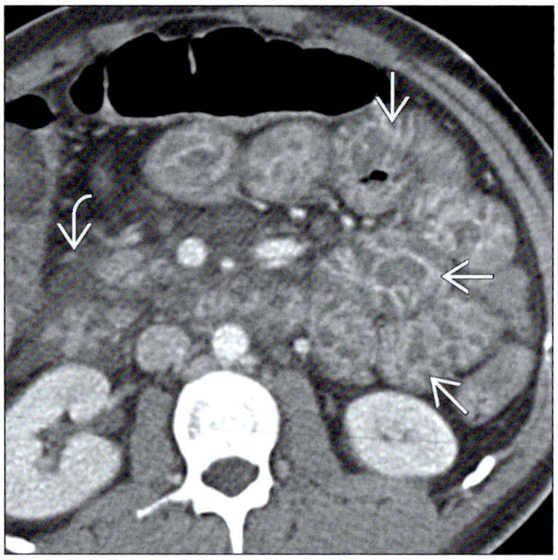

Axial CECT demonstrates luminal distension of multiple small bowel loops with low-attenuation fluid, thickened walls, and intense mucosal hyperenhancement ➡ with intraperitoneal fluid ↪.

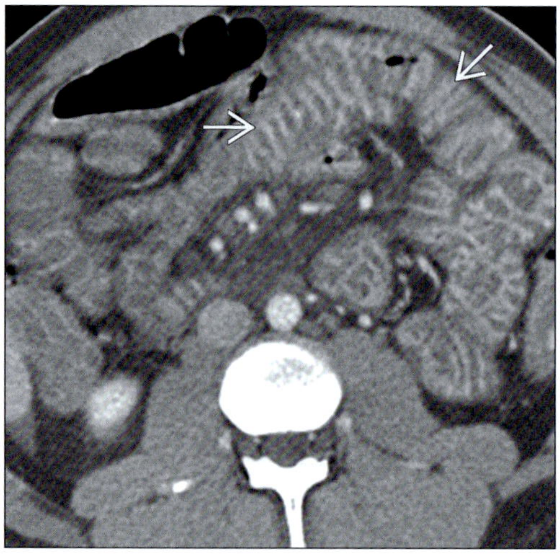

Axial CECT demonstrates significantly thickened small bowel wall with mucosal hyperenhancement ➡.

CLINICAL SCENARIO

History

- 50-year-old hypotensive patient involved in motor vehicle collision

IMAGE INTERPRETATION

Classic Sign

- CECT demonstrates thickened small bowel wall with intense mucosal hyperenhancement, consistent with shock bowel

BACKGROUND

General

- Shock bowel is most widely reported and familiar CT sign of hypovolemic shock in trauma patients
- Although classically associated with trauma, other etiologies include neurogenic shock from head or spinal injury, sepsis, blood loss, and cardiac arrest
- It is characterized by bowel segments with marked submucosal edema and intense mucosal enhancement
- Due to hypovolemia resulting in insufficient oxygen delivery to bowel
- Patients typically have severe hypotension
- Correcting underlying abnormality results in rapid resolution

Relevant Physiology

- Systemic hypotension results in mesenteric arterial vasoconstriction and mesenteric venous constriction
- Alters permeability of bowel, causing interstitial leakage of fluid and contrast material → intense enhancement of mucosa and submucosal edematous wall thickening
- Ischemia results in interruption of intestinal peristalsis → bowel dilatation
- Failure of mucosa to perform normal function of fluid resorption → dilated, fluid-filled small bowel

IMAGING FEATURES

General

- Findings are solely described on contrast-enhanced CT
- Ultrasound demonstrates nonspecific findings seen in trauma patients
- MR imaging is time consuming and subject to motion artifacts; not practical in emergency setting

Contrast-Enhanced CT

- Best imaging modality for detection
- Intense enhancement of bowel mucosa
- Bowel wall thickening with submucosal edema
- Fluid-filled bowel ± luminal distention
- Intraperitoneal free fluid could be seen
- Referred to as CT hypotension complex when associated with collapsed IVC and aorta, abnormal pancreatic enhancement, peripancreatic fluid, &/or poorly enhancing spleen and delayed nephrograms
- CT findings typically resolve within 24 hours of stabilization

Key Teaching Points

- Shock bowel results from systemic hypotension with characteristic imaging features
- Although trauma is predominant etiology, other causes should be entertained in a nontrauma setting
- Distinguishing shock bowel from bowel trauma and other forms of bowel injury has important prognostic and therapeutic implications

RELATED REFERENCES

1. Ames JT et al: CT hypotension complex (shock bowel) is not always due to traumatic hypovolemic shock. AJR Am J Roentgenol. 192(5):W230-5, 2009
2. Lubner M et al: CT evaluation of shock viscera: a pictorial review. Emerg Radiol. 15(1):1-11, 2008
3. Tarrant AM et al: A pictorial review of hypovolaemic shock in adults. Br J Radiol. 81(963):252-7, 2008

CHRONIC INTESTINAL PSEUDO-OBSTRUCTION

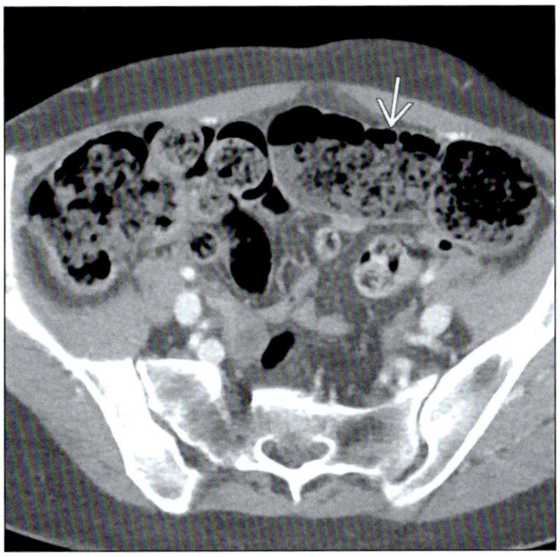

Axial CECT shows a dilated small bowel loop ➡. There was gradual transition to normal-caliber small bowel on both the proximal and the distal end of the involved loop.

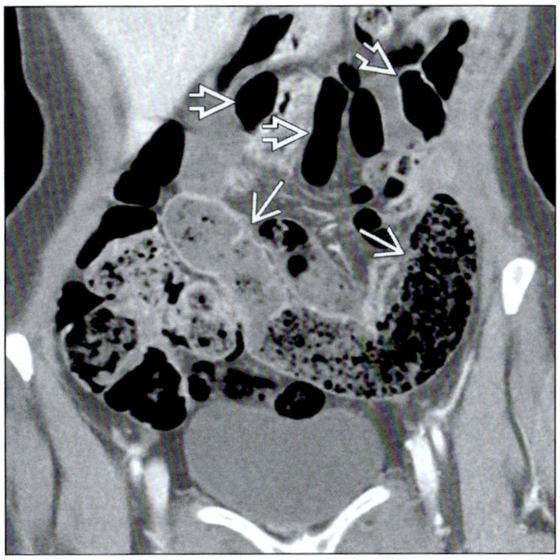

Coronal CECT shows the dilated small bowel loop ➡ containing fecal-like material (small bowel feces sign). More proximal loops ⇨ appear normal in caliber.

CLINICAL SCENARIO

History

- 42-year-old woman with long history of systemic lupus erythematosus (SLE) presenting with history of chronic abdominal pain, nausea, and vomiting

IMAGE INTERPRETATION

Pitfalls

- Clinical presentation and imaging appearance can lead to diagnosis of mechanical intestinal obstruction

Actual Diagnosis

- SLE-related chronic intestinal pseudo-obstruction (CIPO)

Clues to Correct diagnosis

- Clinical image of small bowel obstruction in patient with history of SLE
- Gradual transition from dilated to normal bowel without discernible obstructing lesions
- Often associated with dilatation of ureters and common bile duct

BACKGROUND

Epidemiology

- Rare complication of SLE

General

- Ineffective intestinal propulsion
- Signs and symptoms similar to mechanical bowel obstruction include
  - Abdominal distension, pain, nausea, vomiting, obstipation, and sluggish bowel sounds
  - Symptoms are severely disabling and patients often have severe weight loss secondary to malnutrition
- CIPO can manifest as complication of disease or, less commonly, as initial presentation
- Associated with high morbidity and mortality if treatment is not initiated promptly

Relevant Pathology

- CIPO is characterized by ineffective intestinal propulsion without any mechanical obstruction
- Caused by involvement of visceral smooth muscle and enteric nervous system
- Probable underlying pathophysiology is of intestinal vasculitis of visceral smooth muscles leading to damage and hypomotility

Treatment

- Combination of high-dose intravenous corticosteroids, immunosuppressant, and supportive treatment
- Prompt improvement usually following steroid treatment

IMAGING FEATURES

Plain Radiography

- Dilated small bowel similar to mechanical bowel obstruction

CT

- Dilated small bowel
- Gradual transition to normal small bowel without obstructing lesions

RELATED REFERENCES

1. Khairullah S et al: Chronic intestinal pseudo-obstruction: a rare first manifestation of systemic lupus erythematosus. Lupus. 22(9):957-60, 2013
2. Park FD et al: Generalized megaviscera of lupus: refractory intestinal pseudo-obstruction, ureterohydronephrosis and megacholedochus. World J Gastroenterol. 15(28):3555-9, 2009

DOUGHNUT SIGN: INTUSSUSCEPTION

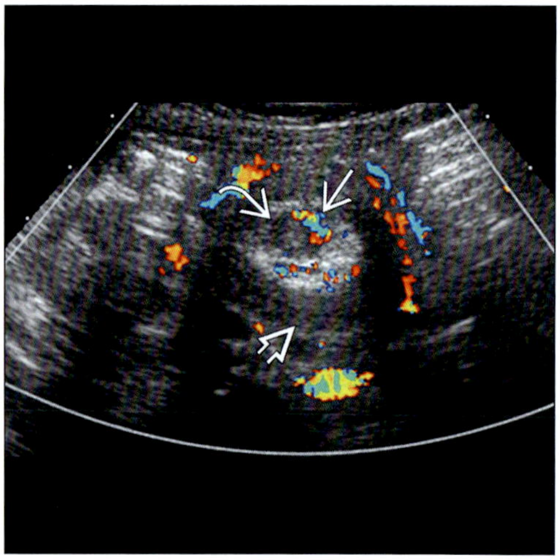

Color Doppler US demonstrates echogenic central layer (intussusceptum) and outer hypoechoic layer (intussuscipiens), with hyperechoic mesenteric fat/vessels interposed in-between.

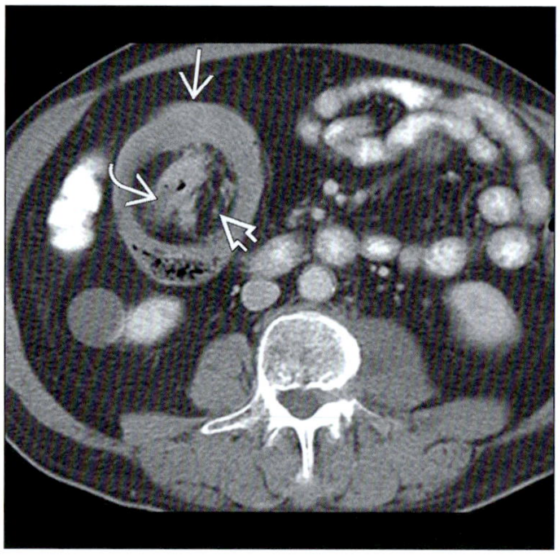

Axial CECT demonstrate a target sign of intussusception: Outer layer represents intussuscipiens and inner layer represents the intussusceptum with interposed mesenteric fat.

CLINICAL SCENARIO

History

- 50-year-old man with right lower quadrant pain

IMAGE INTERPRETATION

Classic Sign

- Segment of bowel (intussusceptum) invaginates into another segment of bowel (intussuscipiens)
- Mesenteric fat and vessels are seen interposed between intussusceptum and intussuscipiens
- US demonstrates concentric alternating echogenic and hypoechoic bands (doughnut sign)

BACKGROUND

Epidemiology

- 95% occur in children after first 3 months of life
- 2nd most common cause of acute abdomen in children
- 1-5% of bowel obstructions in adults
- Ileoileal > ileocolic > colocolic

Relevant Physiology

- Invaginating bowel loop and mesentery (intussusceptum) in a contiguous bowel (intussuscipiens)
- 2 types: Lead point and nonlead point intussusception
- **Lead point intussusception**: Typically long, large-caliber segment with proximal bowel obstruction
  - Any pathology (e.g., mass, inflammation) propelled forward by peristalsis
  - > 50% colon intussusceptions have a lead point
  - Gastrointestinal tract malignancy most common (60% of cases)
    - Colon: Carcinoma (most common), metastasis, lymphoma, lipoma, and adenomatous polyp
    - Small bowel: Lipoma, adenomatous polyp, Meckel diverticulum, lymphoma, and adenocarcinoma
  - Alters normal peristaltic activity and initiates invagination of 1 segment into other
- **Nonlead point intussusception**: Usually incidental (but can be seen with celiac or Crohn disease), more common in small bowel & more often transient
  - Dysrhythmic contractions contribute to nonlead point intussusception
  - In children, typically no lead point; likely related to enlarged lymphoid tissue after infection
- Mesentery involvement can lead to compromised venous return → edema, wall thickening; eventually arterial supply is compromised → ischemia

IMAGING FEATURES

Fluoroscopy

- Upper GI series may show coil spring appearance with barium trapped between folds of 2 components
- Barium enema: Colocolic or ileocolic → cup-shaped filling defect or spiral or coil spring appearance

US

- Hay fork or pseudokidney sign on longitudinal view
- Doughnut sign seen on transverse view
  - Hypoechoic rim (edematous bowel) surrounding hyperechoic area (mesenteric fat)

CT

- Most sensitive and can detect lead point
- Longitudinal: Sausage-shaped mass with visible layers (hypodense mesenteric fat, hyperdense bowel wall)
- Transverse: Target sign (layers of fat and bowel wall creating bowel-within-bowel appearance)
- Reniform mass (edema or mural thickening) secondary to vascular compromise
- Intestinal obstruction may be present

MR

- Best seen on T2WI (bowel-within-bowel appearance)

RELATED REFERENCES

1. Marinis A et al: Intussusception of the bowel in adults: a review. World J Gastroenterol. 15(4):407-11, 2009

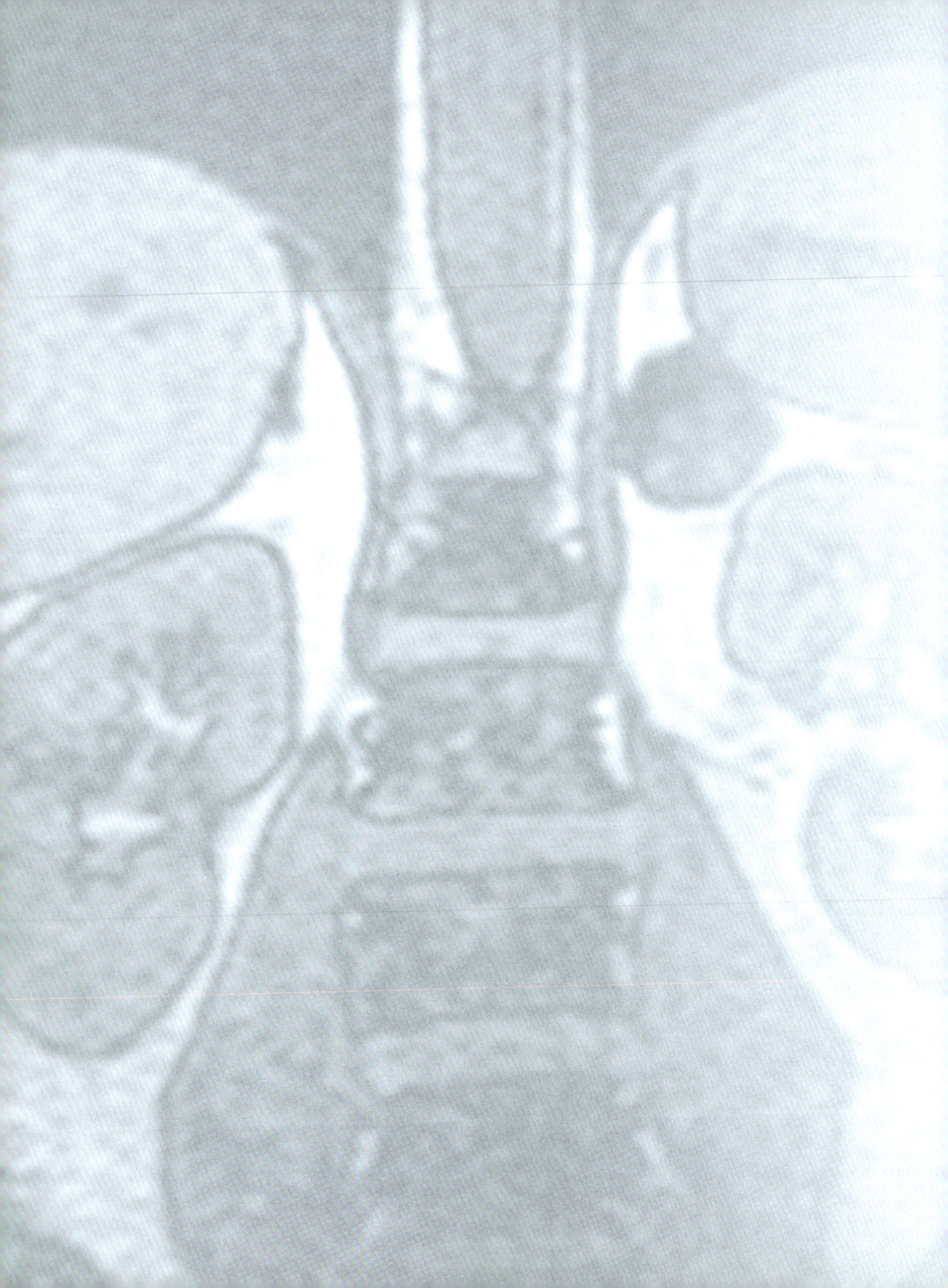

SECTION 7
Adrenal Gland

Benign Conditions Simulating Malignancy

Pitfalls in Adenoma Evaluation

Fat-Related Pitfalls

PSEUDOCYST MIMICKING ADRENAL CC

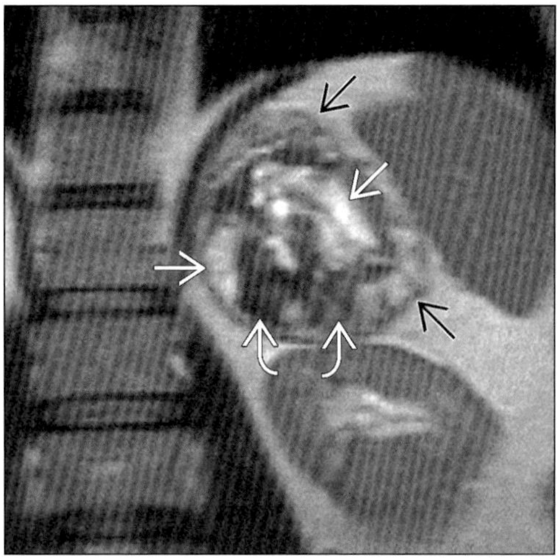

Coronal T2WI MR shows a well-circumscribed, ovoid-shaped, heterogeneous left adrenal mass ⇒ demonstrating mixed signal intensity with hypointense ➦ and hyperintense ➡ areas.

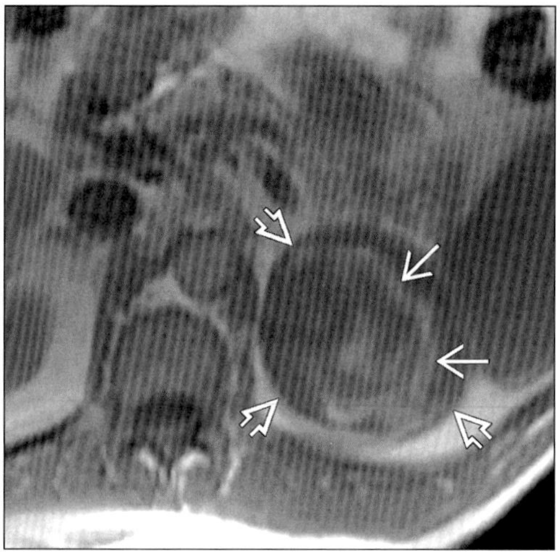

Axial in-phase MR demonstrates a well-circumscribed left adrenal mass ➡ with linear areas of high signal intensity ➡ representing blood.

CLINICAL SCENARIO

History
- 48-year-old man with abdominal pain

IMAGE INTERPRETATION

Pitfalls
- Can mimic malignant adrenal mass, e.g., adrenal cortical carcinoma (ACC)

Actual Diagnosis
- Adrenal pseudocyst

Clues to Correct Diagnosis
- Difficult diagnosis, as features of pseudocyst can overlap with those of malignancy
- Definite diagnosis relies on surgical pathology
  - However, some features may help in differentiation
    - Unlike ACC, pseudocyst is well circumscribed and does not invade vasculature or adjacent organs
    - If adrenal cyst or hemorrhage were noted on previous imaging, pseudocyst can be suspected
- Differentiation can be made by PET as pseudocyst does not exhibit FDG uptake but ACC is typically FDG avid

BACKGROUND

General
- Adrenal cystic lesions are classified as pseudocyst, epithelial cyst, endothelial cyst, and parasitic cyst
- Pseudocyst is 2nd most common adrenal cystic lesion
- Can be symptomatic

Epidemiology
- Uncommon (prevalence: 0.064%)

Relevant Pathophysiology
- 2 hypotheses: Pseudocysts develop secondary to either
  - Hemorrhage in parenchyma or cyst
    - Hemorrhage can be idiopathic or secondary to stress (e.g., neonatal), diathesis, and coagulopathy
  - Vascular malformations or obstructed lymphatics
- Pseudocysts typically have fibrous capsule

IMAGING FEATURES

US
- Well-circumscribed heterogeneous mass

CT
- Uni- or multilocular mass
- Mixed solid components reflect organized hematoma
- Occasional mural, septal, or dystrophic calcifications
- No significant enhancement
  - Possible mild faint enhancement secondary to hyalinized degeneration or fibrosis
- Thin capsule, which may enhance on delayed phase

MR
- T1WI: Heterogeneous, but predominantly hypointense
- T2WI: Heterogeneous, but predominantly hyperintense
- No central enhancement with occasional septations
- No intracellular lipid

PET/CT
- No FDG uptake (if avid, suspect malignancy)

Key Teaching Points
- Pseudocysts may be indistinguishable from malignancy
- Suspect diagnosis of pseudocyst if
  - Prior imaging shows adrenal cyst or hemorrhage
  - Well-circumscribed margins with no invasion of surrounding structures or vasculature
  - No enhancement or FDG uptake

RELATED REFERENCES

1. Cantisani V et al: A giant hemorragic adrenal pseudocyst: contrast-enhanced examination (CEUS) and computed tomography (CT) features. Eur Rev Med Pharmacol Sci. 17(18):2546-50, 2013

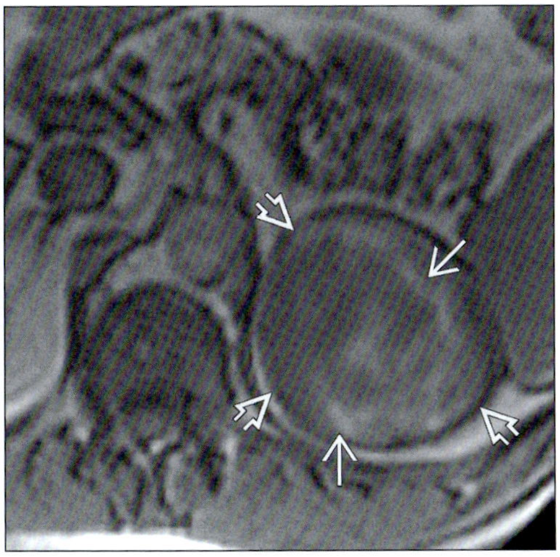

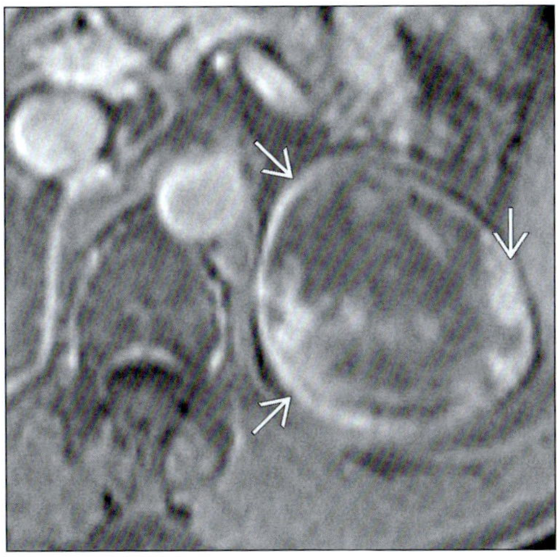

(Left) *Axial out-of-phase image shows heterogeneous signal of the left adrenal mass with areas of high signal intensity and no identifiable signal drop compared to the previous in-phase image.* ***(Right)*** *Axial T1WI C+ MR demonstrates heterogeneous appearance of the mass with faint peripheral enhancement.*

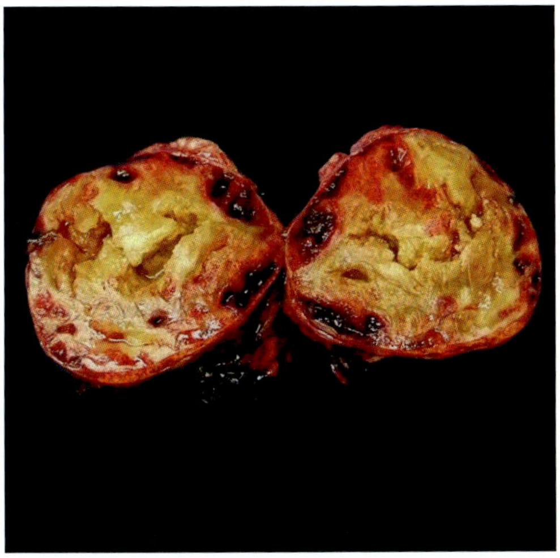

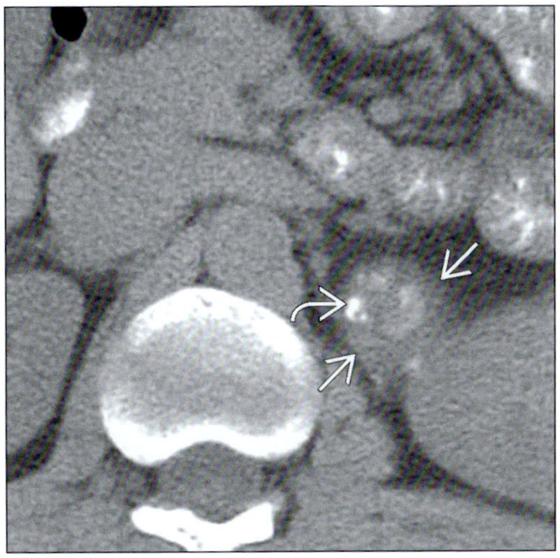

(Left) *Gross pathological specimen demonstrates the complicated adrenal pseudocyst with areas of hemorrhage and hyalinized degeneration.* ***(Right)*** *Axial NECT shows a left adrenal pseudocyst demonstrating fluid attenuation with dystrophic calcifications.*

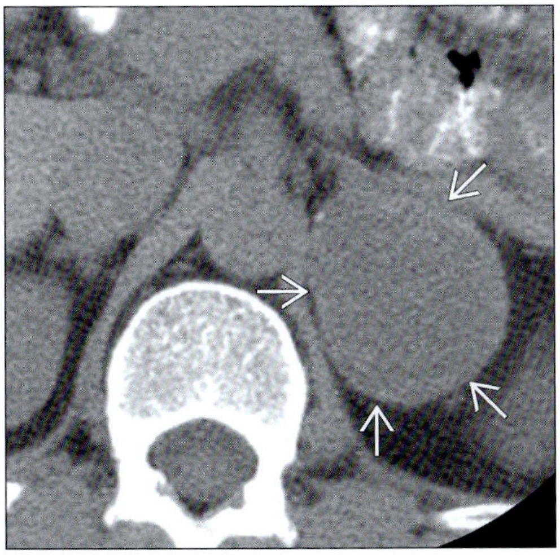

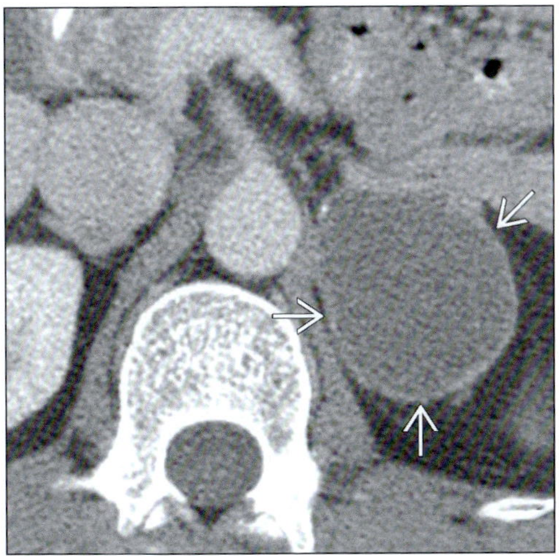

(Left) *Axial NECT in a different patient demonstrates a well-circumscribed, smoothly marginated, fluid attenuation, ovoid left adrenal mass.* ***(Right)*** *Axial CECT in the same patient demonstrates faint peripheral enhancement of the mass, compatible with pathologically proven pseudocyst.*

ADRENAL GANGLIONEUROMA

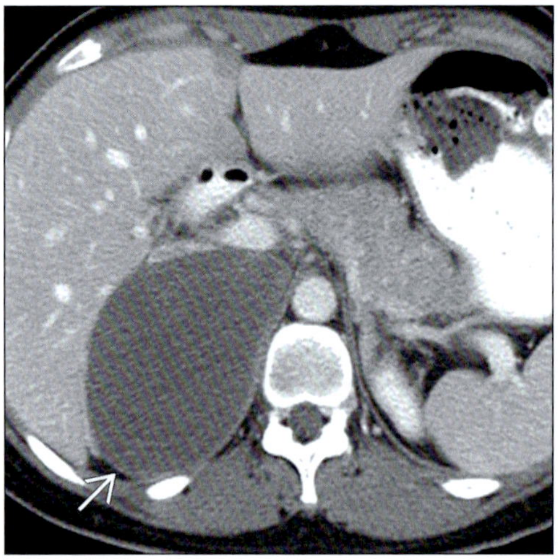

Axial CECT in the venous phase demonstrates a large, well-circumscribed mass lesion measuring 9 x 7 cm ➔ within the right adrenal region exhibiting slight enhancement.

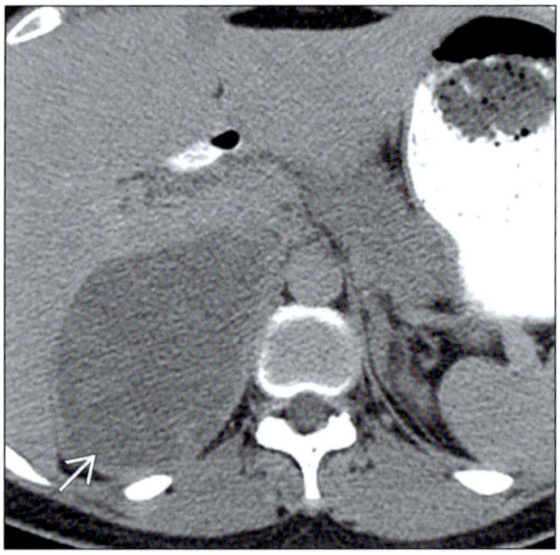

Axial CECT in the delayed phase demonstrates a large, well-circumscribed mass lesion with progressive enhancement ➔ involving the right adrenal gland.

CLINICAL SCENARIO

History

- 32-year-old woman with right upper quadrant pain

IMAGE INTERPRETATION

Pitfalls

- Could be misinterpreted as adrenal malignancy due to large size & enhancement

Actual Diagnosis

- Adrenal ganglioneuroma

Clues to Correct Diagnosis

- Margins of mass are smooth
- Relatively low attenuation on NECT
- Enhances slightly on venous phase post contrast and progressively enhances on delayed phase
- No washout is seen
- Moderately increased signal intensity on T2WI
- Urine and plasma catecholamines are negative

BACKGROUND

General

- Benign differentiated tumor from neural crest cells
- May arise de novo or from neuroblastomas
- Retroperitoneum & posterior mediastinum are common locations
- May be mixed with pheochromocytomas, nerve sheath tumors, neuroblastomas, or myelolipomas

Epidemiology

- Caucasians are more commonly affected
- Median age: 31 years

Relevant Pathology

- Large ganglion cells & Schwann cells admixed with bland spindled cells
- Myxoid tissue in background (calcifications in 30-60%)
- Incidentally found on imaging (63%), abdominal/back pain (33%)

IMAGING FEATURES

US

- Heterogeneous but predominantly hypoechoic

CT

- Median size: 8 cm, typically near-fluid attenuation on NECT with progressive enhancement (no washout)
- Nonenhanced: 25-40 HU
- Minimal post-contrast enhancement: ~ 40 HU
- Delayed enhancement: ~ 66 HU
- Occasional calcifications

MR

- T1: Slightly to moderately hypointense
- T2: Heterogeneous, slightly to moderately hyperintense
- No intracellular lipid; no drop of signal on out of phase

PET/CT

- Low FDG uptake higher than background (SUVmax = 4)
- Mild uptake on MIBG

Key Teaching Point

- Adrenal ganglioneuroma is a rare benign neoplasm
- Imaging characteristics overlap with other malignant adrenal tumors; however, the diagnosis is suspected if
  - Near-fluid attenuation on NECT
  - Slight post-contrast enhancement
  - Progressive delayed enhancement (no washout)
  - Normal catecholamine, aldosterone, & cortisol levels

RELATED REFERENCES

1. Shawa H et al: Adrenal ganglioneuroma: features and outcomes of 27 cases at a referral cancer centre. Clin Endocrinol (Oxf). 80(3):342-7, 2014
2. Alessi S et al: Ganglioneuroblastoma: Case report and review of the literature. J Ultrasound. 14(2):84-8, 2011

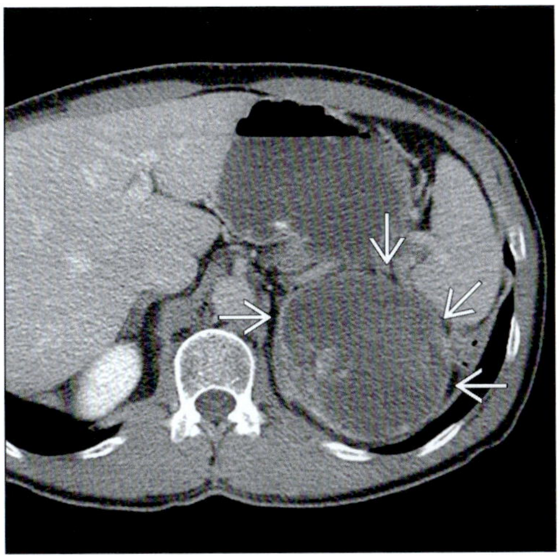

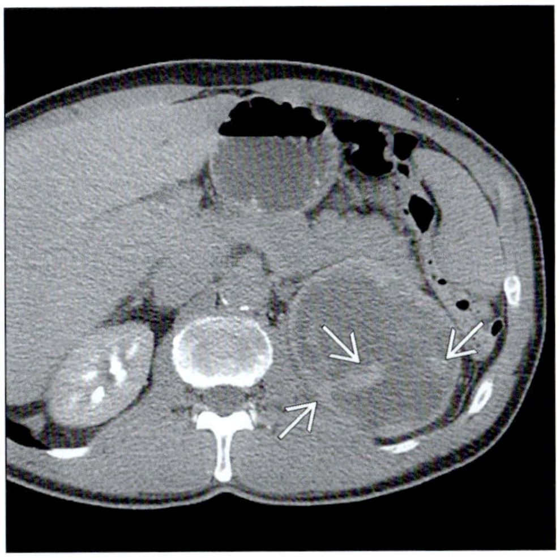

(Left) *Axial CECT in venous phase demonstrates clear intervening fat planes* ➡ *between the mass and surrounding organs.* ***(Right)*** *Axial CECT in delayed phase demonstrates thin peripheral nodular areas of enhancement* ➡ *and a large central area of necrosis.*

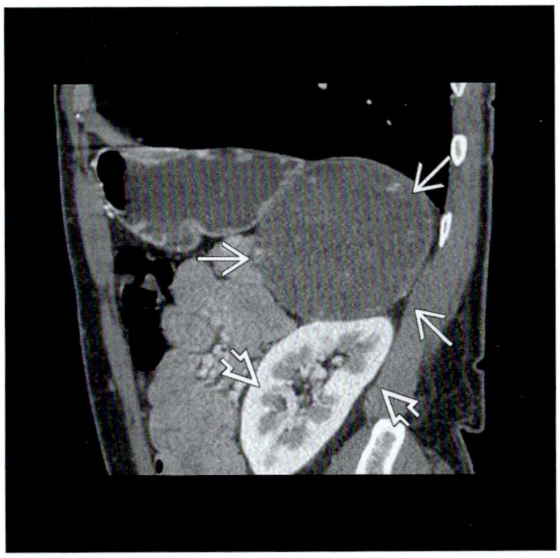

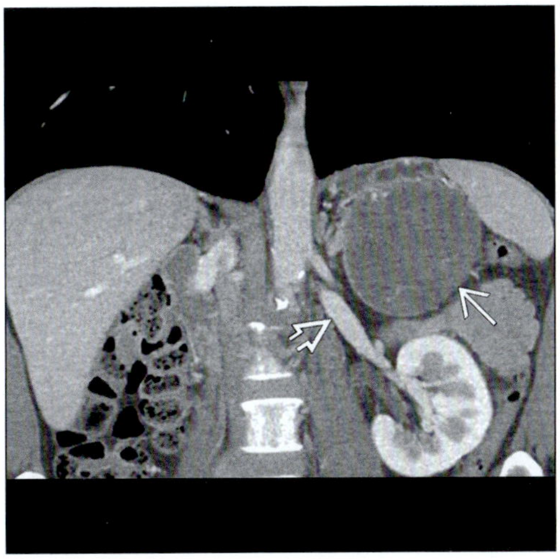

(Left) *Sagittal reformatted CECT in the venous phase demonstrates downward displacement of the left kidney* ➡ *by the large necrotic adrenal mass* ➡*.* ***(Right)*** *Coronal reformatted CECT in the venous phase demonstrates a patent left renal vein* ➡ *with no evidence of vascular invasion by the large left adrenal necrotic mass* ➡*.*

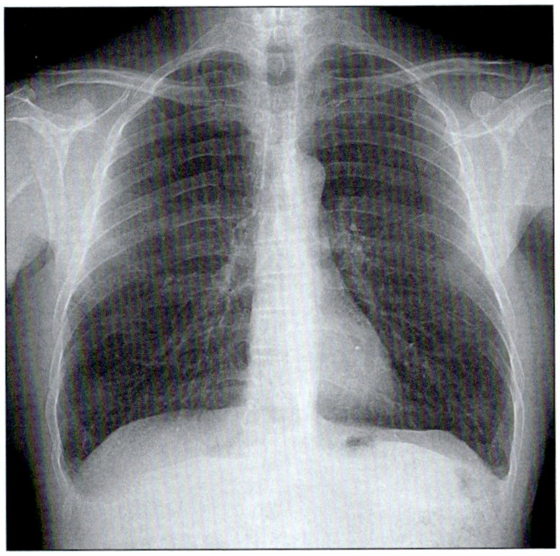

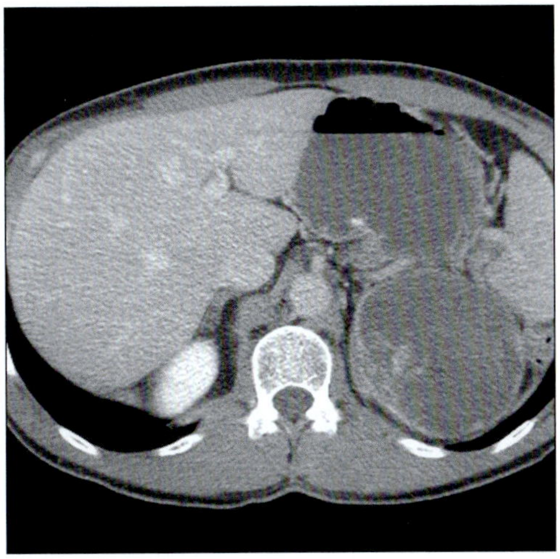

(Left) *Frontal view of plain radiographic examination of the chest demonstrates no definite evidence of metastatic disease.* ***(Right)*** *Axial CECT scan of the abdomen in venous phase demonstrates normal homogeneous texture of the liver without evidence of focal metastatic lesions. Imaging of the rest of abdomen and pelvis demonstrated no evidence of metastases elsewhere.*

SIMPLE CYST MIMICKING LIPID-RICH ADENOMA

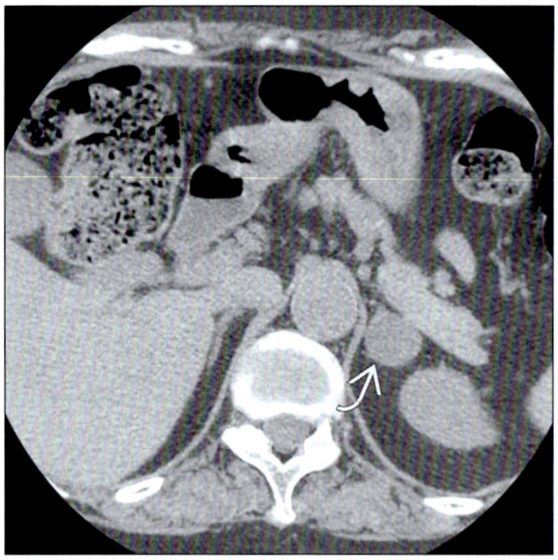

Axial NECT demonstrates a well-circumscribed nodule involving the left adrenal gland ➔, demonstrating an attenuation value of 8 HU (similar to lipid-rich adenoma on NECT).

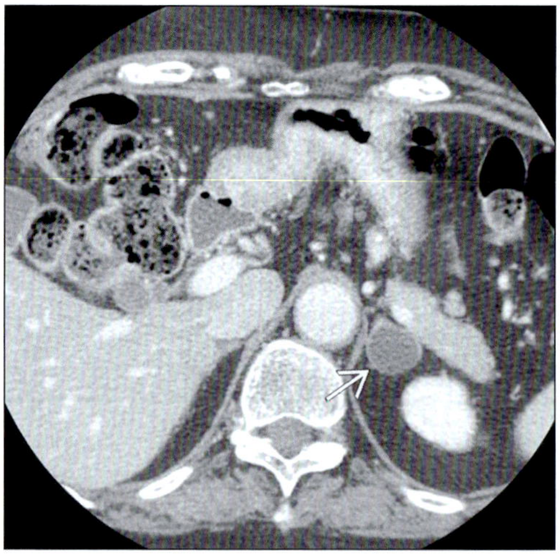

Axial CECT in venous phase demonstrates no intralesional enhancement with a thin rim of enhancement peripherally ➔.

CLINICAL SCENARIO

Clinical History
- 34-year-old woman with abdominal pain

IMAGE INTERPRETATION

Pitfalls
- Can be mistaken for an adrenal adenoma on NECT

Actual Diagnosis
- Simple adrenal cyst

Clues to Correct Diagnosis
- Attenuation value of < 20 HU on noncontrast CT
- No intralesional enhancement on CECT (opposite to adenoma which enhances)
- Nearly imperceptible thin wall with no nodularity
- Possible wall calcifications
- Easy diagnosis on MR (markedly ↑ SI on T2WI & lack of signal loss on out-of-phase compared to in-phase)

BACKGROUND

Epidemiology
- Prevalence of 0.064% to 0.18%
- Most common between 3rd & 5th decades
- F:M = 3:1
- Left and right glands equally involved

Relevant Pathology
- 4 histologic subtypes
  - Endothelial (45%)
    - Lymphangioma from ectatic lymphatic vessels
    - Adrenal hemangiomas
  - Epithelial (9%)
  - Pseudocysts (39%)
    - No lining cells
    - Result from prior hemorrhage (from vascular neoplasms or primary adrenal neoplasms, or infarction of normal adrenal gland)
  - Parasitic (7%)
    - Most commonly echinococcal

IMAGING FEATURES

US
- Anechoic with posterior acoustic enhancement
- May have internal echoes if bleeds

CT
- NECT: Hypodense < 20 HU
- CECT: No internal enhancement
- May have peripheral thin wall enhancement
- 15-69% have mural calcification
- Cyst wall may be thickened, indicative of reactive changes, most commonly from hemorrhage

MR
- T1W1: Hypointense (similar to fluid)
- T2WI: Hyperintense (similar to fluid)
- No signal loss on OP compared to IP
- T1WI C+: No significant enhancement

PET/CT
- No abnormal FDG uptake

Key Teaching Points
- Adrenal cyst may be mistaken for adenoma on NECT
- On CECT, no enhancement (opposite to adenoma)

RELATED REFERENCES

1. Johnson PT et al: Adrenal imaging with MDCT: Nonneoplastic disease. AJR Am J Roentgenol. 193(4):1128-35, 2009
2. Dunnick NR et al: Imaging of adrenal incidentalomas: current status. AJR Am J Roentgenol. 179(3):559-68, 2002
3. Rozenblit A et al: Cystic adrenal lesions: CT features. Radiology. 201(2):541-8, 1996

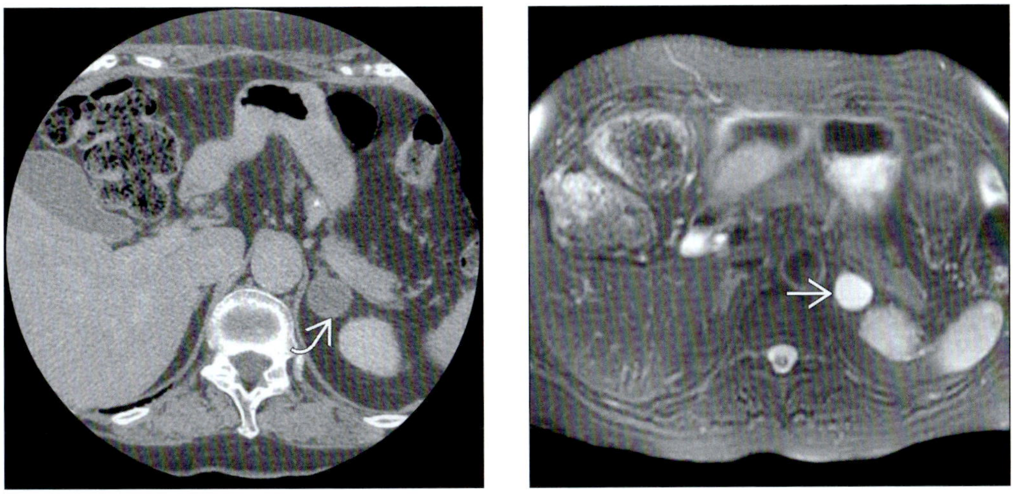

(Left) *Axial CECT in delayed phase demonstrates persistent appearance of nonenhancing lesion, with a thin rim of enhancement peripherally* ↷*.* ***(Right)*** *Axial T2WI FS MR demonstrates marked ↑ signal intensity of the lesion* → *(similar to fluid signal intensity).*

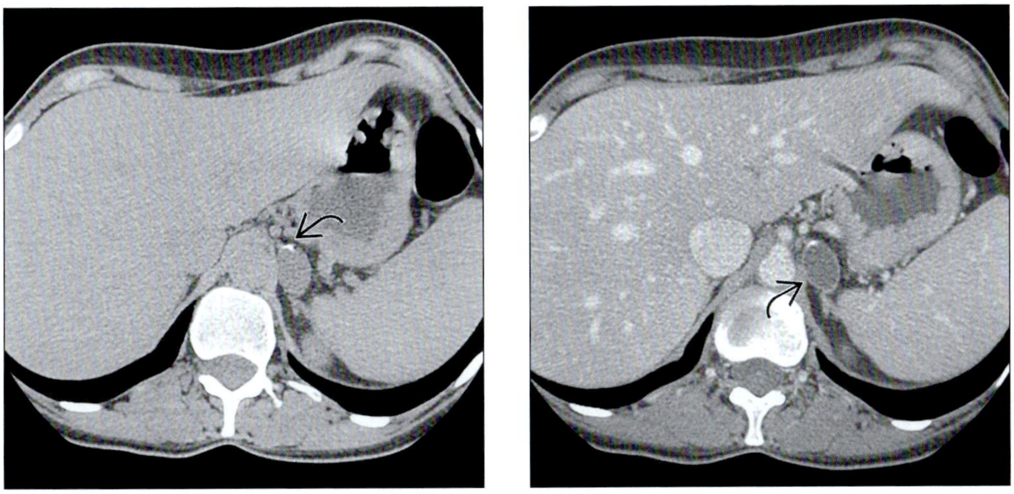

(Left) *Axial NECT in a different patient demonstrates a small, low-attenuation nodule involving the left adrenal gland with a tiny focus of mural calcification* ↷*.* ***(Right)*** *Axial CECT in venous phase demonstrates no intralesional enhancement with a thin rim of enhancement peripherally* ↷*.*

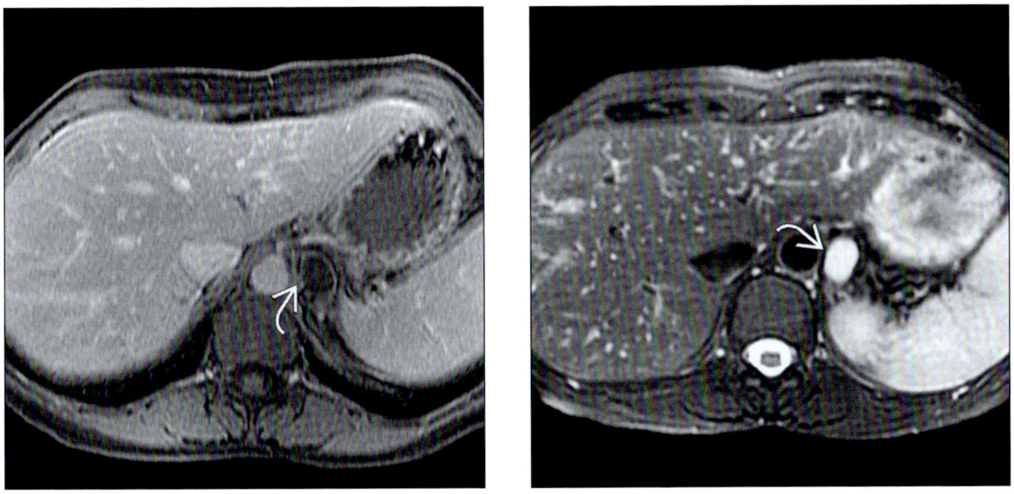

(Left) *Axial T1WI C+ FS MR demonstrates an oval-shaped nodule within the left adrenal gland demonstrating low signal intensity with a thin wall* ↷*.* ***(Right)*** *Axial T2WI MR demonstrates market signal intensity of the left adrenal nodule* ↷*, consistent with fluid signal intensity characteristic for simple cyst.*

LIPID-POOR ADRENAL ADENOMA

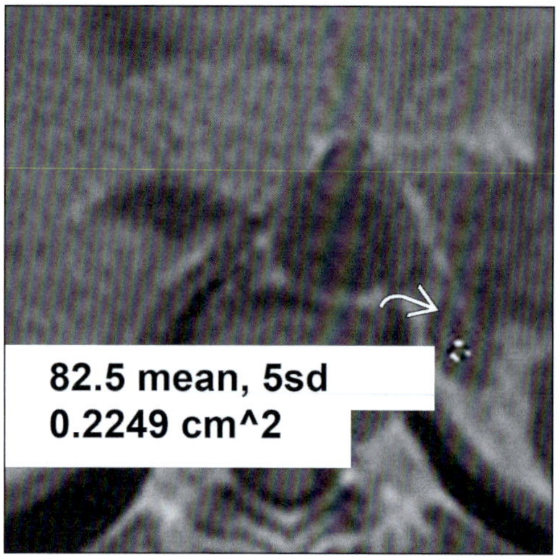

Axial T1WI in-phase MR shows a left adrenal, well-circumscribed, oval mass ➡ demonstrating a signal intensity value of 82.5.

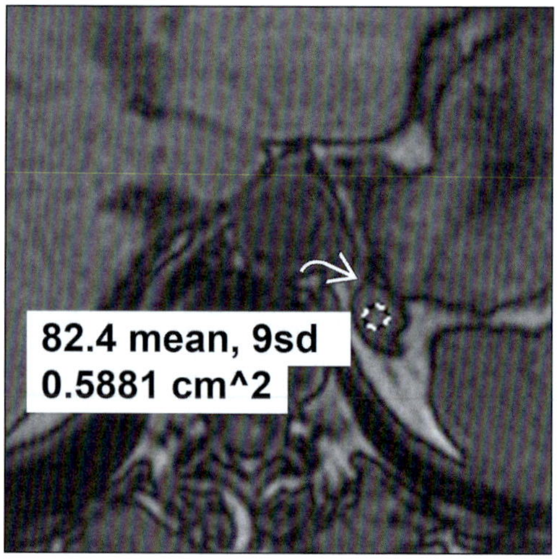

Axial T1WI out-of-phase MR shows no signal drop of the left adrenal mass ➡, which demonstrates a signal intensity similar to that of the IP.

CLINICAL SCENARIO

History

- 44-year-old man presenting for MR to evaluate focal hepatic lesion seen on ultrasound

IMAGE INTERPRETATION

Pitfalls

- Some lipid-poor adenomas may not be characterized by MR and can thus be mistaken for metastasis

Actual Diagnosis

- Lipid-poor adrenal adenoma

Clues to Correct Diagnosis

- On CT, lipid-poor adenoma demonstrates > 60% absolute enhancement washout in 15-minute delayed phase, while metastasis does not wash out
- Chemical shift MR has limited ability to characterize adrenal lipid-poor adenomas (> 10 HU on NECT)

BACKGROUND

General

- On NECT, both lipid poor adenomas and metastases exhibit attenuation values > 10 HU
- Chemical shift MR can characterize only 60% of adrenal lipid-poor adenomas
- Specifically, MR has limited value in characterizing lipid-poor adenomas with attenuation values > 30 HU

IMAGING FEATURES

CT

- Most reliable imaging modality for characterizing adrenal masses
- Unenhanced attenuation value of < 10 HU is characteristic of lipid-rich adenoma
- Contrast enhancement washout helps in characterizing adrenal masses with precontrast attenuation values > 10 HU
- Absolute enhancement washout (AEW) > 60% or relative enhancement washout (REW) > 40% are diagnostic for lipid-poor adenoma

MR

- Most important sequence in characterizing adrenal masses is chemical shift in-phase (IP) and out-of-phase (OP) sequences
- Lipid-rich and most lipid-poor adenomas demonstrate signal loss on OP compared to IP pulse sequences
  - However, MR has been reported to have limited value in characterizing some lipid-poor adenomas

Key Teaching Points

- CT washout is the most sensitive technique for differentiating adenomas from nonadenomas
- Absolute enhancement washout > 60% and relative washout > 40% are highly accurate for diagnosing adrenal adenomas
- Lipid-rich and most lipid-poor adenomas demonstrate signal loss on OP compared to IP pulse sequences
- MR has limited value in characterizing some lipid-poor adenomas

RELATED REFERENCES

1. Haider MA et al: Chemical shift MR imaging of hyperattenuating (>10 HU) adrenal masses: does it still have a role? Radiology. 231(3):711-6, 2004
2. Israel GM et al: Comparison of unenhanced CT and chemical shift MRI in evaluating lipid-rich adrenal adenomas. AJR Am J Roentgenol. 183(1):215-9, 2004
3. Caoili EM et al: Adrenal masses: characterization with combined unenhanced and delayed enhanced CT. Radiology. 222(3):629-33, 2002

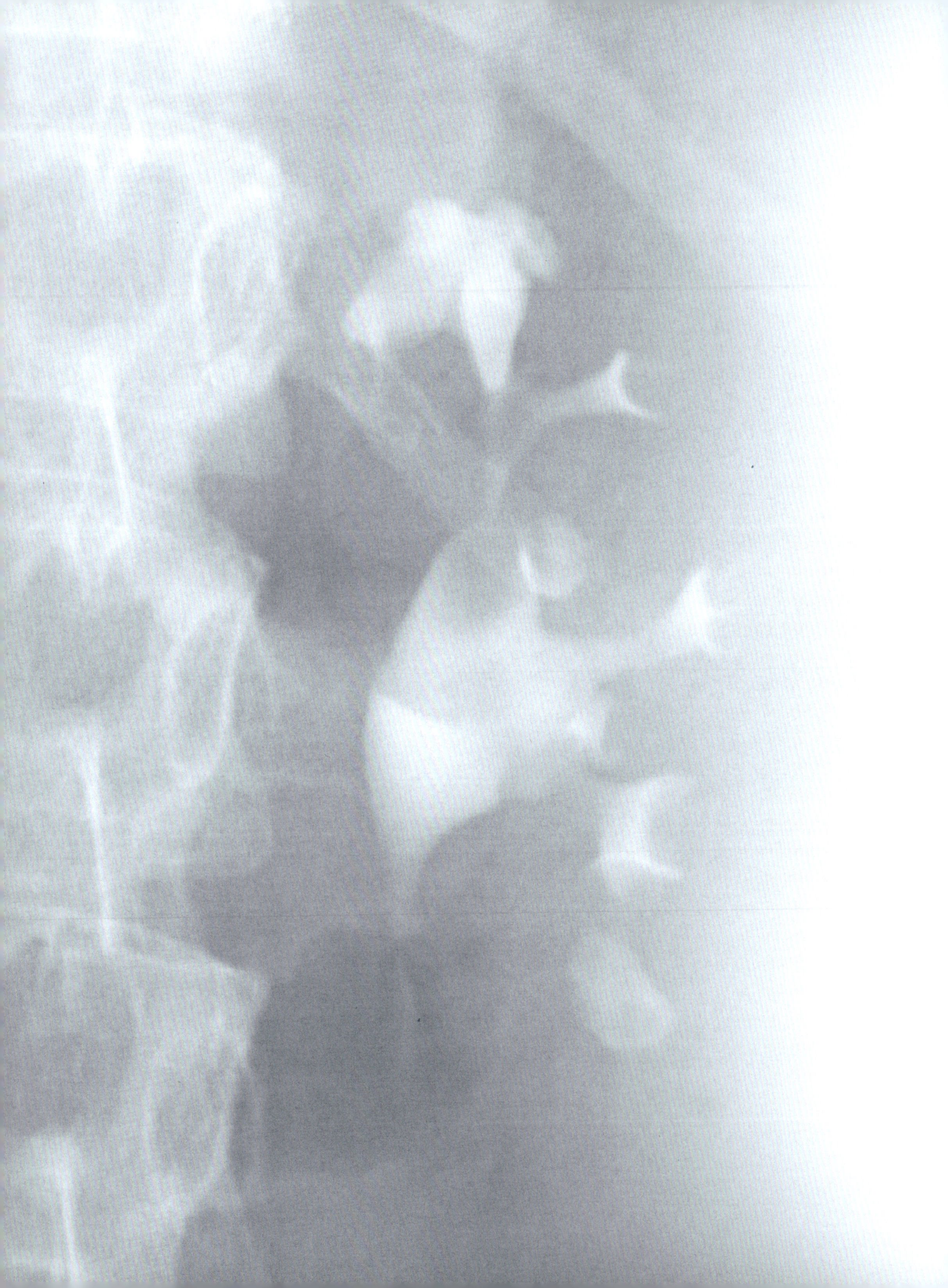

SECTION 8
Kidney

Benign Conditions Simulating Malignancy

Malignant Lesions Mimicking Benign Conditions

Renal Cystic Disease Pitfalls

Classic Signs and Appearances

RENAL VASCULAR LESIONS MIMICKING NEOPLASM

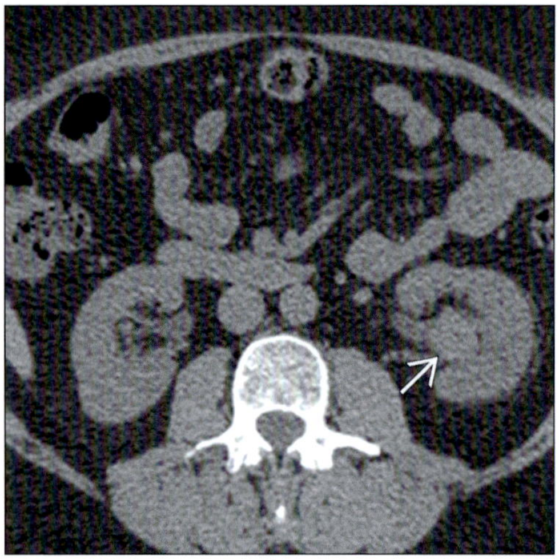

Axial NECT demonstrates a well-circumscribed lesion ➡ exhibiting soft tissue attenuation, making it suspicious for a solid neoplasm such as renal cell carcinoma.

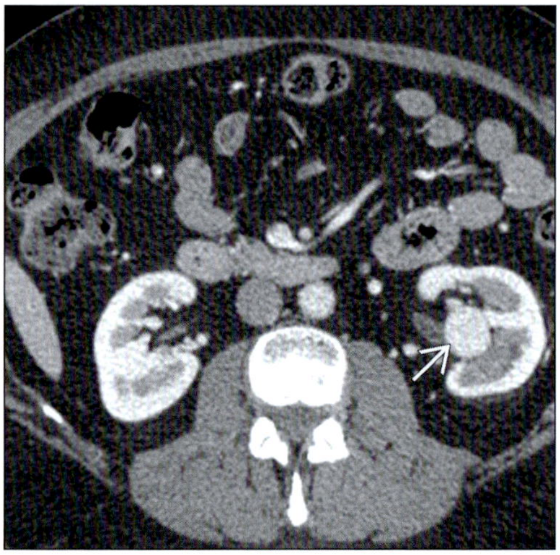

Axial CECT demonstrates significant enhancement of the well-circumscribed lesion ➡, a pattern that could be misinterpreted for a solid enhancing neoplasm such as renal cell carcinoma.

CLINICAL SCENARIO

History

- 40-year-old man with left flank pain

IMAGE INTERPRETATION

Pitfalls

- Renal vascular lesions can be mistaken for enhancing renal masses
- Examples of these lesions include
  - Renal artery true aneurysms
  - Arteriovenous communications, including
    - Arteriovenous fistulas
    - Vascular malformations

Actual Diagnosis

- Left renal artery aneurysm

Clues to Correct Diagnosis

- Mass-like lesions, which follow enhancement pattern of vasculature
  - Renal artery aneurysm has same attenuation values of abdominal aorta on all phases
  - CT or MR angiography can depict communication of aneurysm to main renal artery or its branches
- Signal flow void on all MR pulse sequences
- Color Doppler
  - Turbulent flow is seen with pseudoaneurysm
  - Arterialization pattern in venous flow with arteriovenous malformation

BACKGROUND

General

- Renal artery pseudoaneurysms represent contained arterial injury communicating with artery
- Arteriovenous malformations (AVM) & fistulas (AVF) represent abnormal communications between intrarenal arterial and venous systems
- Gross hematuria is the most common presentation

Epidemiology

- Renal artery aneurysms occur in 0.01-0.1% of population
- Renal artery aneurysms account for 22% of visceral aneurysms
- Biopsy (40%) is most common etiology for acquired renal vascular lesions (pseudoaneurysm & AVF)
- Arteriovenous fistulas account for majority (2/3 of cases) of arteriovenous communications

Relevant Pathophysiology

- Most common causes of aneurysms of renal artery
  - Atherosclerosis (most common)
  - Less common causes include
    - Medial fibroplasia
    - Vasculitis such as polyarteritis nodosa
    - Mesenchymal diseases (e.g., neurofibromatosis and Ehlers-Danlos syndrome)
  - Morphologically, renal artery aneurysms can be divided into
    - Saccular in main renal artery or main branch and likely occur 2° to atherosclerosis
    - Fusiform likely caused by medial fibroplasia
    - Dissecting commonly involves main renal artery but may also extend to its branches
    - Intrarenal, which can be associated with vasculitis, atherosclerosis, trauma, inflammation and tumors
- Renal pseudoaneurysms represent injury to all 3 layers of artery and can occur secondary to
  - Trauma (contained rupture of arterial wall communicating with lumen)
  - Inflammation (such as mycotic aneurysm)
- Arteriovenous communications can be
  - Acquired fistulas are connections between arterial and venous systems
    - Traumatic: Caused by penetrating trauma or biopsy neoplastic and spontaneous less common
    - Neoplastic etiologies and spontaneous arteriovenous fistulas (AVF) are less common
  - Congenital arteriovenous malformation (AVM) is least common

- Congenital cirsoid-type AVMs represent multiple communicating vascular channels creating mass-like appearance adjacent to collecting system

Clinical Background

- Aneurysms
  - Majority are asymptomatic, often discovered incidentally on imaging
  - Hypertension can occur in majority of renal artery aneurysms
- Arteriovenous communications
  - Bruit on auscultation
  - Cardiomegaly or congestive heart failure occur in 50% of symptomatic patients
  - Arteriovenous fistula can lead to ischemia in distal renal parenchyma → renin-mediated hypertension and poor renal function
  - Hematuria

IMAGING FEATURES

US

- Aneurysm
  - Well-circumscribed anechoic mass
    - Thrombus (if present) can result in variable echogenicities
- Arteriovenous communications
  - Serpentine anechoic areas

Color Doppler

- Aneurysm/pseudoaneurysm
  - Turbulent flow
  - Bidirectional blood flow (to-and-fro pattern)
- AVM
  - Turbulent flow
  - Arterial waveform in venous flow
  - Dilated draining vein
  - Localized tissue vibrations

CT

- NECT
  - Vascular calcification in congenital or longstanding type
  - Hyperattenuation if complicated by hemorrhage or clot
- CECT
  - Aneurysm/pseudoaneurysm
    - Well-circumscribed mass-like lesion
    - Follow attenuation of arterial vessels on all phases after contrast administration
    - Reconstructed images and CT angiogram demonstrate communication with renal artery or its branches
  - Arteriovenous communications
    - Demonstrate draining and feeding vessels (frequently dilated)
    - Early enhancement of renal vein
    - Multiphasic technique including arterial and venous postcontrast phases is necessary for diagnosis
    - Decreased enhancement of parenchyma could be seen distal to arteriovenous malformation (due to shunting of blood through fistula)

MR

- T1WI
  - Signal flow void well-circumscribed (aneurysm) or serpentine structure (arteriovenous malformation)
- T2WI
  - Signal void appearance similar to T1WI
- T1WI C+
  - Aneurysm demonstrates enhancement similar to arterial vasculature
  - MR angiography demonstrates communication of aneurysm to renal artery
    - Feeding artery and draining vein of AVF/AVM could be also demonstrated on MRA
- DWI: No restricted diffusion
- Pulsation artifacts could be seen in pseudoaneurysm

Angiography

- Pseudoaneurysm
  - Outpouching from renal artery or its branches
  - Therapeutic embolization or stenting could be utilized for management of symptomatic aneurysms
- AVM
  - Multiple small, tortuous, dilated vessels
  - Early visualization of renal vein and IVC
  - Therapeutic transarterial catheter embolization could be performed in symptomatic cases

PET/CT

- No abnormal uptake

Key Teaching Points

- Renal vascular malformations may appear mass-like and be mistaken for hypervascular masses
- Majority of vascular malformations are acquired and should be considered if recent clinical history of recent renal biopsy or trauma
- Multiphasic contrast-enhanced CT or MR should be utilized to evaluate for similar enhancement and abnormal communication with arterial vasculature
- Color Doppler ultrasound detects turbulent flow in pseudoaneurysm and arterial waveforms in venous flow in renal AVMs

RELATED REFERENCES

1. Cura M et al: Vascular malformations and arteriovenous fistulas of the kidney. Acta Radiol. 51(2):144-9, 2010
2. Sofocleous CT et al: Angiographic findings and embolotherapy in renal arterial trauma. Cardiovasc Intervent Radiol. 28(1):39-47, 2005
3. Surlan M et al: The role of interventional radiology in management of patients with end-stage renal disease. Eur J Radiol. 46(2):96-114, 2003
4. Kawashima A et al: CT evaluation of renovascular disease. Radiographics. 20(5):1321-40, 2000
5. Phadke RV et al: Iatrogenic renal vascular injuries and their radiological management. Clin Radiol. 52(2):119-23, 1997
6. Tarkington MA et al: Spectrum of renal vascular malformation. Urology. 38(4):297-300, 1991

RENAL VASCULAR LESIONS MIMICKING NEOPLASM

*(**Left**) Axial CECT in arterial phase demonstrates a well-circumscribed, enhancing, mass-like lesion →. (**Right**) Coronal reformatted CT angiography demonstrates a focally dilated structure → communicating with the left renal artery ↪ compatible with pseudoaneurysm.*

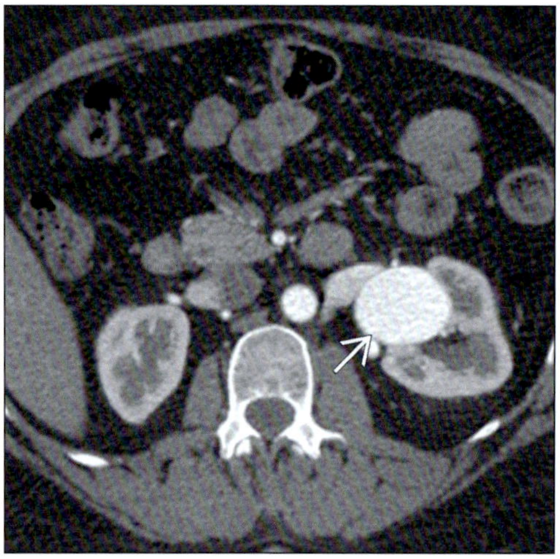

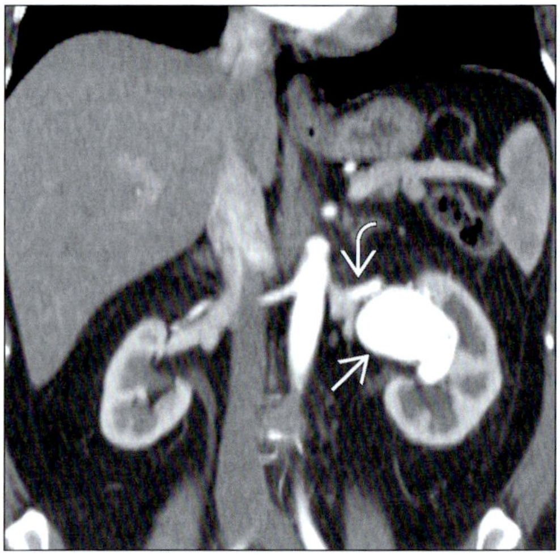

*(**Left**) Axial CECT demonstrates an enhancing nodule → within the posterior aspect of left kidney, related to the posterior margin of a cyst. (**Right**) Catheter angiography of a posterior middle branch of the left renal artery (same patient) demonstrates contrast filling of a peripheral pseudoaneurysm →.*

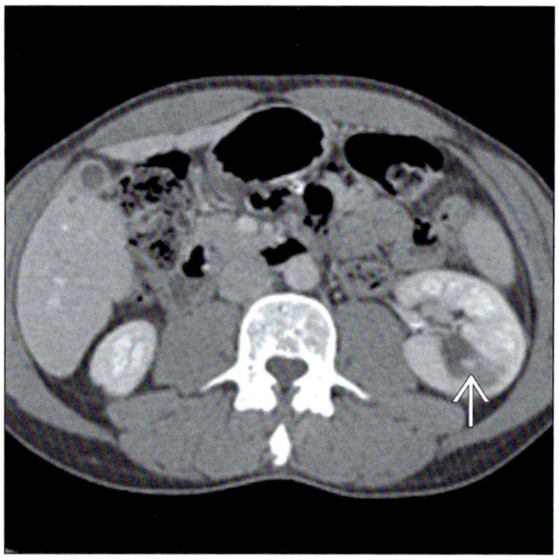

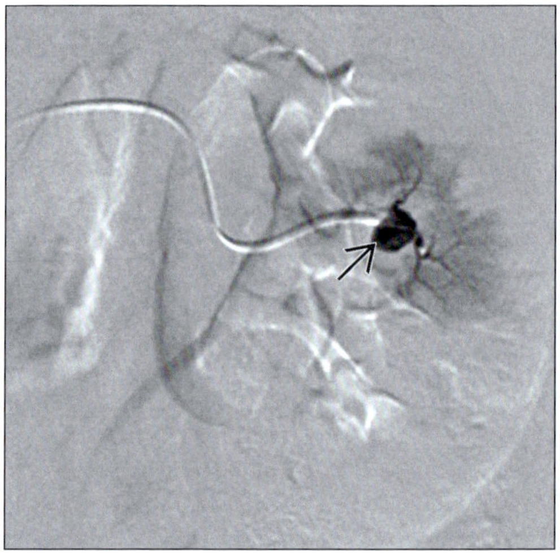

*(**Left**) Grayscale ultrasound of the left kidney (same patient) demonstrates a complex cystic lesion with a secondary cystic area along one wall →. Echogenic material is seen between the 2 cysts. (**Right**) Color Doppler ultrasound demonstrates turbulent flow within the smaller internal focus, characteristic of a pseudoaneurysm.*

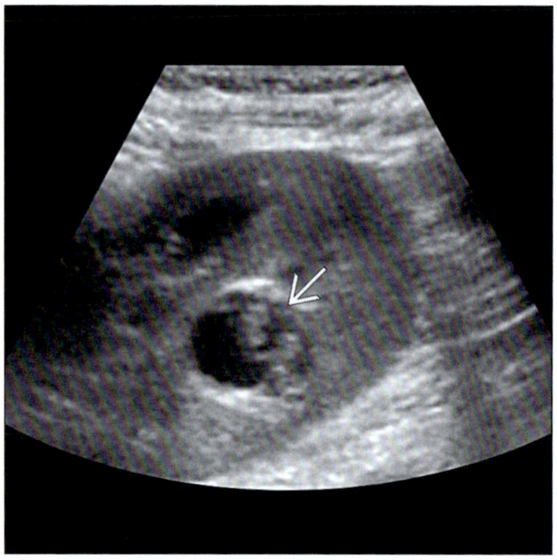

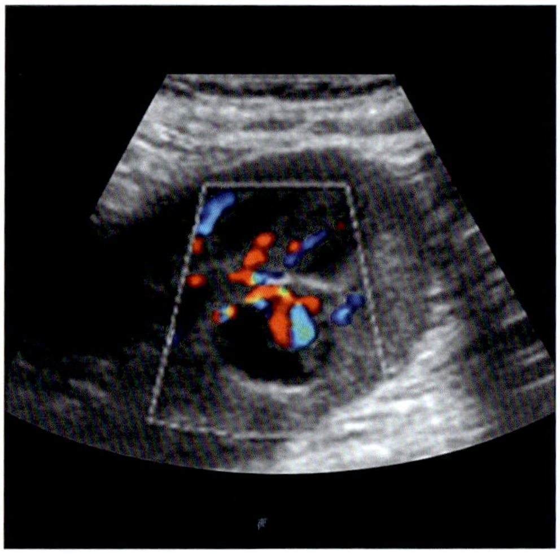

RCC CONTAINING MACROSCOPIC FAT

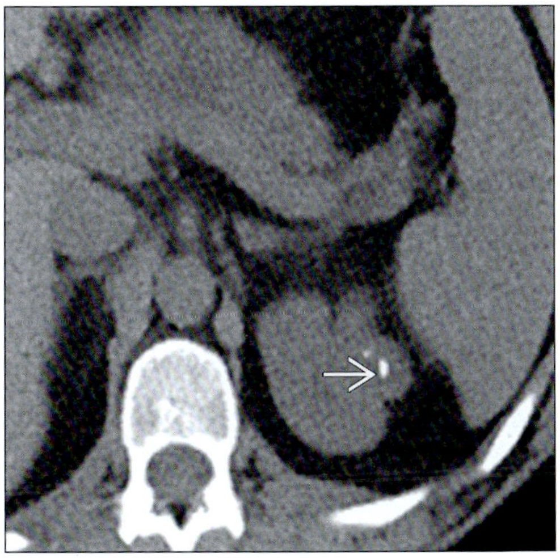

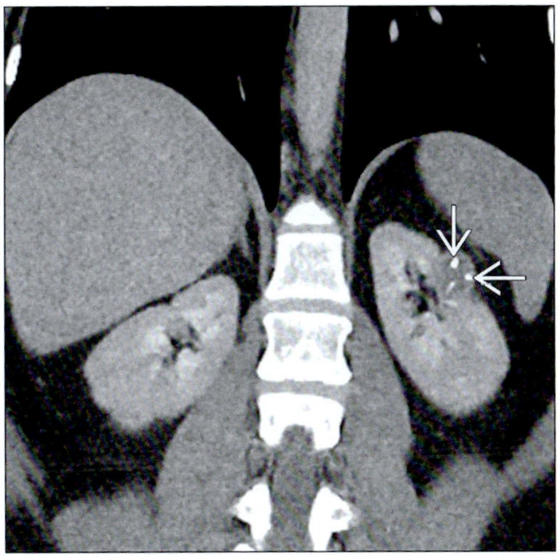

***(Left)** Axial NECT demonstrates a left renal exophytic mass containing foci of calcification* ➡*. **(Right)** Coronal reformatted CECT in delayed phase demonstrates a few foci of calcification* ➡ *within a left renal mass.*

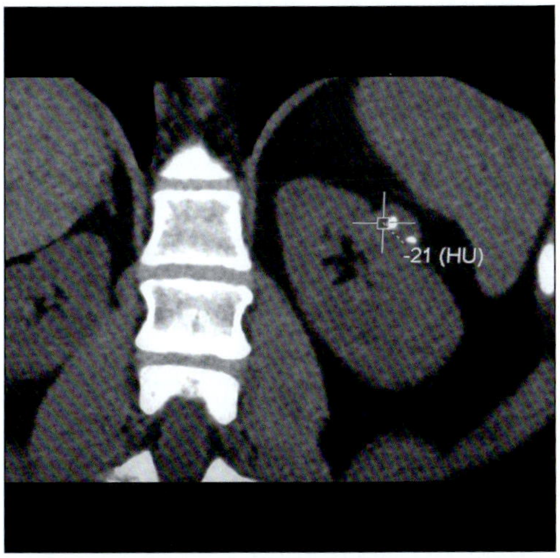

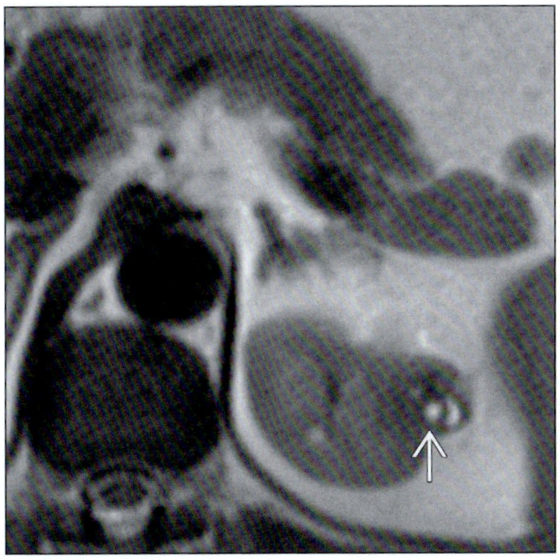

***(Left)** Coronal reformatted NECT demonstrates the point of interest in the hypoattenuating area next to the calcification, revealing a value of -21 HU, consistent with fat. **(Right)** Axial T2WI single-shot turbo spin-echo MR demonstrates a small focus of high signal intensity* ➡*. This could represent either fat or blood. It is imperative to compare with a fat-suppressed sequence to confirm the presence of fat.*

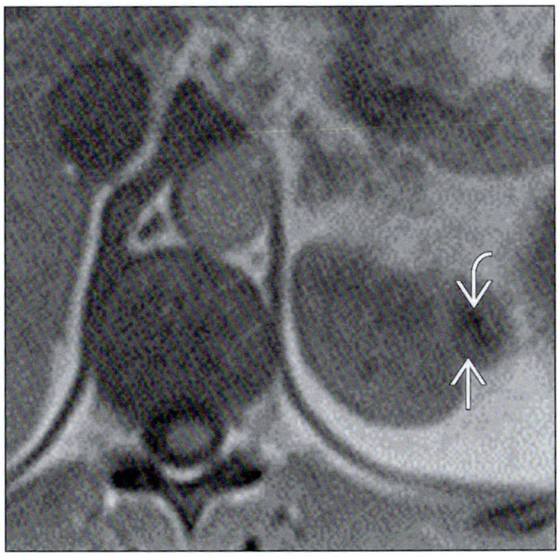

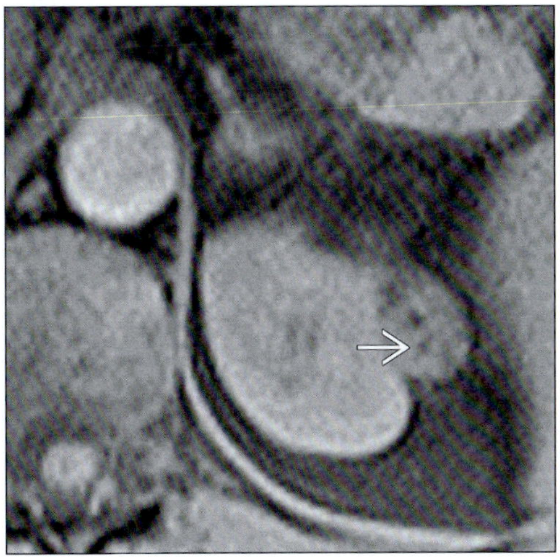

***(Left)** Axial in-phase, non-fat-saturated T1WI MR demonstrates a small focus of higher signal intensity, representing a fat lobule* ➡ *next to the low signal intensity calcification* ↪*. **(Right)** Axial T1WI C+ FS MR demonstrates a low signal intensity* ➡*, which represents macroscopic fat losing signal intensity on this fat-saturated sequence. Other hypointense areas in the lesion either represent calcification or areas of cystic degeneration.*

CLEAR CELL RCC CONTAINING INTRACELLULAR LIPID

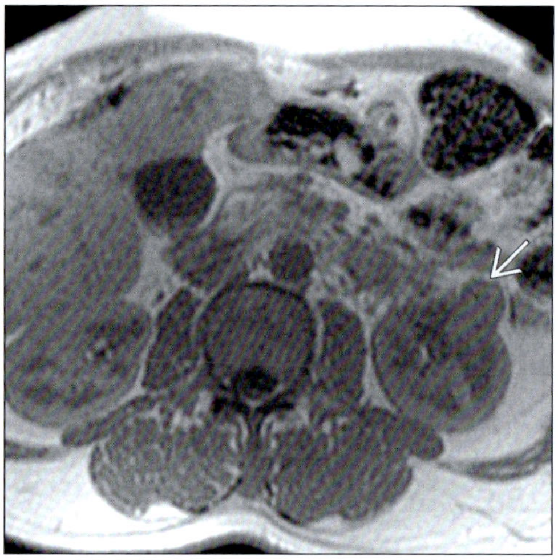

Axial in-phase gradient-echo MR reveals an exophytic well-circumscribed mass ➔ involving the left renal cortex.

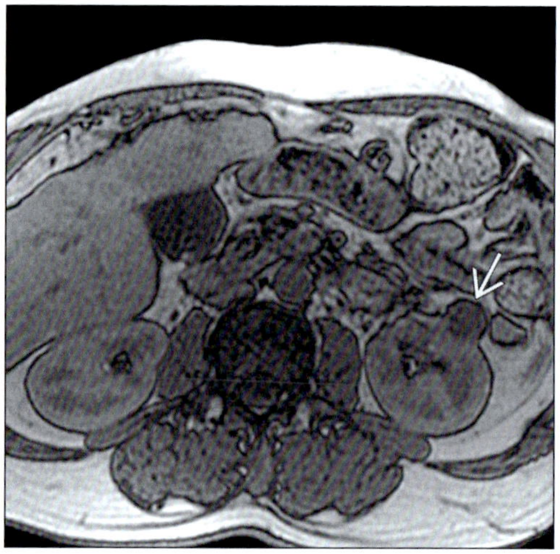

Axial out-of-phase gradient-echo MR reveals drop of signal intensity within the left renal mass ➔, indicating the presence of intracellular lipid.

CLINICAL SCENARIO

History

- 63-year-old man presents for further characterization of left renal mass incidentally noted on CT

IMAGE INTERPRETATION

Pitfalls

- Cortical-based renal mass with signal drop on out-of-phase (OP) compared to in-phase (IP) is suggestive of microscopic (intracellular) instead of macroscopic fat
  - Therefore, suggests clear cell RCC rather than angiomyolipoma (AML); although a few cases of angiomyolipoma can contain intracellular lipid

Actual Diagnosis

- Clear cell renal carcinoma (CCRCC)

Clues to Correct Diagnosis

- Mass demonstrates signal drop on OP compared to IP consistent with intracellular lipid
- No India ink artifact in mass or at interface between mass and kidney
  - Otherwise, India ink artifact is suggestive of macroscopic fat characteristic for angiomyolipoma
- Intense arterial enhancement & significant delayed contrast washout
- While nonspecific, presence of restriction on DWI is suggestive of a highly cellular mass

BACKGROUND

General

- CCRCC is the most common histological type of RCC
- Usually, CCRCC is characterized by clear cytoplasm
- Clear cytoplasm reflects presence of glycogen, phospholipids, and cholesterol ester
- CCRCC is also characterized by variable presence of granular eosinophilic cells

Epidemiology

- Average age of diagnosis is 60-64 years
- 7% are diagnosed in patients < 40 years of age
- Incidence is higher for African Americans

IMAGING FEATURES

US

- Solid, cystic, or complex
- Most commonly hyperechoic but could be isoechoic or hypoechoic
- May have calcifications as opposed to AML, which rarely has calcifications
- Doppler signal or contrast-enhanced sonography demonstrates increased vascularity

CT

- Variable attenuation relative to renal parenchyma
- Most CCRCC avidly enhances on arterial phase
- Occasional amorphous calcifications

MR

- T1WI: Most commonly isointense to skeletal muscles
- T2WI: Likely hyperintense to skeletal muscles
- T1WI C+: Typically shows marked enhancement on arterial phase & washout on delayed phase
- Signal drop on OP compared to IP if clear cells are predominant epithelial cell component
- DWI: Typically restricts diffusion

PET/CT

- FDG avid except necrotic or hemorrhagic components

RELATED REFERENCES

1. Karlo CA et al: MR imaging of renal cortical tumours: qualitative and quantitative chemical shift imaging parameters. Eur Radiol. 23(6):1738-44, 2013
2. Israel GM et al: The use of opposed-phase chemical shift MRI in the diagnosis of renal angiomyolipomas. AJR Am J Roentgenol. 184(6):1868-72, 2005

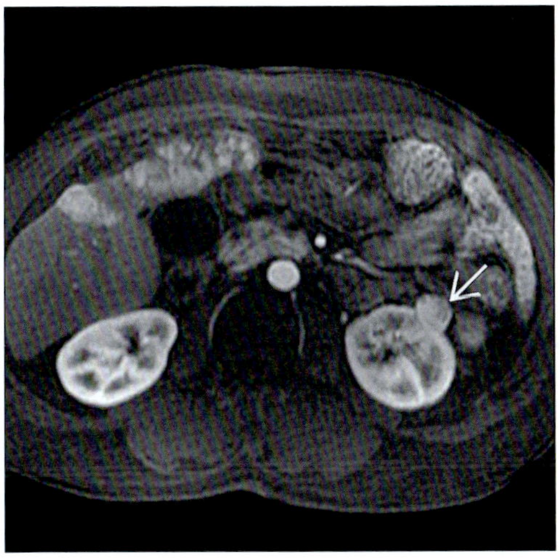

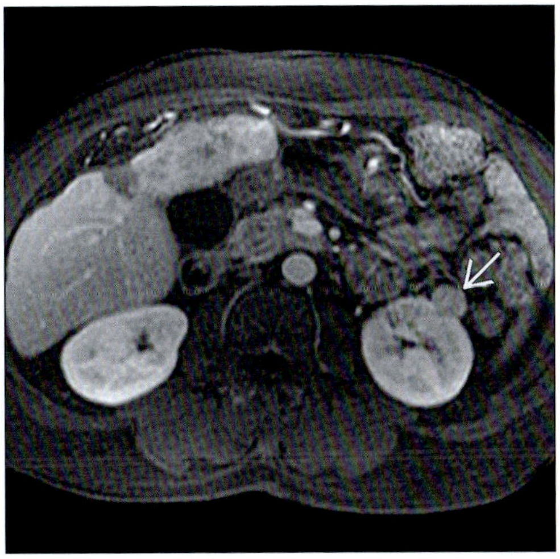

(Left) *Axial T1WI C+ MR in arterial phase demonstrates marked enhancement of the left renal mass ➡.* ***(Right)*** *Axial T1WI C+ MR in venous phase shows some washout of the left renal mass ➡.*

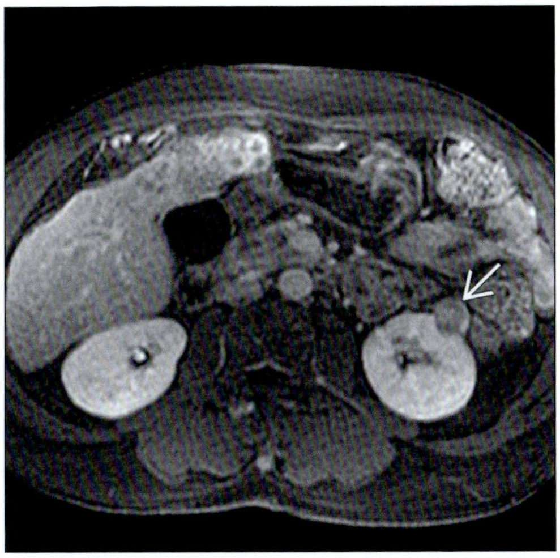

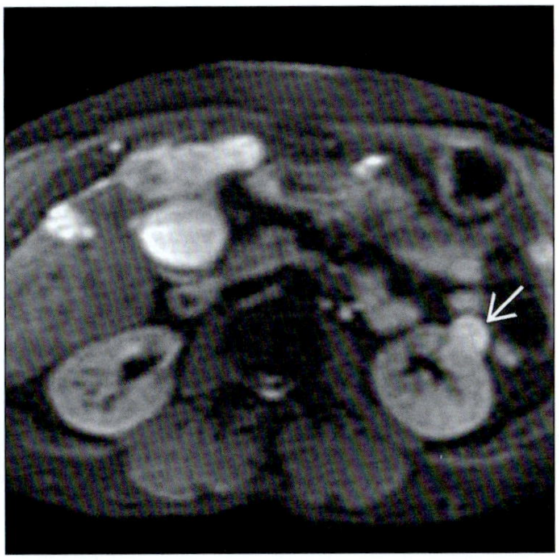

(Left) *Axial T1WI C+ MR in the late nephrographic-excretory phase shows further significant washout of the left renal mass ➡.* ***(Right)*** *Axial diffusion-weighted MR (b value = 500) demonstrates increased signal intensity ➡ due to restricted diffusion.*

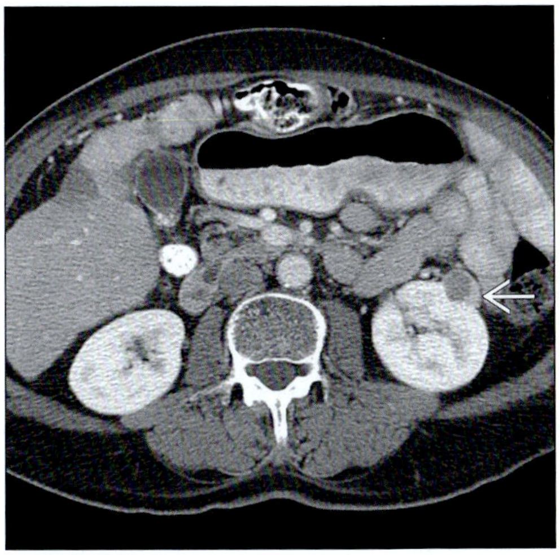

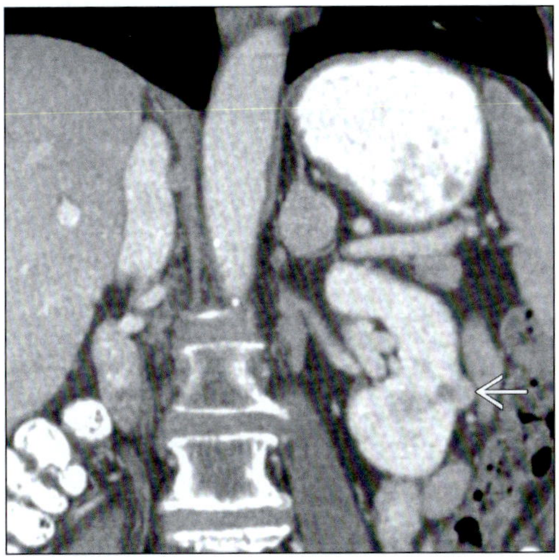

(Left) *Axial CECT in the late nephrographic-excretory phase shows the mass to be relatively lower attenuation than the surrounding cortex with a thickened wall ➡.* ***(Right)*** *Coronal reformatted CECT in the late nephrographic-excretory phase shows the mass to be hypodense compared to surrounding enhancing cortex with a thickened wall ➡.*

ECHOGENIC RCC

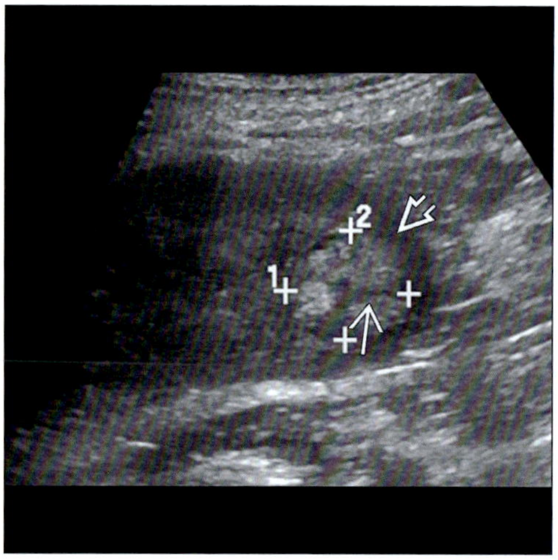

Grayscale ultrasound examination demonstrates a focal hyperechoic renal mass ➪ with thin internal linear areas ➔.

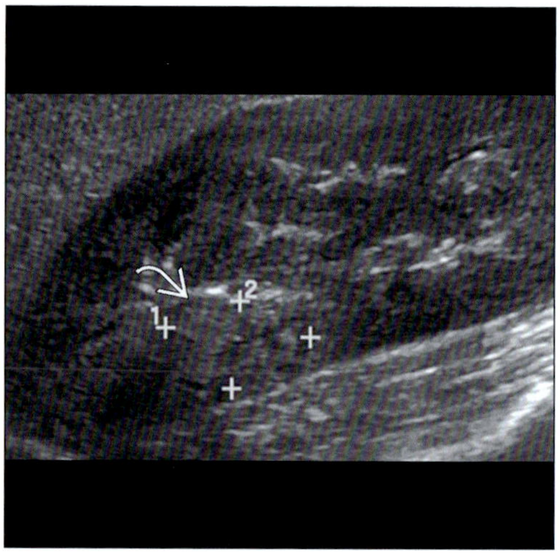

Longitudinal grayscale ultrasound examination shows a left hyperechoic renal mass (between calipers) with a thin hypoechoic rim ➪.

CLINICAL SCENARIO

History

- 33-year-old man with bilateral flank pain and recent dysuria

IMAGE INTERPRETATION

Pitfalls

- Hyperechoic renal cell carcinoma (RCC) can be mistaken for angiomyolipoma

Actual Diagnosis

- Renal cell carcinoma

Clues to Correct Diagnosis

- Hypoechoic rim surrounding renal lesion and intratumoral cysts (if present) are specific for RCC
- Presence of shadowing is specific for angiomyolipoma

BACKGROUND

Relevant Pathology

- 30% of RCC were reported to be echogenic
- Most renal tumors with homogeneous architecture are hyperechoic
  - Tumors with inhomogeneous architecture because of bleeding, degeneration, or cysts are hypoechoic
- No definite correlation between tumor echogenicity and cellular differentiation

IMAGING FEATURES

General

- Hyperechoic renal lesions should be further evaluated with CT or MR to differentiate between RCC and angiomyolipoma

US

- RCC usually displays wide spectrum of echogenicities
  - Usually, small RCC is hyperechoic relative to renal parenchyma and mimics renal angiomyolipoma, while larger RCCs are hypoechoic

CT

- RCC typically exhibits soft tissue attenuation
  - Larger lesions frequently have areas of necrosis
  - About 30% demonstrate calcification
- In general, small lesions enhance homogeneously, whereas larger lesions have irregular enhancement due to areas of necrosis
  - Clear cell subtype may show stronger enhancement

MR

- RCC appears heterogeneous due to necrosis, hemorrhage, and solid components on T1WI, but T2WI appearances depend on histology (clear cell RCC is hyperintense, while papillary RCC is hypointense)
- T1WI C+ often shows prompt arterial enhancement
- DWI has been helpful in characterizing small renal lesions, which may be inflammatory or malignant in nature
- MR is also useful for imaging renal vein and IVC tumor thrombus

Angiography

- Tumor vascularity is closely correlated with tumor architecture; most hypervascular tumors are solid, while hypovascular tumors are usually papillary, tubular, multilocular, or solid tumors with hemorrhage or necrosis

RELATED REFERENCES

1. Farrelly C et al: Do all non-calcified echogenic renal lesions found on ultrasound need further evaluation with CT? Abdom Imaging. 33(1):44-7, 2008
2. Ng CS et al: Renal cell carcinoma: diagnosis, staging, and surveillance. AJR Am J Roentgenol. 191(4):1220-32, 2008
3. Yamashita Y et al: Small renal cell carcinoma: pathologic and radiologic correlation. Radiology. 184(2):493-8, 1992

PAPILLARY RCC MIMICKING SIMPLE CYST

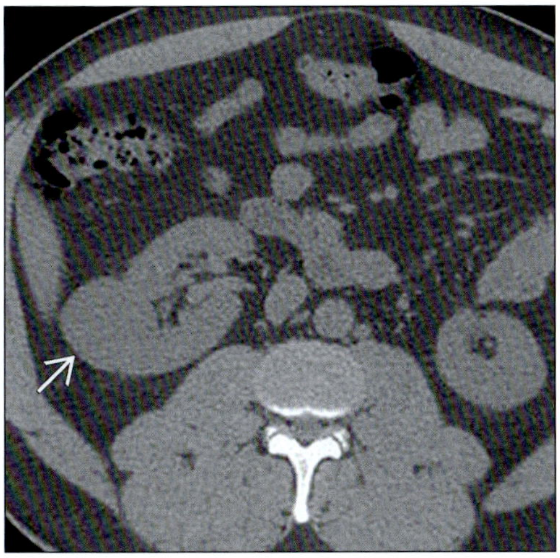

Axial NECT demonstrates a well-circumscribed rounded mass lesion ➡, which is isodense compared to the renal parenchyma.

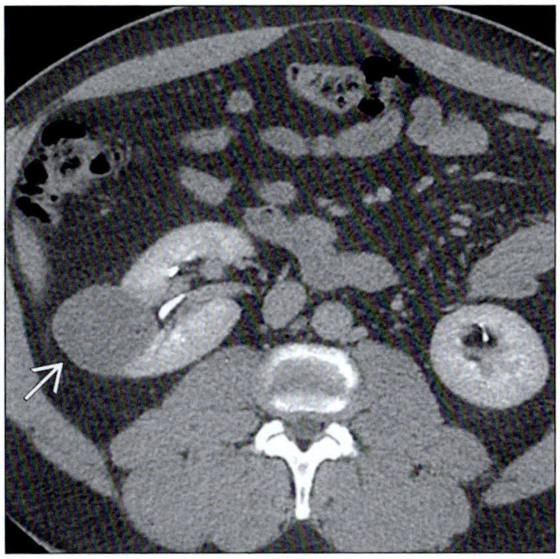

Axial CECT demonstrates a well-circumscribed mass exophytic the interpolar region, which appears hypodense ➡ with slight enhancement compared to the enhancing renal parenchyma.

CLINICAL SCENARIO

History

- 52-year-old man with recent onset of right back pain

IMAGE INTERPRETATION

Pitfalls

- Relatively low attenuation on NECT and slight post-contrast enhancement can be misdiagnosed as hyperdense (hemorrhagic or complicated) cyst

Actual Diagnosis

- Papillary renal cell carcinoma (pRCC)

Clues to Correct Diagnosis

- Unenhanced attenuation > 10 HU
- Simple cysts do not enhance > 10 HU from precontrast to post contrast
- Unclear if pseudoenhancement of cyst or true neoplasm: Suggest other modality (US or MR)

BACKGROUND

General

- 2nd most common RCC subtype after clear cell (cRCC), accounting for 13-15% of all RCCs

Epidemiology

- 3rd-8th decades of life
- M:F ratio ranges from 2:1 to 3.9:1
- Although most pRCCs are unilateral, it is most common multifocal or bilateral renal tumor

Relevant Pathology

- 2 morphologic types of pRCC
  - Type 1: Papillae covered by a single layer of cuboidal or low columnar cells with scanty cytoplasm and low-grade nuclei
  - Type 2: Higher nuclear grade, > 1 layer of cells with abundant eosinophilic cytoplasm
    - Type 2 has worse prognosis than type 1 tumors
- Sarcomatoid dedifferentiation is seen in 5% of pRCCs; associated with worse prognosis

IMAGING FEATURES

US

- Useful in differentiating cystic from solid masses, particularly for lesions that show borderline enhancement at CT and for high-attenuation lesions that show little or no enhancement at CT
- No specific characteristics on US other than solid mass

CT

- NECT: Calcification is seen slightly more than in cRCC
- CECT: pRCC enhances to lesser degree than does cRCC in all post-contrast phases
  - Difference in degree of enhancement between pRCC and cRCC is due to differences in intratumoral vascularity, measured in terms of microvessel density
- On CT, pRCC is more likely to be homogeneous in comparison with cRCC, particularly in tumors < 3 cm in diameter

MR

- T1WI: Low signal intensity and pseudocapsule
- T2WI: Low signal intensity and pseudocapsule
- T1WI C+: Enhancement is less intense in pRCC than in cRCC

RELATED REFERENCES

1. Zhang J et al: Solid renal cortical tumors: differentiation with CT. Radiology. 244(2):494-504, 2007
2. Herts BR et al: Enhancement characteristics of papillary renal neoplasms revealed on triphasic helical CT of the kidneys. AJR Am J Roentgenol. 178(2):367-72, 2002
3. Delahunt B et al: Morphologic typing of papillary renal cell carcinoma: comparison of growth kinetics and patient survival in 66 cases. Hum Pathol. 32(6):590-5, 2001

RENAL MEDULLARY CARCINOMA

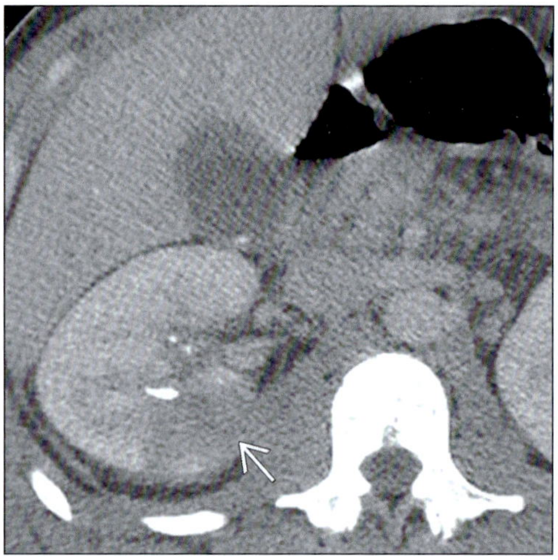

Axial CECT in delayed phase demonstrates an ill-defined infiltrative mass ➔ involving the medial aspect of the right kidney, predominantly centered in the medulla with extension into adjacent cortex.

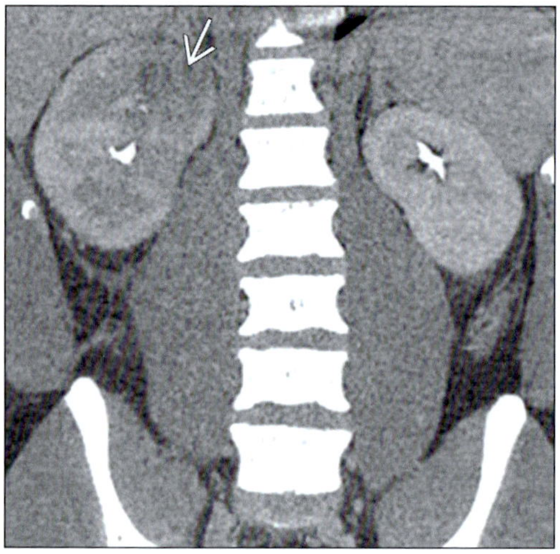

Coronal reformatting of CECT in delayed phase shows the infiltrative ill-defined mass ➔ located predominantly within the upper pole and centered within the medulla with extension into the adjacent cortex.

CLINICAL SCENARIO

History

- 24-year-old African American man presenting with cough and blood stained sputum for 5 months
- 10 lb weight loss in last 5 months
- Bilateral flank pain and intermittent hematuria for 5 months

Relevant Laboratory Tests

- Sickle cell trait

IMAGE INTERPRETATION

Pitfalls

- Can be mistaken for acute bacterial pyelonephritis, lymphoma, or urothelial malignancy, given central location

Actual Diagnosis

- Renal medullary carcinoma

Clues to Correct Diagnosis

- Infiltrative ill-defined mass
- Centrally located mass (centered on medulla)
- Preserved renal shape
- In patients with sickle cell trait

BACKGROUND

General

- 1st described in 1995 (previously called collecting duct carcinoma)

Epidemiology

- Very rare; ~ 50 cases reported in USA
- Occurs almost exclusively in patients with sickle cell trait
- Highly aggressive with direct local invasion and distant metastases
- Clinical presentation: Painless hematuria
- Mean duration of survival: 15 weeks

Relevant Anatomy

- Predilection for right kidney (70%)

Relevant Physiology

- Highly aggressive, very rare tumor of renal medulla (arises in calyceal transitional epithelium)

IMAGING FEATURES

Excretory Urography

- Preserved contour of kidney
- Ill definition of 1 or more calyx, may result in amputated or phantom calyx

CT

- Central infiltrative tumor growth → caliectasis without pelviectasis
- Fistula between necrotic cavity and collecting system
- Infiltration from renal medulla to renal cortex → renal enlargement and preservation of reniform shape
- Heterogeneous enhancement (necrosis)
- Infiltration into peripelvic or perinephric fat
- Renal vein and IVC tumor extension
- Direct extension to retroperitoneal structures and ipsilateral adrenal gland
- Metastases to lung, liver, and lymph nodes

Angiographic Findings

- Hypovascular mass

RELATED REFERENCES

1. Blitman NM et al: Renal medullary carcinoma: CT and MRI features. AJR Am J Roentgenol. 185(1):268-72, 2005
2. Choyke PL et al: Hereditary renal cancers. Radiology. 226(1):33-46, 2003
3. Khan A et al: Renal medullary carcinoma: sonographic, computed tomography, magnetic resonance and angiographic findings. Eur J Radiol. 35(1):1-7, 2000
4. Davidson AJ et al: Renal medullary carcinoma associated with sickle cell trait: radiologic findings. Radiology. 195(1):83-5, 1995

RENAL LYMPHANGIOMATOSIS

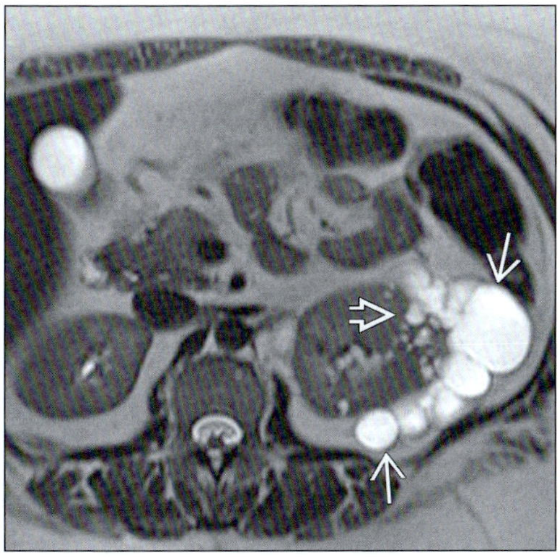

Axial T2WI MR shows multiple cysts ➡ of different sizes within the left perinephric space. There are small renal parenchymal cysts ⇨ in a segmental distribution.

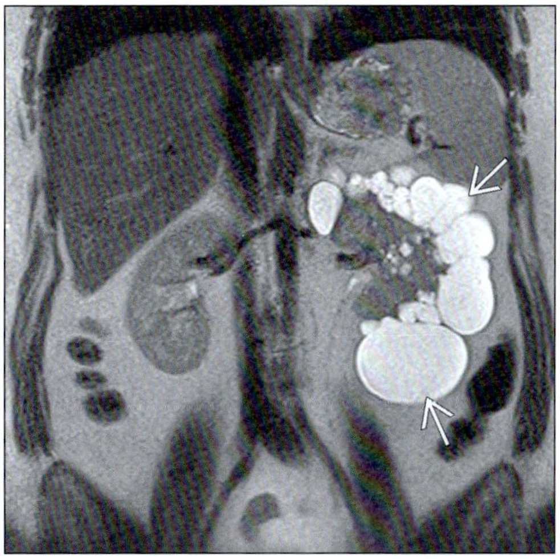

Coronal T2WI MR shows multiple cysts ➡ of different sizes surrounding the kidney within the left perinephric space. The right kidney appears normal.

CLINICAL SCENARIO

History

- 30-year-old asymptomatic woman with abnormal findings on lumbar spine MR

IMAGE INTERPRETATION

Pitfalls

- Multicystic left perinephric lesion may be misinterpreted as polycystic renal diseases, urinoma, and cystic renal neoplasms

Actual Diagnosis

- Renal lymphangiomatosis (lymphangiectasia)

Clues to Correct Diagnosis

- Location within perinephric space
- Associated dilated, fluid-filled tubular structures within retroperitoneum or penetrating renal parenchyma towards renal sinus

BACKGROUND

Epidemiology

- Rare
- 2/3 present in adults
- No sex predilection

Etiology

- Developmental anomaly of perirenal lymphatic system
- Some lesions are neoplastic with distinct karyotypic abnormalities such as monosomy X, trisomy 7q, and defects in *VHL* gene

Clinical Presentation

- Most are asymptomatic
- May present with flank pain, abdominal mass, and occasionally hematuria
- Variable natural history, with spontaneous regression in some cases

Relevant Pathology

- Macroscopically
  - Characterized by ectatic perinephric, peripelvic and intraparenchymal lymphatic vessels
  - Well-encapsulated multicystic mass containing fluid
- Microscopically
  - Multiple communicating cysts are lined with flattened endothelial cells
  - Fibrous septa are present that may contain entrapped renal tubules, lymphoid cells, and smooth muscle elements

IMAGING FEATURES

General Features

- Multicystic mass in renal sinus or in perinephric region
- Usually unilateral, may be bilateral
- Linear tortuous fluid-filled structures may be identified in retroperitoneum, which are suggestive of dilated lymphatic channels

US

- Anechoic or hypoechoic cyst contents

CT

- Cyst content is fluid attenuation
  - High attenuation may occur due to hemorrhage

MR

- Fluid content is typically hypointense on T1WI and hyperintense on T2WI
  - Signal intensity varies depending on presence of hemorrhage, debris, and protein content

RELATED REFERENCES

1. Hakeem A et al: Computed tomography findings in bilateral perinephric lymphangiomatosis. Urol Ann. 2(1):26-8, 2010
2. Katabathina VS et al: Mesenchymal neoplasms of the kidney in adults: imaging spectrum with radiologic-pathologic correlation. Radiographics. 30(6):1525-40, 2010

CALYCEAL DIVERTICULUM

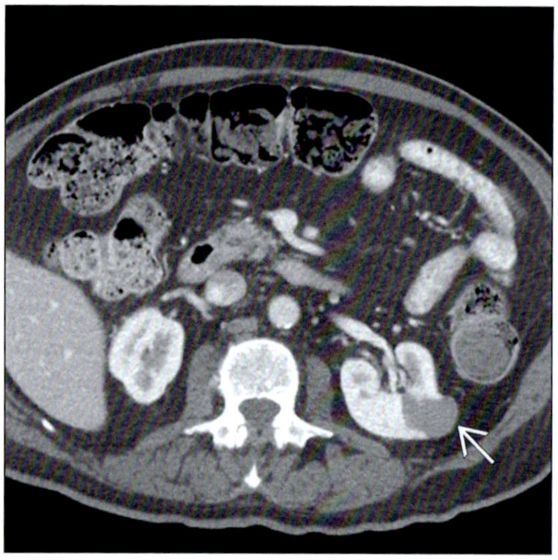

Axial CECT in venous phase demonstrates a well-circumscribed, exophytic lesion ➔ involving the left kidney exhibiting attenuation value of 59 HU, raising suspicion of solid enhancing neoplasm.

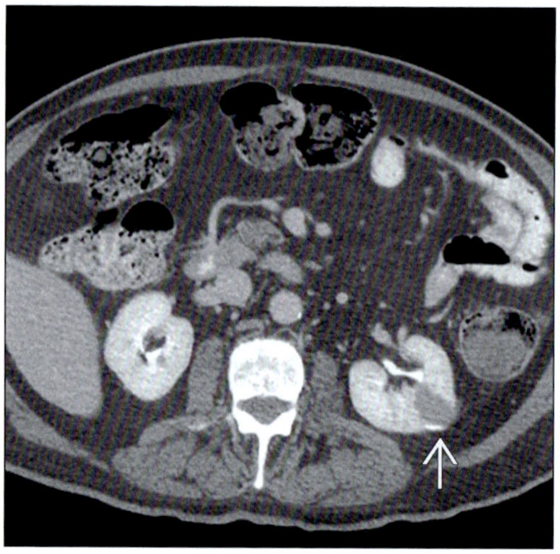

Axial CECT in delayed phase demonstrates layering excreted contrast within the lesion ➔ indicating communication with the collecting system, diagnostic of calyceal diverticulum.

CLINICAL SCENARIO

History

- 75-year-old man with metastatic melanoma

IMAGE INTERPRETATION

Pitfalls

- Can be misinterpreted as renal mass (e.g., renal cell carcinoma, metastasis, simple or complex cyst)

Actual Diagnosis

- Calyceal diverticulum (CD)

Clues to Correct Diagnosis

- Filling with excreted contrast on delayed CECT
- Layering urolithiasis or milk of calcium, if present

BACKGROUND

General

- Cyst-like cavitary outpouching within renal parenchyma communicating with collecting system

Epidemiology

- Incidence: 4.5%; CD is bilateral in 3%
- Stone formation in 1/2 of cases
- Urinary stasis within diverticulum → recurrent urinary tract infections or stone formation within diverticulum → symptoms such as flank pain and hematuria

Relevant Anatomy

- CD communicates with collecting system through narrow infundibulum
  - Thus, it is lined by transitional epithelium and surrounded by muscularis mucosa
  - 2 types
    - More common: Communicates with minor calyx, more commonly located at upper pole
    - Less common: Communicates with major calyx or renal pelvis

Etiology

- More commonly congenital or less likely acquired resulting from infection or passage of small stone

IMAGING FEATURES

Plain Radiography

- Radiopaque calculi may be seen

Ultrasound

- Cystic lesion closely related to renal sinus
  - Can be misinterpreted as complex cystic lesion
- In 1/2 of cases, layered calculi or milk of calcium can be present and seen as mobile echogenic foci

Intravenous Urography (IVU)

- Delayed imaging can depict connection to renal pelvis or calyx
  - Contrast surrounds stone
- Retrograde pyelography can be utilized if IVU failed to depict CD; however, CD cannot be visualized if infundibulum is obstructed by calculus, which can mimic complex cystic mass

CT

- NECT: Fluid attenuation lesion (0.5-2 cm) with dense urolithiasis (in 50% of cases)
- CECT: Demonstrates post-contrast enhancement; thus, may simulate enhancing mass
- On delayed phase, lesion fills with excreted contrast, which has similar density to collecting system
- Coronal & sagittal reformatted images can depict location of CD in relation to pelvicalyceal system

RELATED REFERENCES

1. Pareek A et al: Calyceal diverticulum: a benign imitator of serious pathology. BMJ Case Rep. 2014, 2014
2. Stunell H et al: The imaging appearances of calyceal diverticula complicated by uroliathasis. Br J Radiol. 83(994):888-94, 2010

CLAW SIGN

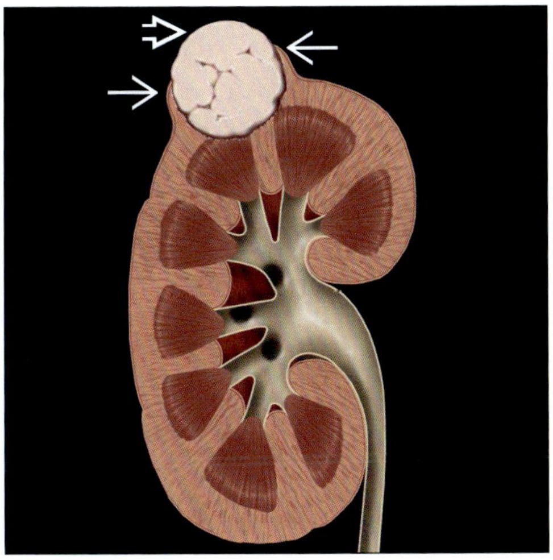

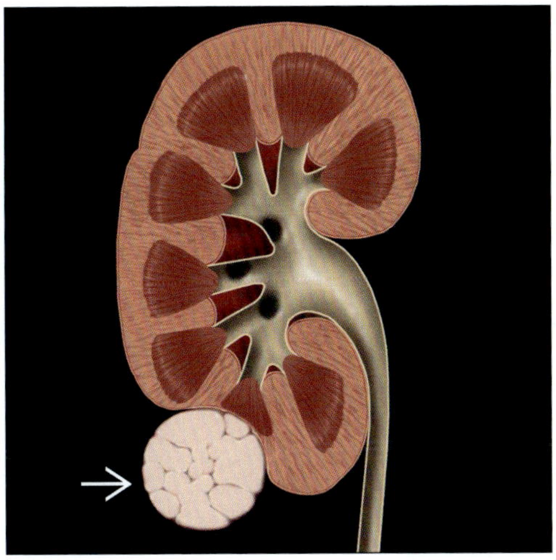

(Left) *Graphic shows sharp angles of renal parenchyma, giving the appearance of a claw due to an intrarenal mass.* ***(Right)*** *Graphic shows an extrarenal mass indenting the renal parenchyma.*

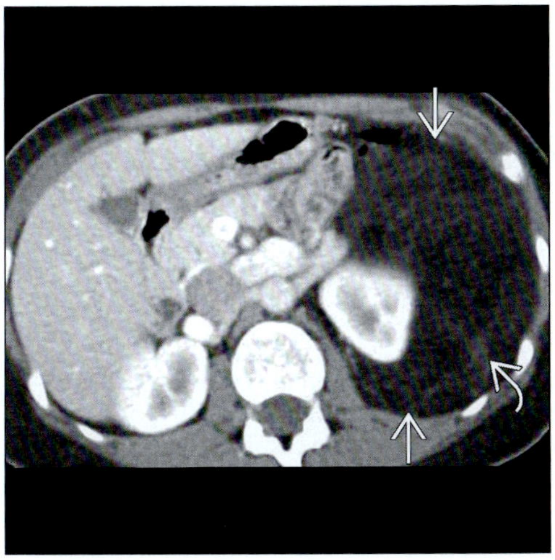

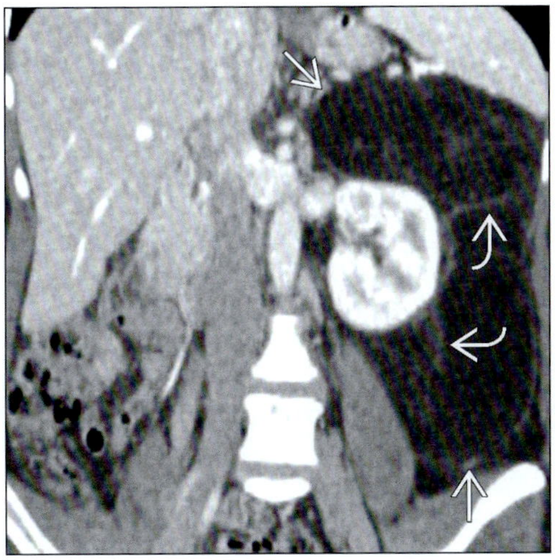

(Left) *Axial CECT shows a large left retroperitoneal pararenal mass with fat and soft tissue components, displacing the kidney anteromedially. This extrarenal mass does not demonstrate the claw sign.* ***(Right)*** *Coronal reformatted CECT shows a large left retroperitoneal mass lateral to the left kidney. The mass is predominantly fatty and contains thin soft tissue areas; this was surgically proven to represent liposarcoma.*

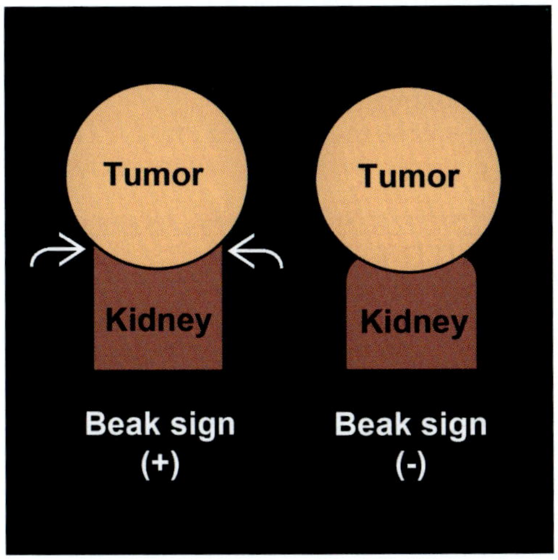

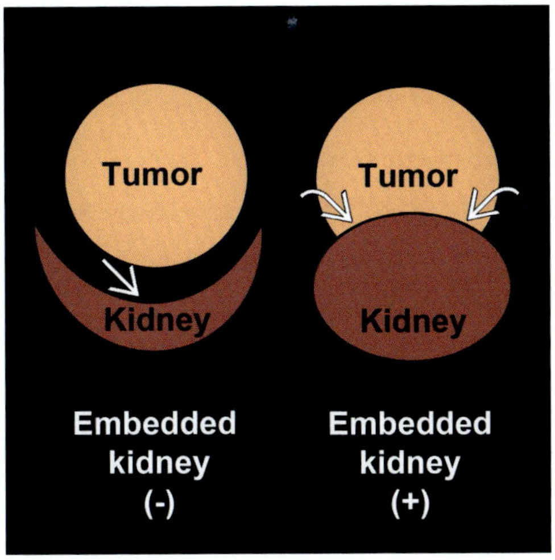

(Left) *Illustration shows the beak sign. Renal tissue is seen forming the shape of bird's beak on its contact surface with the intrarenal mass, with absence of the beak sign in the case of an extrarenal mass.* ***(Right)*** *Illustration shows the embedded kidney sign. In the case of an intrarenal mass, the kidney appears to be embedded in the tumor, while the extrarenal mass compresses the kidney with absence of the embedded kidney sign.*

RENAL CORTICAL T2 LOW SIGNAL INTENSITY

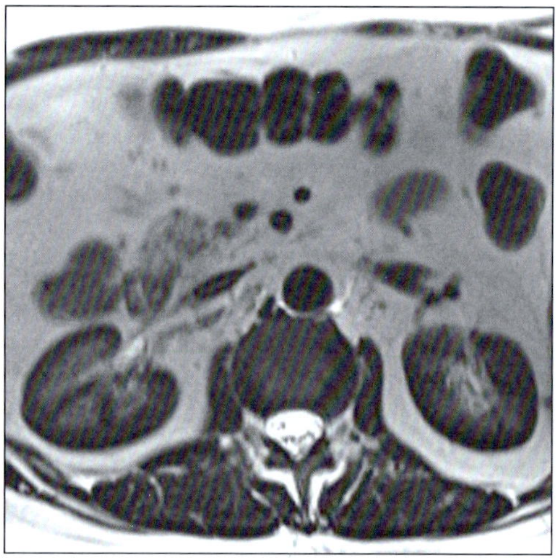

Axial T2WI MR in a 35-year-old man with history of paroxysmal nocturnal hemoglobinuria shows diffuse decrease in the signal intensity of the renal cortices with normal signal intensity of the renal medulla.

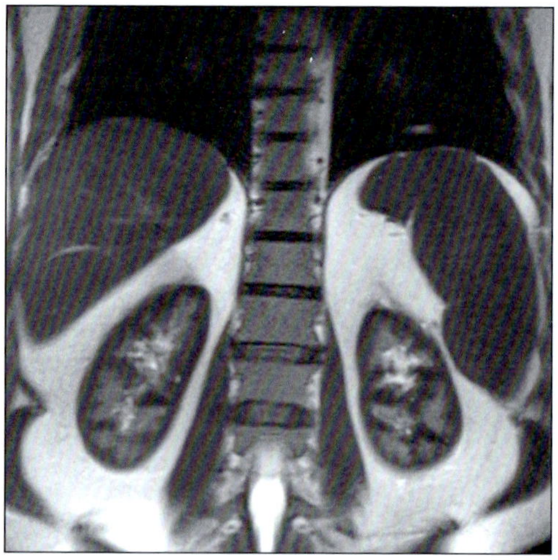

Coronal T2WI MR in the same patient shows diffuse decrease in signal intensity of renal cortices with normal signal intensity of renal medulla. Normally, there is poor differentiation of cortex and medulla on T2WI.

IMAGE INTERPRETATION

Radiographic Finding

- Diffuse decrease in cortical signal intensity on T2WI

Causes

- **Hemolysis**
  - Paroxysmal nocturnal hemoglobinuria (PNH)
    - Acquired myelodysplastic, hematopoietic stem cell disorder due to ↑ sensitivity to complement → in acute or chronic intravascular hemolysis
    - Occurs predominantly in adults
    - Factors that precipitate hemolysis include infections, reactions to drugs, transfusion, surgery, and exercise
  - Mechanical hemolysis due to prosthetic valves
  - Sickle cell disease
- **Renal cortical necrosis**

Differential Diagnosis

- PNH
  - Low signal intensity in renal cortex on T1 and T2WI
    - Medulla is usually spared
  - Lower signal intensity on in-phase compared to opposed-phase images
  - Liver and spleen are usually spared
    - May be involved due to repeated transfusions
  - NECT can show high attenuation of renal parenchyma
- Mechanical hemolysis due to prosthetic valves
  - Indistinguishable from PNH
- Sickle cell disease
  - Renal changes are indistinguishable from PNH
  - Low signal intensity of spleen on T2WI due to extravascular hemolysis
    - Low signal intensity of liver or pancreas can be seen only in patients who have received multiple blood transfusions
- Renal cortical necrosis
  - Cortical calcifications can be seen in patients with cortical necrosis on CT

BACKGROUND

Normal Renal MR

- T1WI
  - Low or medium signal intensity
  - Relatively good differentiation between cortex and medulla
    - Renal cortex is slightly hyperintense with respect to medulla
- T2WI
  - Intermediate signal intensity
  - No differentiation between cortex and medulla

Relevant Physiology

- Low signal intensity of renal cortex could be secondary to hemosiderin, hemorrhage, calcifications, or fibrosis
- With hemolytic disorders, iron resulting from extravascular hemolysis is mainly deposited in liver and spleen
- Intravascular hemolysis does not result in hemosiderin accumulation elsewhere in body
  - PNH and mechanical damage from heart valves → intravascular hemolysis → release of free hemoglobin
    - Free HB forms a complex molecule with haptoglobin and hemopexin
    - When plasma haptoglobin becomes saturated, free hemoglobin is filtered by glomeruli and is partially reabsorbed in proximal tubules
    - Part of the iron will be incorporated into hemosiderin deposits and the rest will be excreted

RELATED REFERENCES

1. Rimola J et al: The kidney in paroxysmal nocturnal haemoglobinuria: MRI findings. Br J Radiol. 77(923):953-6, 2004
2. Jeong JY et al: Atypical low-signal-intensity renal parenchyma: causes and patterns. Radiographics. 22(4):833-46, 2002

RENAL CORTICAL T2 LOW SIGNAL INTENSITY

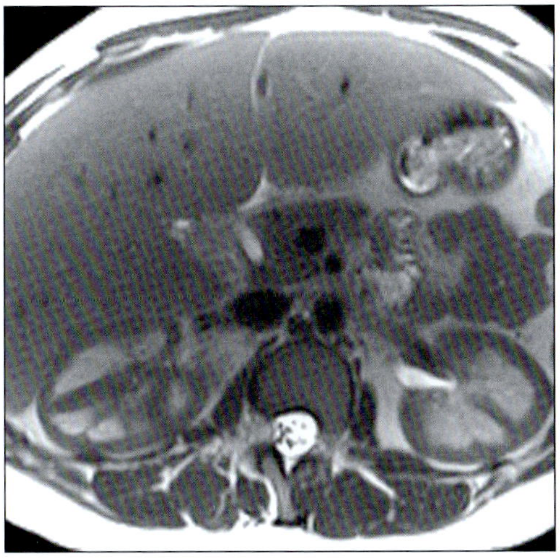

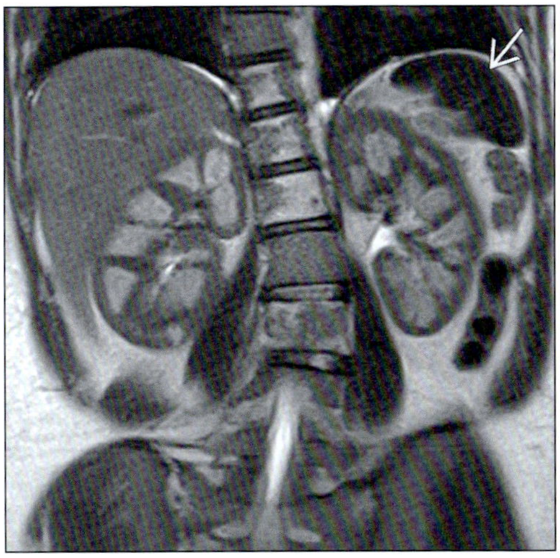

(Left) *Axial T2WI MR in a 25-year-old man with a history of sickle cell anemia shows diffuse decrease in the signal intensity of the renal cortices with normal signal intensity of the renal medulla.* ***(Right)*** *Coronal T2WI MR in the same patient shows diffuse decrease in the signal intensity of the renal cortices with normal signal intensity of the renal medulla. Note the small spleen displaying very low signal intensity →.*

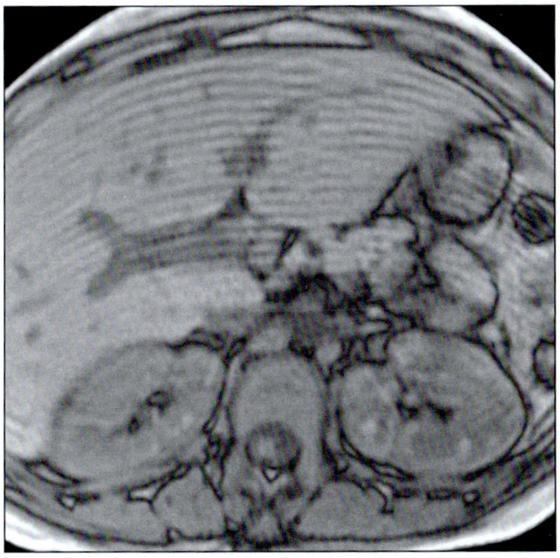

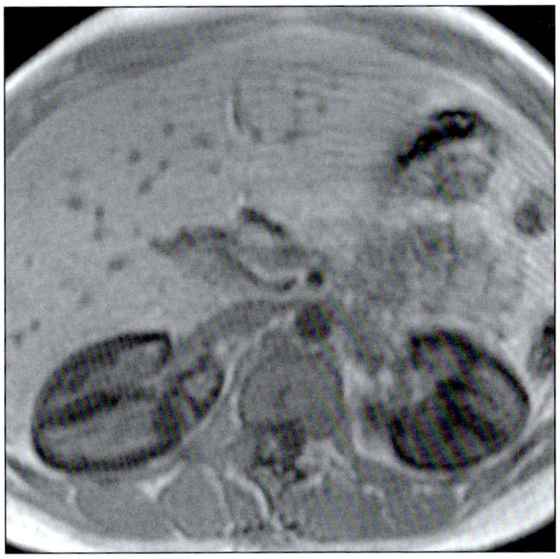

(Left) *Axial opposed-phase T1WI MR shows relatively normal appearance of the renal cortex.* ***(Right)*** *Axial in-phase T1WI MR shows significant drop of signal in the renal cortices bilaterally due to hemosiderin deposition. The loss of signal on in-phase images is the result of longer echo time (TE). Note the sparing of the liver and pancreas, which can be seen only in patients who have received multiple blood transfusions.*

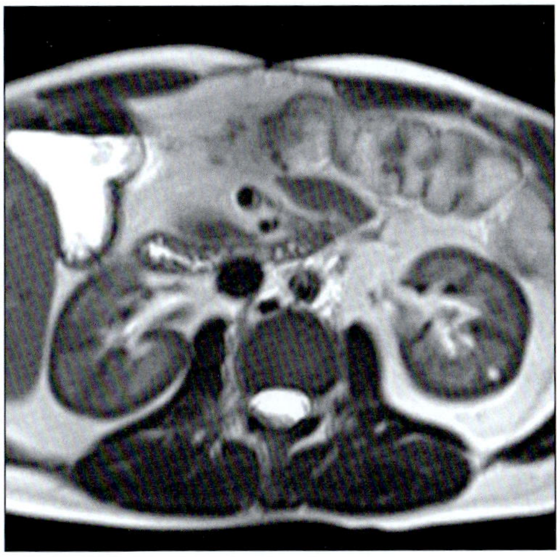

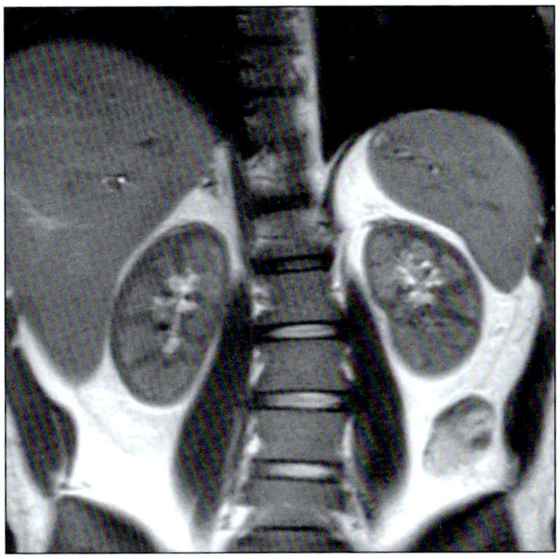

(Left) *Axial T2WI MR in a 30-year-old woman with a history of acute cortical necrosis following postpartum hemorrhage shows diffuse decrease in the signal intensity of the renal cortices with normal signal intensity of the renal medulla.* ***(Right)*** *Coronal T2WI MR in the same patient shows diffuse decrease in the signal intensity of the renal cortices with normal signal intensity of the renal medulla. No calcifications were seen on abdominal CECT.*

BEAR PAW SIGN

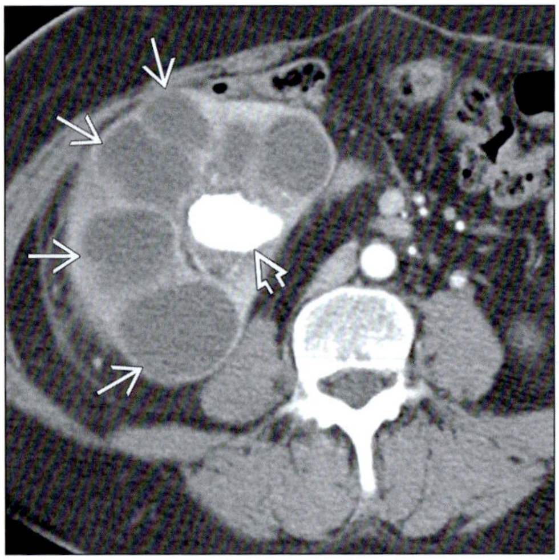

Axial CECT demonstrates a centrally obstructing stone ➩ with replacement of the renal parenchyma by low-attenuation collections ➔ in a "hydronephrotic" pattern. The pattern seen at CT resembles a bear's paw.

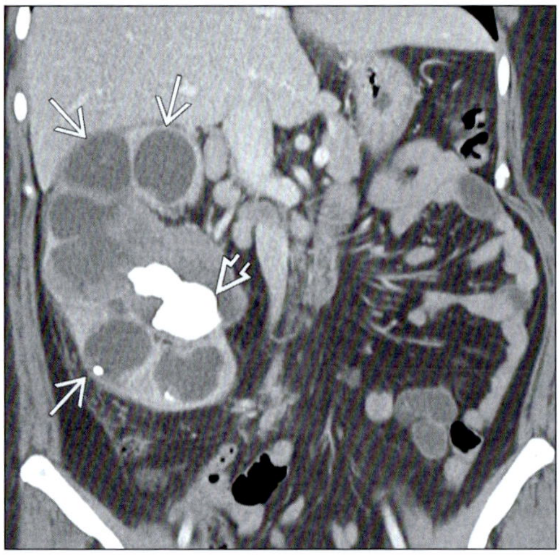

Coronal CECT demonstrates a centrally obstructing stone ➩ with replacement of the renal parenchyma by low-attenuation collections ➔ in a "hydronephrotic" pattern. Note the marked thinning of renal parenchyma.

CLINICAL SCENARIO

Appearance

- Renal parenchyma is replaced by hypoattenuating mass-like structures arranged in a "hydronephrotic" pattern
  - This appearance on CT scans has been described as bear paw sign

Diagnosis

- Xanthogranulomatous pyelonephritis (XGP)

Other Imaging Findings

- Enlarged kidney with poor renal function
- Simple or staghorn calculi
  - Present in most cases
- May be enhancement in margins of calyces after contrast material administration
- Inflammatory changes in perinephric fat
- May extend to involve perinephric fat and psoas muscles

BACKGROUND

Explanation

- Due to filling of renal calyces with extensive inflammatory infiltrate rather than fluid
  - Percutaneous nephrostomy is not performed in most instances

Epidemiology

- XGP is a rare entity and constitutes < 1% of chronic pyelonephritis
- Females are more commonly involved
- Usually unilateral
  - Right and left kidneys affected with equal frequency
  - Bilateral lesions, although rare, are fatal

Relevant Pathology

- XGP is severe and chronic renal inflammatory condition, generally associated with urinary tract infection and obstructing renal calculi → diffuse or focal kidney destruction
  - Destruction and replacement of renal parenchyma by lipid-laden macrophages (xanthoma cells)
- Believed to result from atypical, incomplete immune response to subacute bacterial infection
- Starts within pelvis and calyces and subsequently spreads into renal parenchyma
  - If uncontrolled, spreads to perirenal tissue
- *Escherichia coli* and *Proteus* species are mostly isolated organisms in urine
- Exact pathogenesis of XGP is still not known
  - A number of predisposing factors have been implicated, including
    - Recurrent urinary tract infection
    - Urinary obstruction
    - Urolithiasis (in 70% of patients with XGP, 1/2 of whom had staghorn calculi)
    - Diabetes mellitus
    - Transplanted kidney
- 2 forms of XGP
  - Diffuse (85%)
  - Localized, segmental (15%)

Clinical Presentation

- Fever, flank pain, and weight loss
- Urinary symptoms can include dysuria, frequency, and hematuria
- Leukocytosis, ↑ C-reactive protein and ↑ ESR

RELATED REFERENCES

1. Craig WD et al: Pyelonephritis: radiologic-pathologic review. Radiographics. 28(1):255-77; quiz 327-8, 2008
2. Dyer RB et al: Classic signs in uroradiology. Radiographics. 24 Suppl 1:S247-80, 2004

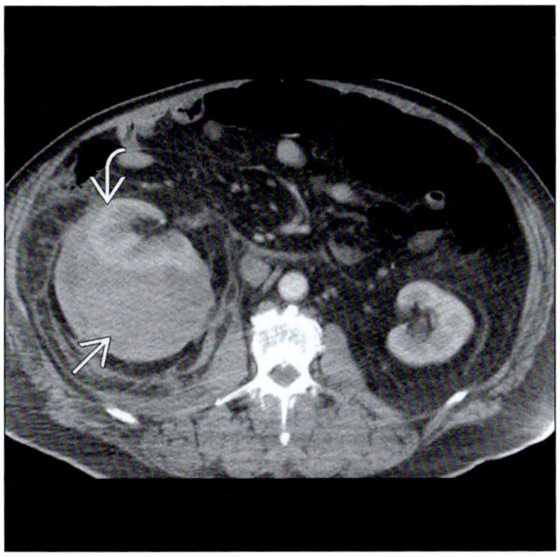

Axial CECT demonstrates a large, heterogeneous collection in the tight perinephric space consistent with a perinephric hematoma, with compression and distortion of the adjacent kidney.

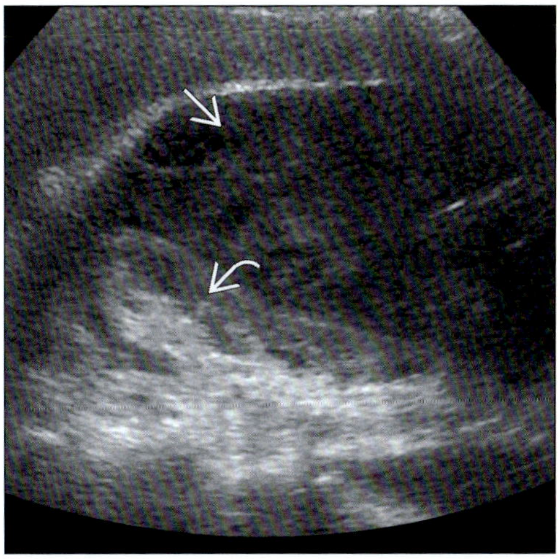

Grayscale ultrasound shows a large, heterogeneous, echogenic perinephric hematoma with compression and distortion of the adjacent kidney.

IMAGE INTERPRETATION

Appearance & Explanation

- Page kidney refers to compression of renal parenchyma by surrounding collection (e.g., hematoma, seroma, urinoma)
- Results in ↓ blood flow and activation of renin-angiotensin system, which leads to ↑ blood pressure
- Phenomenon was first described by Irvine H. Page in 1939 when he discovered that hypertension could be produced in a dog by wrapping 1 or both kidneys in cellophane

Differential Diagnosis

- Page kidney is an important cause of hyperreninemic hypertension that should be included in differential diagnosis of secondary hypertension
- Many causes, including
  - Bleeding due to trauma or intervention (contact sports or motor vehicle accident, postoperative, kidney biopsy)
  - Spontaneous bleeding (warfarin/anticoagulation, tumor, pancreatitis, polyarteritis nodosa)
  - Nonbleeding causes (pararenal lymphocele, large simple cyst, urinoma, perirenal pseudocyst, peritransplant lymphocele)

BACKGROUND

Clinical Presentation

- Flank pain, ecchymoses, and hematuria

Epidemiology

- Initial description in humans was in athletes with renal subcapsular hematoma after flank trauma in 1955
- Has been reported in all age groups (pediatric, adolescent, and adult)

Relevant Pathology

- Collection might be perinephric or subcapsular, with no differences between trauma and nontrauma patients

IMAGING FEATURES

General

- Perinephric or subcapsular fluid collection surrounding kidney of variable attenuation/intensity/echogenicity depending on nature of collection
- Kidney compressed and distorted
- Delayed nephrogram compared to normal kidney may be observed at contrast-enhanced CT and MR
  - Reflects decreased renal perfusion
- Angiography can be used to obtain renin levels from renal veins to confirm hyperreninemia

Ultrasound

- Lymphocele and urinoma appear as anechoic collections
- Hematoma can be heterogeneous and echogenic

CT and MR

- Lymphocele and urinoma appear as simple fluid attenuation/signal intensity
- Complex fluid collection in cases of infection and hematoma
- MR demonstrates blood degradation products in various degrees of evolution

RELATED REFERENCES

1. Smyth A et al: Page kidney: etiology, renal function outcomes and risk for future hypertension. J Clin Hypertens (Greenwich). 14(4):216-21, 2012
2. Dopson SJ et al: Page kidney as a rare cause of hypertension: case report and review of the literature. Am J Kidney Dis. 54(2):334-9, 2009
3. Chamorro HA et al: Multiimaging approach in the diagnosis of Page kidney. AJR Am J Roentgenol. 136(3):620-1, 1981

GAS WITHIN RENAL PARENCHYMA

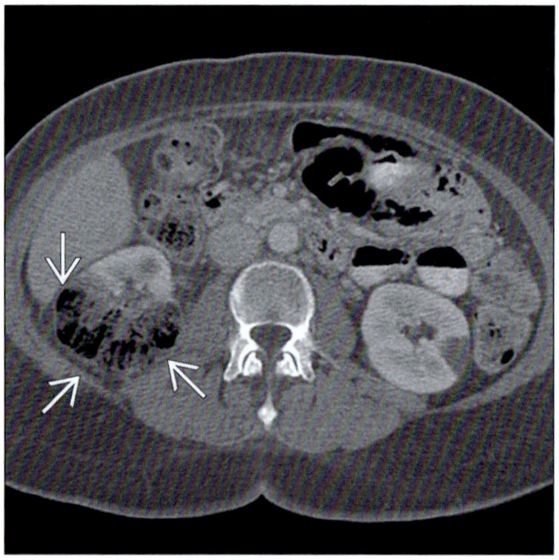

Axial CECT demonstrates replacement of the posterior cortex of the right kidney with gas loculation ➡.

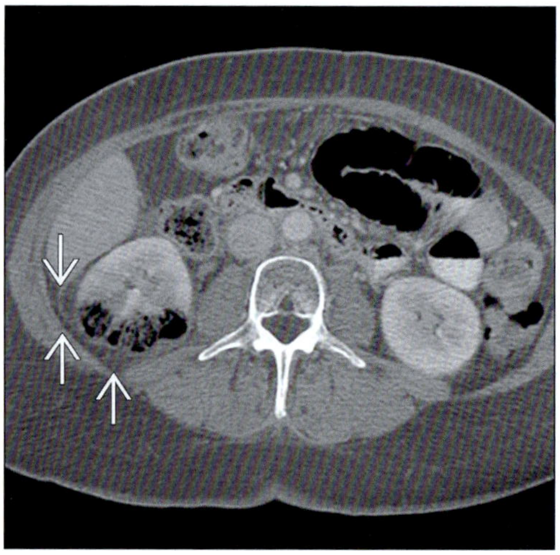

Axial CECT shows significant fat stranding ➡ *in the perirenal space with thickening of the fascial layer.*

CLINICAL SCENARIO

History

- 57-year-old woman with type 2 diabetes mellitus presents to emergency department with vomiting

IMAGE INTERPRETATION

Classic Sign

- Gas in renal parenchyma with destruction is classic for emphysematous pyelonephritis (EP)

BACKGROUND

General

- Necrotizing gas-forming infection of renal parenchyma
- Single or mixed organism infections may occur
  - Most common causative organism is *Escherichia coli* (68%) followed by *Klebsiella pneumoniae* and *Proteus mirabilis*
- Clinically, may present with fever, flank or abdominal pain, thrombocytopenia, and acute renal insufficiency
- Mild; treated conservatively (antibiotics & drainage)
- Surgery (partial or complete nephrectomy): Required in severe cases and for those who fail conservative management

Epidemiology

- Typical age: 50-60
- F > M
- Majority: Poorly controlled DM; others: Obstruction, alcoholism, and immunocompromised

Relevant Pathology

- Macroscopic
  - Cystic appearance with cortical abscesses, papillary necrosis, necrotic renal parenchyma
- Microscopic
  - Nonepithelial lined empty spaces distorting renal parenchyma

IMAGING FEATURES

US

- Echogenic reflectors within renal parenchyma &/or collecting system with posterior reverberation artifact
- Ring-down artifact from air bubbles trapped in fluid
- Difficult to visualize (artifact from perirenal gas)

CT

- Gold standard for evaluation of EP
- 2 types of infections may be classified by CT
  - Type 1 (1/3 of cases, mortality 69%): Parenchymal destruction, mottled gas without fluid collections
  - Type 2 (2/3 of cases, mortality 18%): Renal or perirenal abscesses with gas or collecting system gas
- Huang-Tseng also described a CT classification
  - Type 1: Gas seen in collecting system only
  - Type 2: Gas seen in renal parenchyma only
  - Type 3: Gas or abscess extend to perirenal space
  - Type 4: Bilateral EP, or EP in a solitary kidney

Nuclear Medicine

- Findings overlap with non EP
- Tc-99m DMSA may demonstrate areas of photopenia corresponding to infarcted renal tissue
- Labeled WBC scan may demonstrate focal uptake in renal parenchyma or perirenal abscesses

MR

- Limited sensitivity, signal voids corresponding to gas in renal parenchyma, perirenal, or collecting system

RELATED REFERENCES

1. Akhtar AL et al: AJR teaching file: diabetic patient presenting with right flank pain and fever. AJR Am J Roentgenol. 194(6 Suppl):WS31-3, 2010
2. Craig WD et al: Pyelonephritis: radiologic-pathologic review. Radiographics. 28(1):255-77; quiz 327-8, 2008
3. Huang JJ et al: Emphysematous pyelonephritis: clinicoradiological classification, management, prognosis, and pathogenesis. Arch Intern Med. 160(6):797-805, 2000

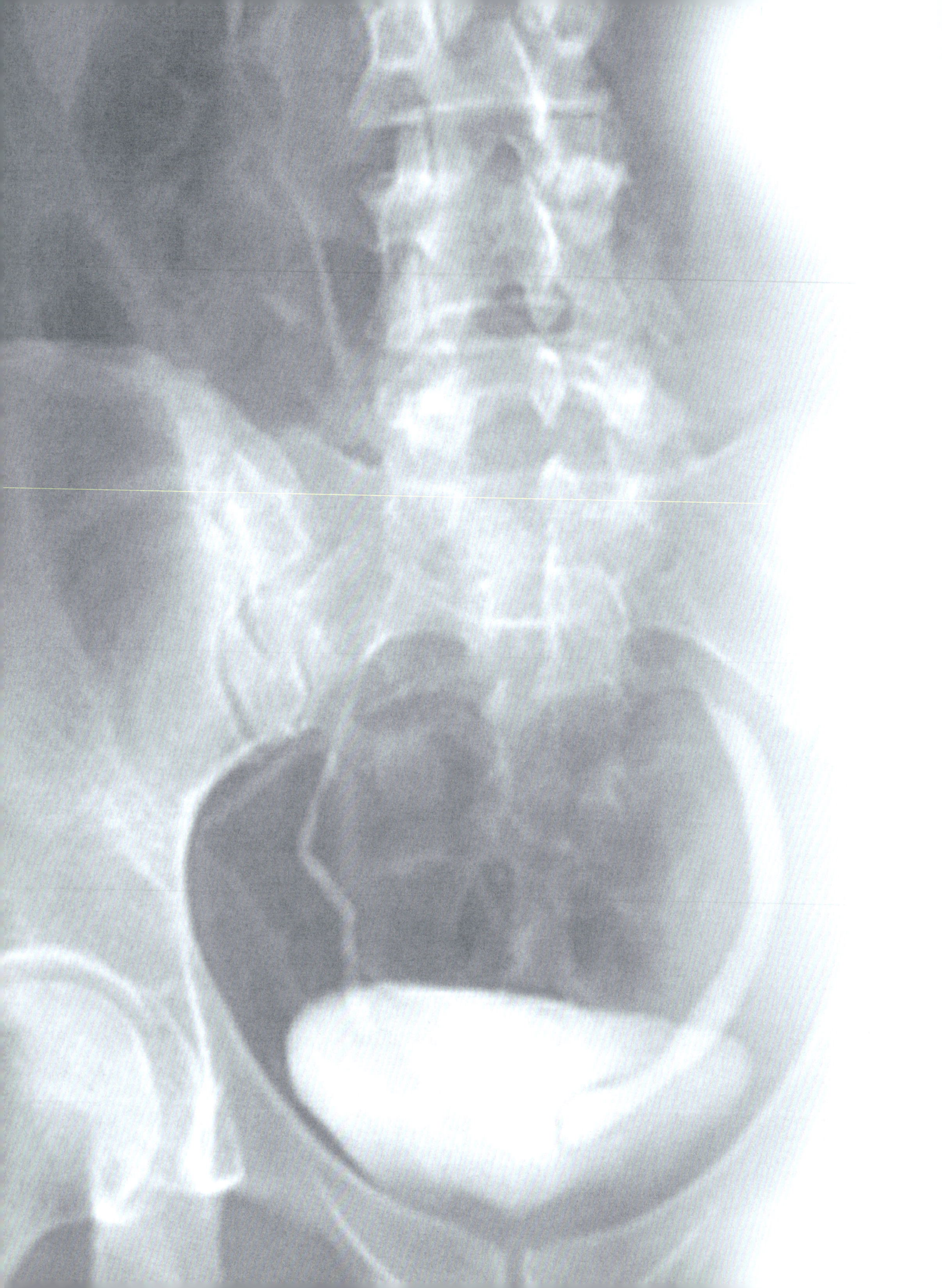

GOBLET SIGN

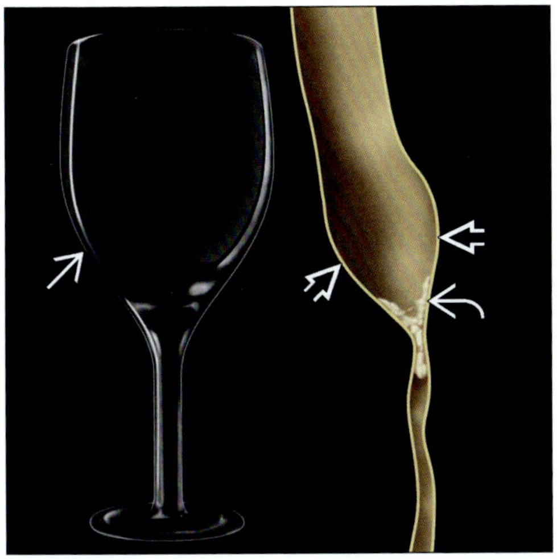

Illustration demonstrates the goblet or champagne glass sign ➡, which may result secondary to urothelial neoplasm ➡, leading to significant dilatation of the proximal ureter ➡.

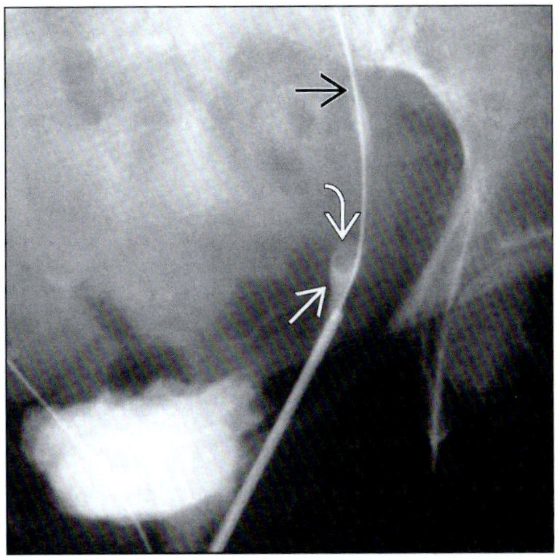

Retrograde ureterogram shows a goblet or champagne glass sign ➡ of ureteral dilatation distal to a filling defect ➡, secondary to transitional cell carcinoma. A catheter is noted in the ureter →.

IMAGE INTERPRETATION

Appearance and Explanation

- Goblet sign (or champagne glass sign) describes appearance of ureteral dilatation below site of intraluminal ureteral filling defect
  - Best seen on retrograde ureterogram
- Implies chronic gradual pathological process allowing lesion to be accommodated in ureter

Differential Diagnosis

- Although primarily described with transitional cell carcinoma, goblet sign may be seen with other processes, including metastatic disease or endometriosis
- Goblet sign allows differentiating these entities from calculus impacted in ureter
  - Calculus should cause distal spasm and narrowing

BACKGROUND

Epidemiology

- Urothelial carcinoma is typically tumor of elderly
- Strong male predilection
- A number of chemical compounds have been responsible for development of this tumor, including tobacco, compounds found in dye/pigment manufacturing, cyclophosphamide, Thorotrast, and phenacetin
- Bilateral in 2-5% of patients

Clinical Presentation

- Usually hematuria and flank pain
- Renal colic mimicking ureterolithiasis

Relevant Pathology

- 2 main morphologic patterns: Papillary (accounts for 60% of urothelial carcinomas and tends to be low grade) and nonpapillary (tends to be high grade)
- Distal ureter is more frequently affected

IMAGING FEATURES

General

- Collecting system can be opacified by contrast in different ways, e.g., intravenous injection (CTU & IVU), direct instillation of contrast into collecting system (antegrade pyelography via nephrostomy or retrograde pyelography via cannulation of ureter via cystoscopy)
- Dilated ureteral segment above filling defect allows coiling of catheter in retrograde catheterization, giving appearance of coiled catheter sign

US

- Little role in diagnosis of ureteral TCC, although may suggest diagnosis by detecting secondary signs like hydronephrosis
- Absent acoustic shadowing allows for differentiation from calculi

CT or Conventional Urography and Direct Pyelography

- CT urography has largely replaced conventional IVU
- Can detect dilated collecting system and demonstrate level of obstruction
- Smaller or polypoid tumor may be seen as filling defects
- CT may demonstrate extraureteral extension
- Intraluminal mass representing ureteral tumor can be differentiated from obstructing calculus by CT in terms of Hounsfield units

RELATED REFERENCES

1. Vikram R et al: Imaging and staging of transitional cell carcinoma: part 2, upper urinary tract. AJR Am J Roentgenol. 192(6):1488-93, 2009
2. Dyer RB et al: Classic signs in uroradiology. Radiographics. 24 Suppl 1:S247-80, 2004

WATERING CAN PERINEUM

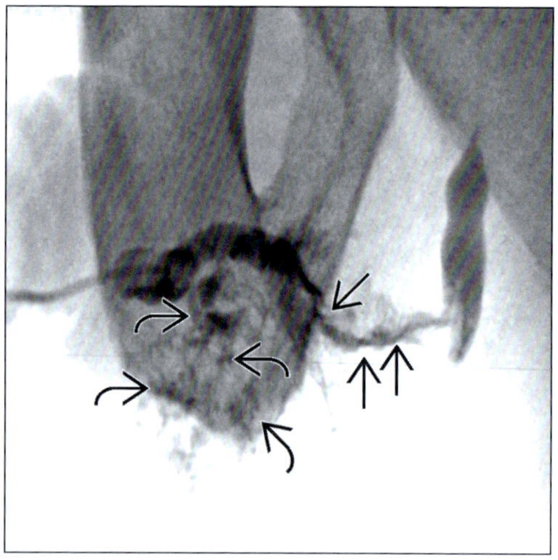

Retrograde urethrogram reveals multiple irregular strictures ➔ involving the penile and bulbar urethra with extensive fistulous tracts ➔ to perineal skin.

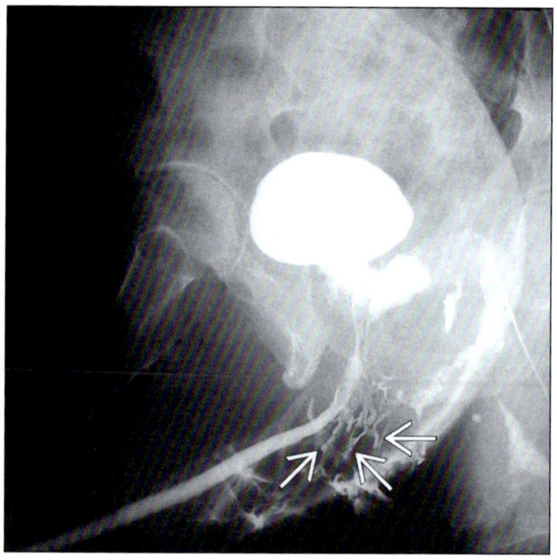

Retrograde urethrogram reveals multiple linear tracts of extraluminal contrast outside the urethra in the perineum, extending to the skin ➔, giving the appearance of a watering can.

CLINICAL SCENARIO

History

- 45-year-old male immigrant with history of genital tuberculosis (TB) complaining of urine dripping from perineum during micturition

IMAGE INTERPRETATION

Classic Sign

- Multiple urethral strictures and urethroperineal fistulas
- Term "watering can" perineum refers to urination through perineum due to multiple urethroperineal fistulas
  - Seen in chronic inflammatory conditions of urethra, e.g., tuberculosis (TB)

BACKGROUND

General

- Watering can appearance can be seen 2° to post inflammatory urethral stricture
  - Most commonly caused by chronic inflammatory urethral strictures due to TB, schistosomiasis, or gonorrhea
- Incidence has greatly decreased due to widespread use of antibiotic for gonorrhea and early detection and management of TB
- Management includes
  - Treating of cause of stricture (e.g., antibiotics or antituberculous agents)
  - Diversion of urine with suprapubic cystostomy
  - Once fistulae have healed, attention is directed to relieving stricture

Epidemiology

- More common in developing countries as a sequela of longstanding neglected inflammatory urethral stricture
- Mean age at presentation is 46 years

Relevant Anatomy

- Anatomically, male urethra is divided into
  - Posterior urethra
    - Prostatic and membranous
    - Most commonly, posterior urethral strictures are secondary to trauma
  - Anterior urethra
    - Bulbar and penile
    - Most commonly, anterior urethral strictures are secondary to infection

Relevant Pathology

- Urethroperineal fistulas are most often consequence of a periurethral abscess
  - In general, initial abscess cavity contracts by means of healing fibrosis, which leaves only the narrow fistulous tract from urethra to perineum
  - Consequently, urination usually occurs through perineal fistulas, which results in so-called watering can perineum

IMAGING FEATURES

Retrograde Urethrogram

- Anterior urethral stricture associated with multiple prostatocutaneous and urethrocutaneous fistulas
- May be difficult to visualize entire urethra, since instilled contrast leaks out of fistulas before opacifying more proximal urethra
  - Fistulography, therefore, may be needed to visualize entire urethra

RELATED REFERENCES

1. Kawashima A et al: Imaging of urethral disease: a pictorial review. Radiographics. 24 Suppl 1:S195-216, 2004
2. Sharfi AR et al: The 'watering-can' perineum: presentation and management. Br J Urol. 80(6):933-6, 1997

SOFT TISSUE RIM SIGN

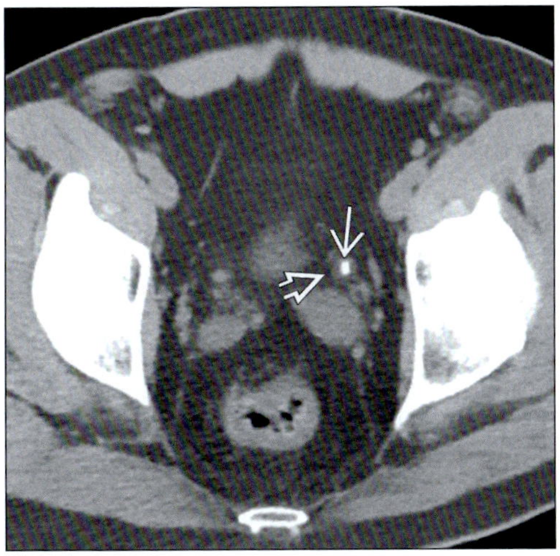

Axial NECT shows a left pelvic calcification ➡ surrounded by a circumferential rim of soft tissue attenuation ➡.

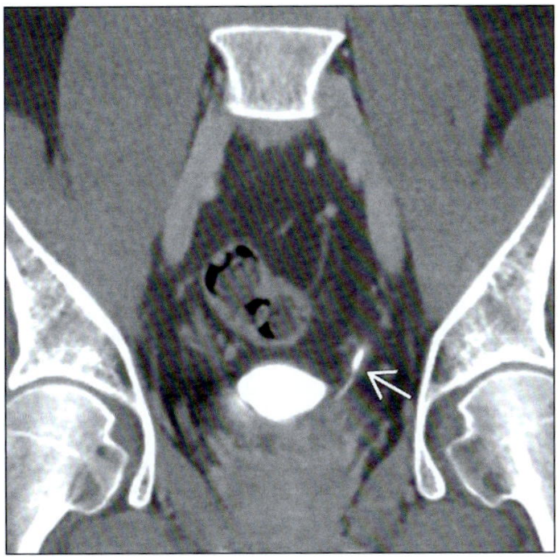

Coronal CECT in the same patient during the pyelographic phase shows contrast within the distal left ureter ➡, obscuring the stone. A rim of soft tissue attenuation surrounds the distal ureter.

IMAGING FEATURES

Appearance

- Circumferential rim of soft tissue attenuation surrounding ureteral calculus on nonenhanced CT studies
- Useful sign in diagnosis of urolithiasis in patients with renal colic

Diagnostic value

- Unlike their appearance on plain radiography, pelvic phleboliths lack radiolucent center on routine clinical CT examinations
- Rim sign can help distinguish stone in ureter from phlebolith in adjacent vein
  - Helpful in pelvis where there is crossing of multiple tubular structures, particularly in elderly patients and those with small amount of pelvic fat
- Soft tissue rim is very uncommon around phlebolith
  - Only 2% of phleboliths show rim sign
- Sensitivity of 77% and specificity reaching 92%
  - Present around 50-76% of ureteric calculi

Limitation

- Rim sign usually does not appear for 4-24 hours after patient becomes symptomatic
  - Will frequently be absent in patients who have acutely obstructed collecting system

Other Signs Observed With Ureteral Calculi

- Other secondary signs that are usually present and suggest that pelvic calcific structure is likely calculus
  - Ureteral dilatation with perinephric stranding of fat
    - Sensitivity: 82%; specificity: 93%
  - Renal enlargement
    - Sensitivity: 71%; specificity: 89%
  - Caliceal ectasis or hydronephrosis
    - Sensitivity: 83%; specificity: 94%
- Rim sign is only rarely identified in absence of any ipsilateral secondary signs
  - Still can be very helpful in absence of equivocal cases when other signs are absent

Signs Observed With Phleboliths

- Comet tail sign
  - Linear or wavy thin soft tissue structure extending from abdominal or pelvic calcification; generally indicates that calcification is phlebolith
    - Positive predictive value: 100%

BACKGROUND

Explanation

- It has been suggested that rim represents edematous ureteral wall surrounding ureteral stone
- Visualization of soft tissue rim sign is dependent on stone size
  - Larger stones (~ 6 mm) tend to thin ureteral wall to greater degree than do smaller stones (~ 4 mm) and are less likely to exhibit rim sign
    - 90% of stones ≤ 4 mm exhibit rim sign
    - Stones ≥ 5 mm do not exhibit rim sign

RELATED REFERENCES

1. Dyer RB et al: Classic signs in uroradiology. Radiographics. 24 Suppl 1:S247-80, 2004
2. Al-Nakshabandi NA: The soft-tissue rim sign. Radiology. 229(1):239-40, 2003
3. Guest AR et al: Assessment of the clinical utility of the rim and comet-tail signs in differentiating ureteral stones from phleboliths. AJR Am J Roentgenol. 177(6):1285-91, 2001
4. Traubici J et al: Distinguishing pelvic phleboliths from distal ureteral stones on routine unenhanced helical CT: is there a radiolucent center? AJR Am J Roentgenol. 172(1):13-7, 1999

FISHHOOK SIGN

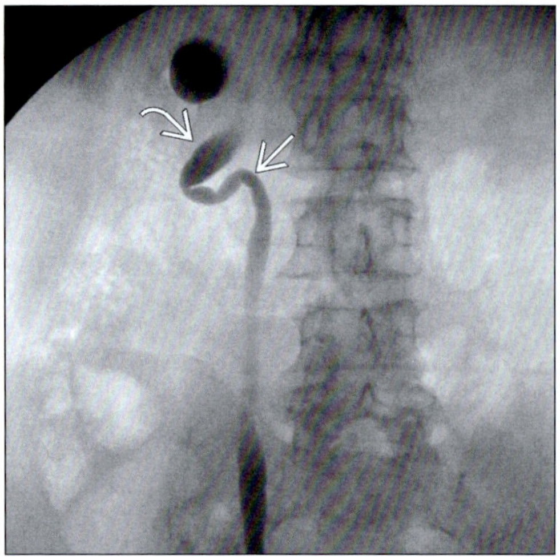

Oblique frontal image of a right retrograde pyelogram demonstrates a medial course of the right ureter with an S or fishhook shape ➔ and mild dilation of the proximal ureter ➔.

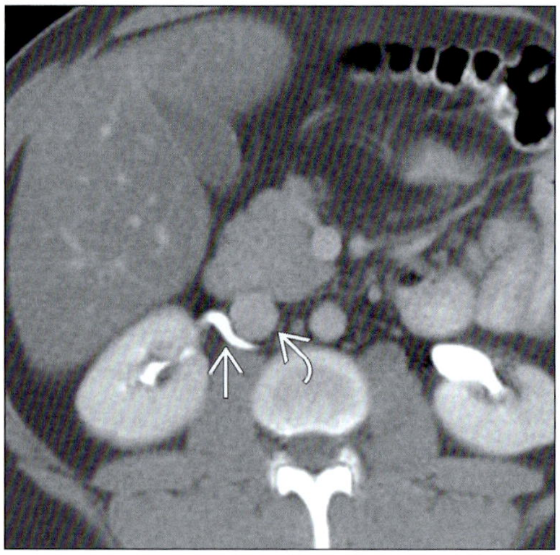

Axial CECT in delayed phase demonstrates the right ureter ➔ coursing posterior to the inferior vena ➔.

CLINICAL SCENARIO

History

- 40-year-old woman with right flank pain

IMAGE INTERPRETATION

Classic Sign

- Fishhook or S-shaped course of proximal ureter is characteristic of retrocaval ureter

BACKGROUND

General

- Type of primary inferior vena cava congenital anomaly that results in right proximal ureter coursing posterior to IVC
- Commonly associated with dilatation of right proximal ureter and right renal collecting system
- Appears as fishhook sign of proximal ureter on frontal radiograph of IVU and coronal CT urogram (CTU)

Epidemiology

- Incidence: 1/1,500 individuals
- Autopsy shows male preponderance
- Typically involves right ureter unless there is a situs inversus or duplicated IVC
- If symptoms arise, they usually occur in 3rd and 4th decades due to hydronephrosis, calculi, or pyelonephritis

Relevant Physiology

- Medial deviation of ureter with compression of IVC may result in hydronephrosis secondary to compression of ureter against psoas muscle
- Other reasons for hydronephrosis include kinking of ureter or adynamic segment of ureter

Relevant Embryology

- Condition is thought to be due to an anomaly related to development of IVC rather than ureter
- Right supracardinal venous system fails to develop while right posterior cardinal vein develops normally

Treatment

- Surgery is indicated for symptomatic patients
  - ○ Relocation of ureter anterior to IVC
- Asymptomatic patients can be followed-up to monitor for complications such as calculi or infection

IMAGING FEATURES

US

- Dilated renal collecting system and proximal right ureter, which may be mistaken for ureteropelvic junction obstruction on ultrasound

CT

- Right proximal ureter courses posterior to IVC and emerges to right of aorta
- Dilation of proximal ureter and collecting system
- Findings of secondary complications such as calculi or pyelonephritis of right kidney

MR

- MR urography shows similar findings to CTU with retrocaval course of right ureter & dilation of proximal ureter collecting system

Renal Scintigraphy

- Tc-99m-labeled agents may show a fishhook- or J-shaped dilated ureter, dilated collecting system, and urinary stasis

RELATED REFERENCES

1. Lee S et al: Retrocaval ureter. Kidney Int. 70(4):615, 2006
2. Salonia A et al: Diagnosis and Treatment of the Circumcaval Ureter. European Urology. 5: 449-462, 2006
3. Uthappa MC et al: Case report: retrocaval ureter: MR appearances. Br J Radiol. 75(890):177-9, 2002
4. Bass JE et al: Spectrum of congenital anomalies of the inferior vena cava: cross-sectional imaging findings. Radiographics. 20(3):639-52, 2000

STRETCH URETHRAL INJURY

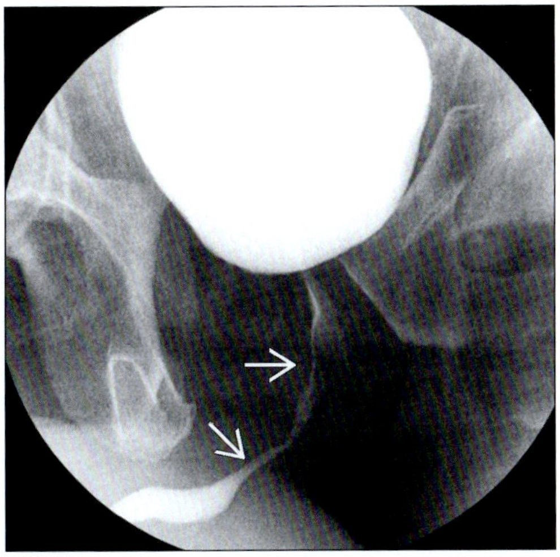

Retrograde urethrogram shows intact but stretched membranous urethra ➡, which exceeds the normal length of 1 cm. Note the upward displacement of bladder neck due to disruption of puboprostatic ligaments.

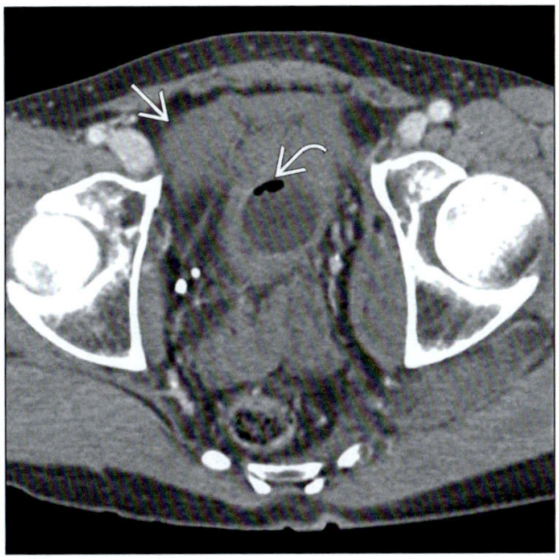

Axial NECT demonstrates hematoma anterior to the urinary bladder ➡. Air ➡ is also noted within the urinary bladder lumen.

CLINICAL SCENARIO

History

- 36-year-old man presenting after fall from 2-story building

IMAGE INTERPRETATION

Classic Sign

- Stretch urethra is indicative of type I injury
  - Intact but stretched and elongated posterior urethra (hence, can be misinterpreted as normal)
  - Bladder neck and prostate are displaced superiorly

BACKGROUND

General

- Urethral injuries are divided into anterior urethral injuries (those involving bulbous and penile urethra) and posterior urethral injuries (those involving membranous and prostatic urethra)
- Anterior urethral injuries are often caused by straddle pelvic injuries and are often isolated
- Posterior urethral injuries are caused by crushing force to pelvis (commonly associated with other organ injuries)
- Clinical signs: Blood at urethral meatus, high-riding prostate at digital rectal examination, and inability to void are not completely sensitive or specific
- Urethral injuries are subdivided into 5 types
  - Type I: Posterior urethra is stretched and elongated but intact, with prostate and bladder apex displaced superiorly due to disruption of puboprostatic ligaments and resulting hematoma
  - Type II: Disruption of urethra occurs above urogenital diaphragm (UGD) in prostatic segment, with intact membranous urethra
  - Type III (most common): Membranous urethra is disrupted with extension of injury to proximal bulbous urethra &/or disruption of UGD
  - Type IV: Bladder neck injury with extension into proximal urethra
    - Type IVa: Injury of bladder base with periurethral extravasation simulating true type IV
  - Type V: Partial or complete anterior urethral injury

Epidemiology

- Posterior urethral injury or bladder rupture is seen in 20% of major pelvic ring disruptions
- Prevalence of urethral injuries in males with pelvic fractures is 24% (6% in women)

Relevant Anatomy

- Male urethra is divided into 4 sections: Prostatic, membranous, bulbous, and penile
  - Posterior urethra: Prostatic and membranous
  - Anterior urethra: Bulbous and penile

IMAGING FEATURES

Retrograde Urethrogram

- Imaging modality of choice
- Posterior urethra is stretched and elongated but intact
- Prostate & bladder apex are displaced superiorly due to disruption of puboprostatic ligaments & hematoma

CT

- Intact stretched urethra
- Associated findings include distortion of prostatic contour and obscuration of preprostatic fat space by hematoma (constellation of findings could be explained by disruption of puboprostatic ligaments, which run in preprostatic fat space)

RELATED REFERENCES

1. Myers JB et al: Management of posterior urethral disruption injuries. Nat Clin Pract Urol. 6(3):154-63, 2009
2. Kawashima A et al: Imaging of urethral disease: a pictorial review. Radiographics. 24 Suppl 1:S195-216, 2004
3. Ali M et al: CT signs of urethral injury. Radiographics. 23(4):951-63; discussion 963-6, 2003

FAT-FLUID LEVEL IN URINARY BLADDER

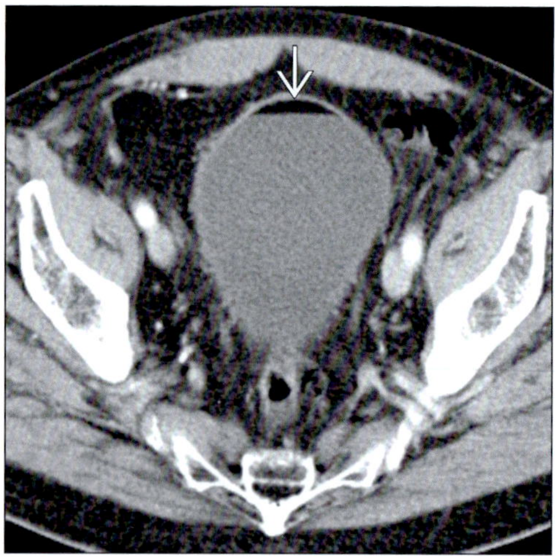

Axial CECT shows low-attenuation material ➡ layering on top of urine, simulating air-fluid level.

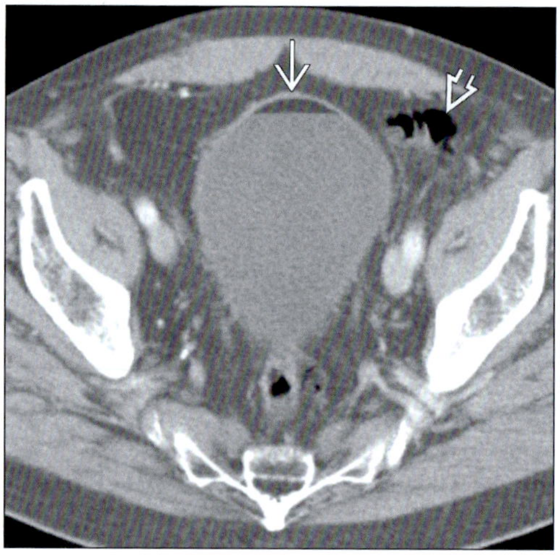

Axial CECT (same image at a wider window setting) confirms the presence of fat ➡ due to chyluria. Compare the fat attenuation within the urinary bladder to air attenuation within bowel ➡.

CLINICAL SCENARIO

History

- 62-year-old man with history of prior thermal ablation of melanoma renal metastasis
  - Now presenting with milky urine

Relevant Laboratory Tests

- Microscopic urine analysis
  - Fatty globules turn orange with Sudan III stain

IMAGE INTERPRETATION

Pitfalls

- Fat-urine level can be dismissed as air within urinary bladder
  - As seen following bladder instrumentation or in patients with enterovesical fistula

Actual Diagnosis

- Chyluria

Clues to Correct Diagnosis

- Using wide window setting can differentiate between fat and gas within urinary bladder
- Measures fat attenuation

BACKGROUND

General

- Tropical or parasitic chyluria
  - Due to filariasis (infestation of *Wuchereria bancrofti*)
    - Can manifest with chyluria, elephantiasis, chylous ascites, or chylothorax
    - ~ 120 million people are infected with filariasis in tropical and subtropical regions of Asia, Africa, Pacific islands, and South America
- Nontropical chyluria
  - Obstruction of thoracic duct (TD) or upper retroperitoneal lymph drainage due to surgical intervention, trauma, and various inflammatory or neoplastic processes
    - Obstruction of TD by masses such as aortic aneurysm or metastatic lymph nodes
  - Postoperative disruption of renal or bladder lymphatics → retrograde flow of chyle into kidneys and its urinary excretion
    - Occurs following partial or radical nephrectomy, radiofrequency ablation of renal tumors, renal transplantation, percutaneous nephrolithotomy, and partial cystectomy
    - May be self-limiting with spontaneous resolution
    - Persistent chyluria → malnutrition and immune deficiency due to chronic loss of lipids, proteins, and fat-soluble vitamins
  - Congenital or post-traumatic lymphorenal fistula
    - Lymphangiomas of kidneys and bladder
    - Renal angiomyolipomas

IMAGING FEATURES

CT

- Fat-fluid level within urinary bladder

MR

- Fat signal intensity floating on top of fluid signal intensity within the urinary bladder
- Can provide diagnostic information about source of chyluria

Lymphangiography or Lymphoscintigraphy

- May be used to determine site of chyle leakage

RELATED REFERENCES

1. Panchal VJ et al: Non-tropical chyluria: CT diagnosis. Abdom Imaging. 37(3):494-500, 2012
2. Miller FH et al: CT diagnosis of chyluria after partial nephrectomy. AJR Am J Roentgenol. 188(1):W25-8, 2007

GAS WITHIN URINARY BLADDER WALL

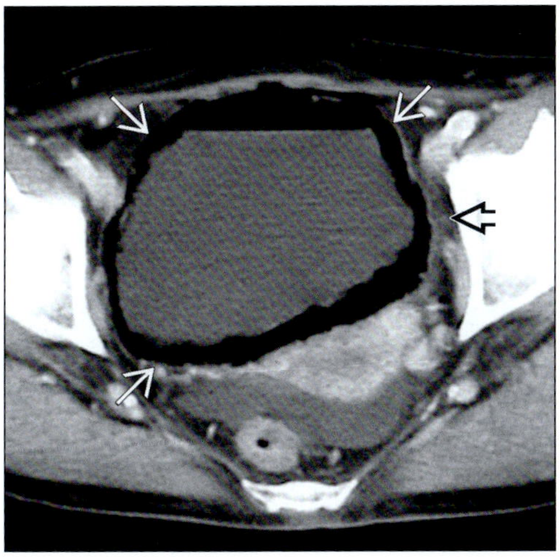

Axial CECT (soft tissue window) demonstrates gas attenuation ➡ within the thickened urinary bladder wall, associated with adjacent stranding ⇨ secondary to inflammation.

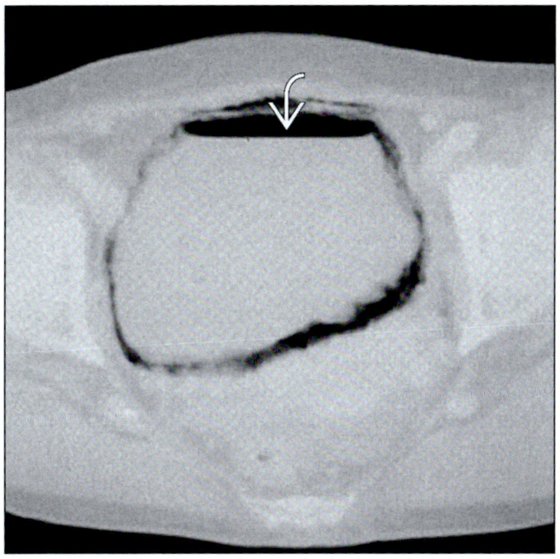

Axial CECT at the same level using lung windows confirms the low attenuation to be gas. Intravesicular air is also demonstrated more clearly on the lung windows with air-fluid level ↷.

CLINICAL SCENARIO

History

- 52-year-old neutropenic woman with acute myeloid leukemia presents with worsening abdominal pain

IMAGE INTERPRETATION

Classic Sign

- Gas within thickened bladder wall in setting of perivesical inflammatory change without demonstrable fistulous connection is classic for emphysematous cystitis

BACKGROUND

General

- Gas-forming infection of bladder wall
- Most common causative organisms: *Escherichia coli* followed by *Enterobacter aerogenes* (other organisms include *Klebsiella*, *Clostridia*, and *Candida* spp.)
- Variable clinical presentation: Dysuria, hematuria, and increasing urinary frequency
  - However, urinary symptoms may be absent and patients may present with nonspecific findings of nausea, abdominal pain, and fever
  - Pneumaturia is uncommon but more specific symptom
- Typically responds well to antibiotic therapy, glycemic control, and ensuring adequate urine drainage

Epidemiology

- F > M; typical age is 50 years and older
- Most common in patients with diabetes mellitus
- Other risk factors: Chronic urinary tract infections, bladder outlet obstruction, neurogenic bladder, alcoholic liver disease, and immunocompromised state

Relevant Physiology

- ↓ host defenses and urine stasis combined with ↑ urine glucose in those with diabetes facilitates infection of bladder
- Glucose and mixed acid fermentation by bacteria → gas formation

Relevant Pathology

- Gross: Mucosal gas-filled cystic blebs
- Microscopic: Empty cavities lined by flattened cells and separated by thin septa in lamina propria
  - Empty cavities range 0.5-3 mm in diameter

IMAGING FEATURES

Plain Radiograph

- Curvilinear or mottled lucency conforming to shape of urinary bladder separate from bowel gas

CT

- Highly sensitive allowing for early detection of intramural or intraluminal gas within bladder
- Bladder wall thickening may be seen
- Inflammatory change may surround bladder
- Excludes other sources of air within bladder, such as vesicovaginal or vesicoenteric fistulas

US

- May demonstrate irregular bladder wall thickening
- Bladder wall &/or lumen may have echogenic reflectors with posterior reverberation ring-down artifacts

RELATED REFERENCES

1. Eken A et al: Emphysematous cystitis: The role of CT imaging and appropriate treatment. Can Urol Assoc J. 7(11-12):E754-6, 2013
2. Grayson DE et al: Emphysematous infections of the abdomen and pelvis: a pictorial review. Radiographics. 22(3):543-61, 2002

MAIDEN WAIST DEFORMITY

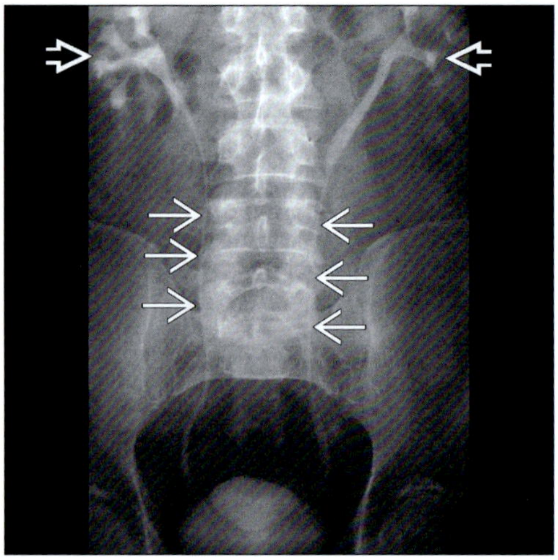

Frontal film of intravenous urography demonstrates narrowing, tapering, and medial deviation of the mid 1/3 of both ureters ➡, with prominence of the pelvicalyceal systems bilaterally ➡.

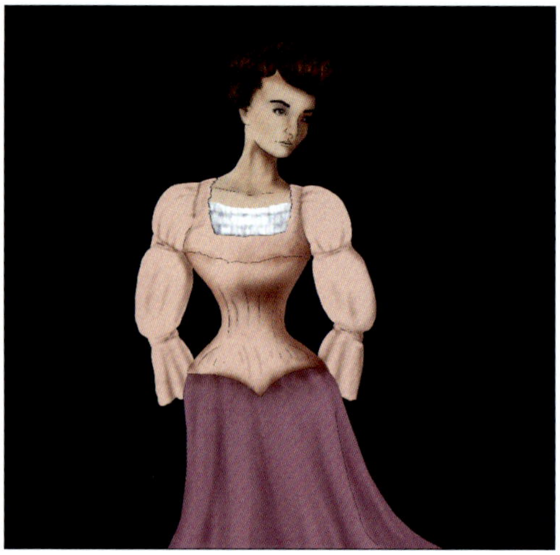

Illustration demonstrates the waistline created by 18th century corsets, which simulates appearance of ureters affected by retroperitoneal fibrosis which taper, narrow, and are drawn medially.

IMAGE INTERPRETATION

Maiden Waist Deformity

- Classic sign for retroperitoneal fibrosis (RPF)
- Seen on intravenous urography
  - Occurs when fibrotic plaque entangles both ureters and draws them medially → change in normal course and caliber of both ureters, which tapers and narrows (resembling a narrow-waisted maiden)

BACKGROUND

General

- RPF: Retroperitoneal fibroinflammatory tissue surrounding infrarenal aorta
- May envelop retroperitoneal structures, such as inferior vena cava (IVC), aorta, and often, ureters
- May also extend distally to surround iliac vessels
- Can obstruct ureters, leading to hydronephrosis, which results in poor renal function

Epidemiology

- 1.38:100,000 people

Etiology

- Idiopathic in majority of cases (70%)
  - Could relate to longstanding periaortic inflammation
  - Can surround abdominal aortic aneurysm
  - Can occur as part of IgG4-related disease
- Secondary to
  - Medications (e.g., β-blockers, methysergide, methyldopa), possibly by acting as haptens, leading to hypersensitivity or autoimmune reaction
  - Tumors (e.g., lymphoma, sarcoma, metastatic disease, and carcinoid tumor [2° to circulating serotonin])
  - Infections, such as tuberculosis and histoplasmosis
  - Post-radiation therapy
  - Trauma, hematoma, and abdominal surgery

Treatment

- Medical treatment with corticosteroid
- Surgery or ureteric stenting to relieve obstruction

IMAGING FEATURES

US

- Low sensitivity as retroperitoneal structures could be obscured by overlying bowel gas

Intravenous Urography

- Delayed excretion of contrast

CT

- Rind of soft tissue surrounding abdominal aorta (sparing posterior aspect)
  - As opposed to lymphoma, which extends posteriorly and elevates aorta from spine
- May extend
  - Laterally, to entangle ureters and surround IVC
  - Inferiorly, to surround iliac vessels
  - Superiorly, in perirenal tissue
- Degree of enhancement correlates with disease activity
  - Enhancement may decrease in response to treatment
- CT urogram delineates ureters in relation to RPF
- In secondary RPF, CT can demonstrate cause (e.g., primary malignancy)

MR

- T1WI: Low signal intensity
- T2WI: Increased signal intensity could correlate with disease activity (decrease in signal intensity may indicate response to treatment)
- MR urogram utilizing heavily T2WI could be used in evaluation of urinary tract in cases of poor renal function (where IV contrast cannot be administered)

RELATED REFERENCES

1. Caiafa RO et al: Retroperitoneal fibrosis: role of imaging in diagnosis and follow-up. Radiographics. 33(2):535-52, 2013
2. Scheel PJ Jr et al: Retroperitoneal fibrosis. Rheum Dis Clin North Am. 39(2):365-81, 2013
3. Dyer RB et al: Classic signs in uroradiology. Radiographics. 24 Suppl 1:S247-80, 2004

MAIDEN WAIST DEFORMITY

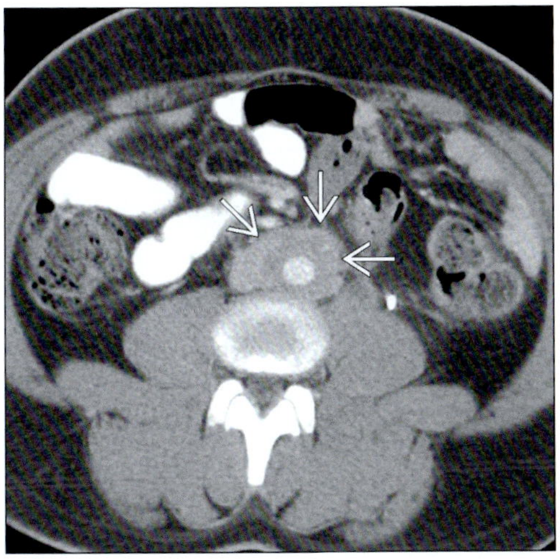

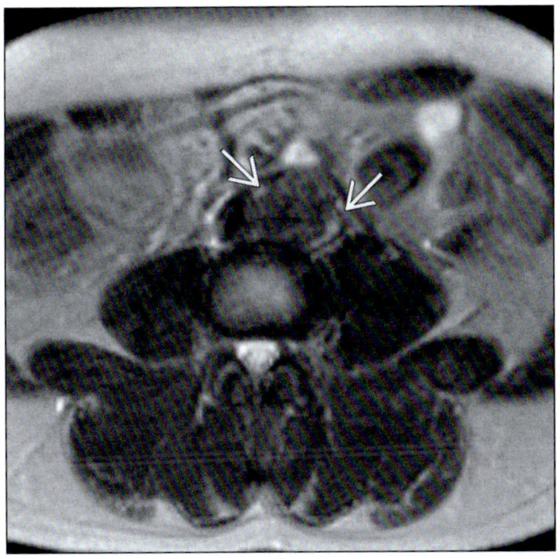

(Left) *Axial CECT demonstrates a rind of enhancing soft tissue attenuation* → *encircling the aorta and exhibiting homogeneous enhancement.* ***(Right)*** *Axial T2WI MR demonstrates slightly increased signal intensity of the periaortic mass* →*.*

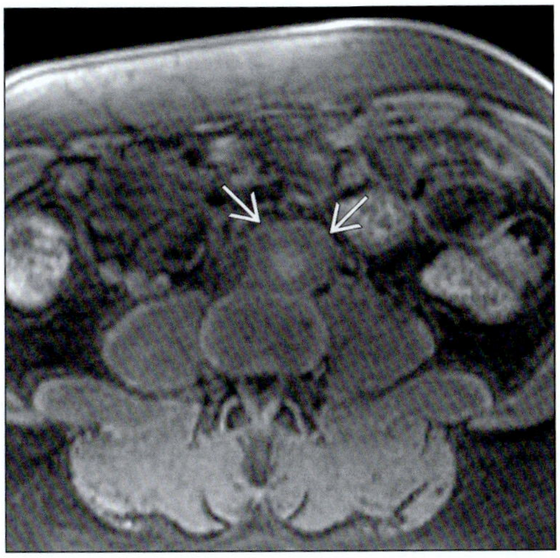

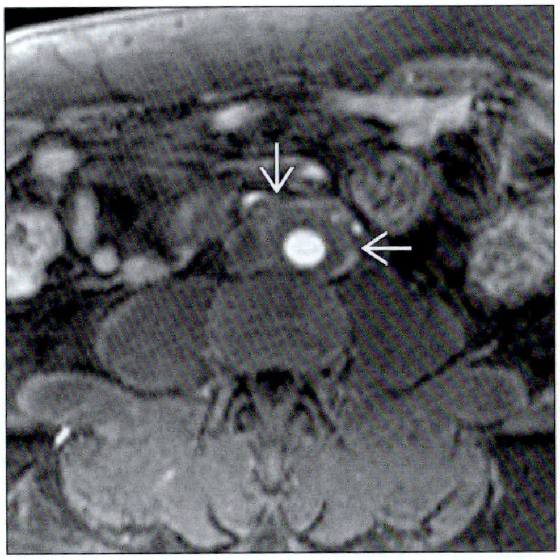

(Left) *Axial T1WI MR demonstrates the well-circumscribed periaortic mass* →*, which exhibits isointense signal.* ***(Right)*** *Axial T1WI C+ MR in arterial phase demonstrates homogeneous subtle enhancement of the well-circumscribed periaortic mass* →*.*

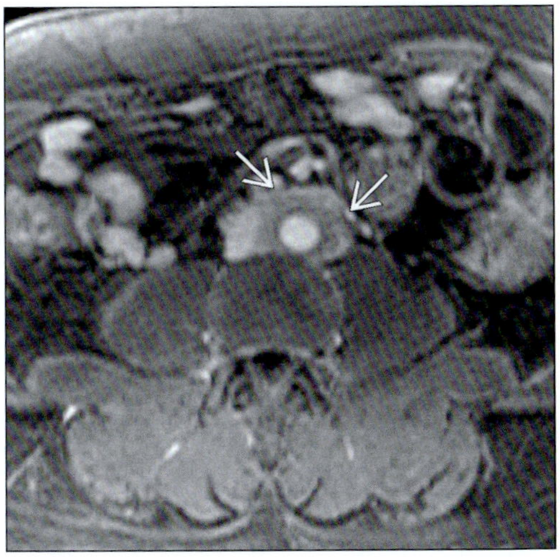

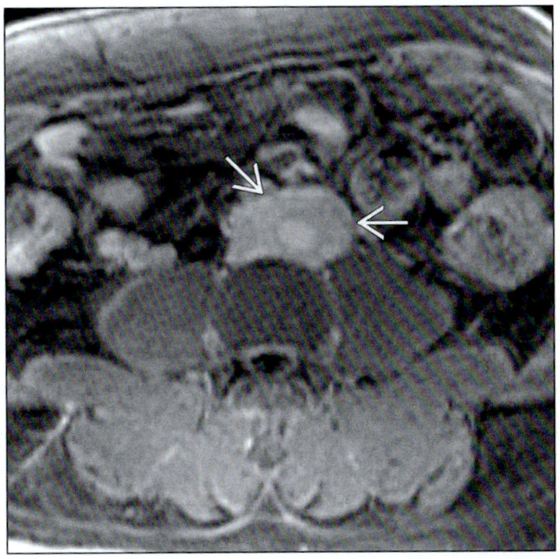

(Left) *Axial T1WI C+ MR in venous phase demonstrates homogeneous, progressive, increased enhancement of the retroperitoneal periaortic mass* →*.* ***(Right)*** *Axial T1WI C+ MR in delayed phase demonstrates increased progressive enhancement of the retroperitoneal mass* →*, most compatible with retroperitoneal fibrosis.*

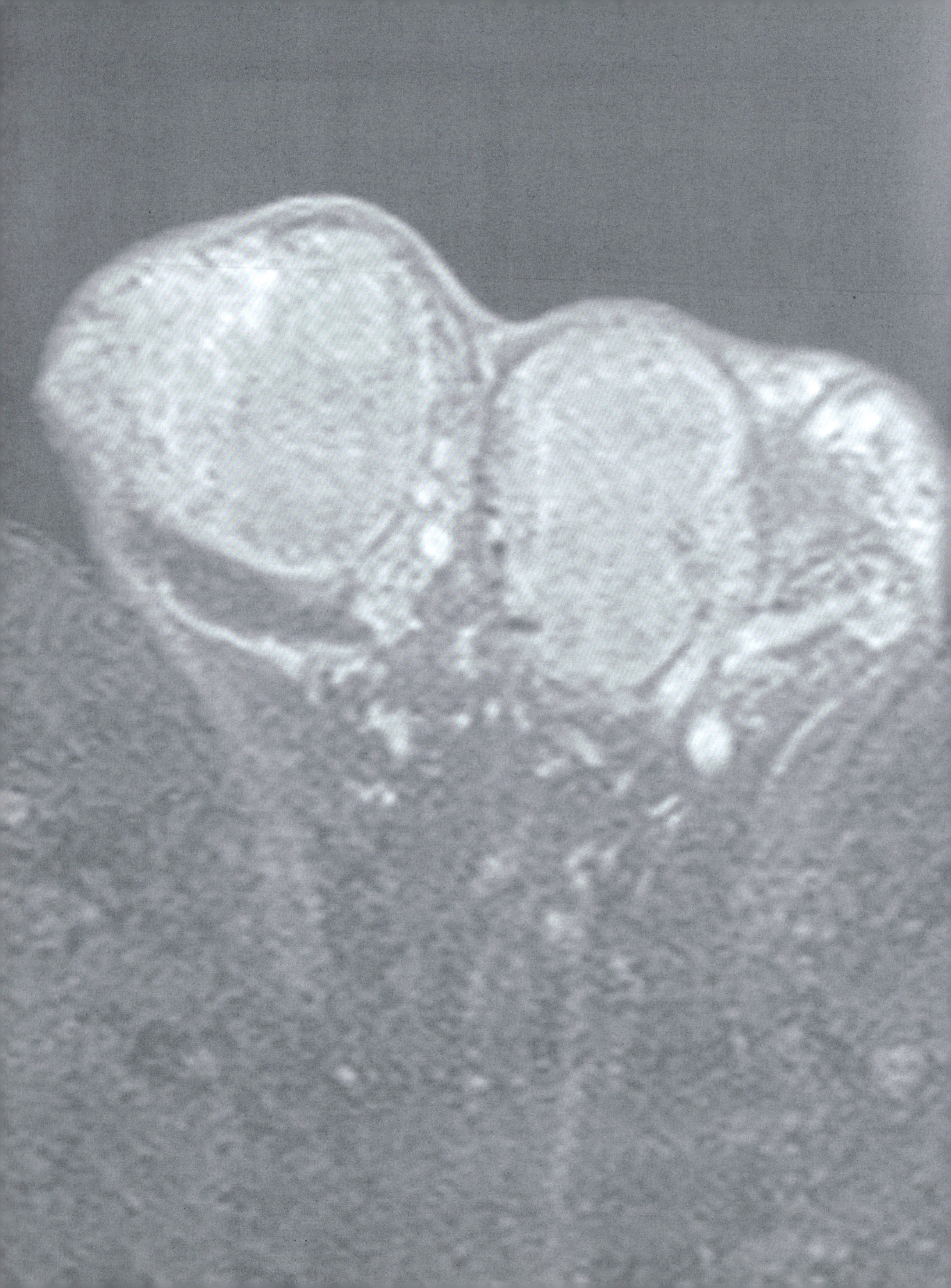

SECTION 10
Scrotum

Benign Lesions Simulating Malignancy

Malignant Lesions Mimicking Benign Conditions

TESTICULAR ADRENAL REST TUMORS

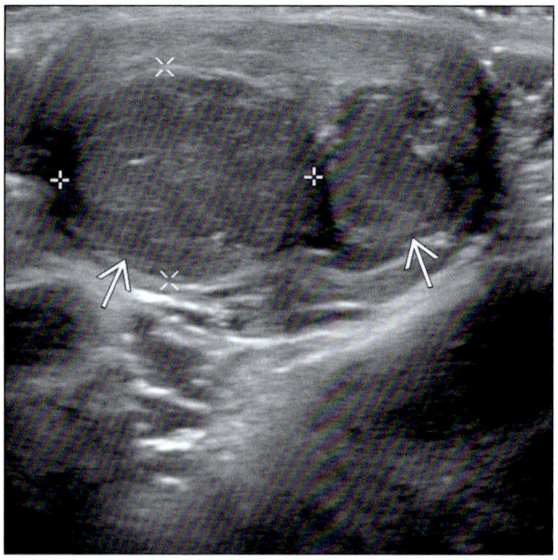

Scrotal ultrasound shows 2 testicular masses ➡. The masses are slightly heterogeneous, predominantly hypoechoic relative to testicular parenchyma. Similar masses were seen in the other testis.

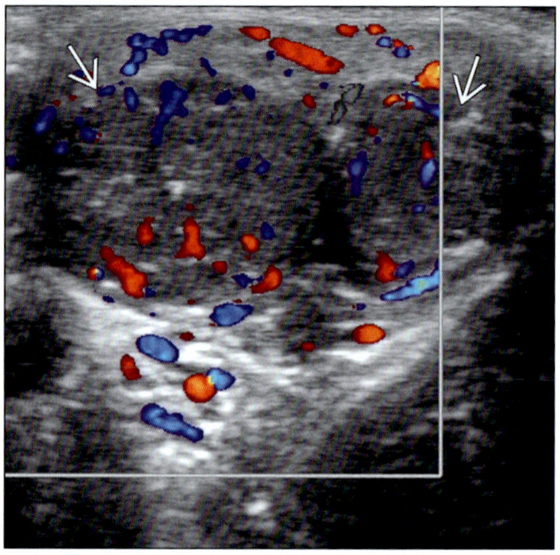

Scrotal color Doppler ultrasound shows 2 testicular hypoechoic masses ➡ with internal vascularity.

CLINICAL SCENARIO

History

- 26-year-old man with history of congenital adrenal hyperplasia presented with palpable testicular masses

IMAGE INTERPRETATION

Pitfalls

- Multiple testicular masses can be mistaken for testicular tumors such as metastases, lymphoma, or leukemia

Actual Diagnosis

- Adrenal rest tumors

Clues to Correct Diagnosis

- History of congenital adrenal hyperplasia
- Typical imaging features of bilateral multiple testicular masses
- Decreased size or complete resolution of lesions with therapy confirms diagnosis

BACKGROUND

General

- Congenital adrenal hyperplasia is an autosomal recessive disease characterized by deficiency of adrenocortical enzymes, notably 21-hydroxylase
  - Deficiency of adrenocortical enzyme (21-hydroxylase) → ↓ glucocorticoid synthesis → ↑ adrenocorticotrophic hormone (ACTH)
- ↑ ACTH levels → benign testicular tumor due to hyperplasia of adrenal remnants
- Embryologic origin of adrenal rests is still obscure
  - Testicular adrenal rests can normally be found in testis and surrounding tissues in 7.5-15% of neonates and 1.6% of adults
    - Usually < 5 mm in size

Epidemiology

- Most patients with congenital adrenal hyperplasia are diagnosed at birth or early adulthood
- Testicular adrenal rests have been reported in as many as 29% of patients
  - Most cases are bilateral

IMAGING FEATURES

US

- Typically involve mediastinum testis and do not distort shape of testis
- Both hypoechoic and hyperechoic nodules may be associated with acoustic shadowing
- Color Doppler US
  - Variable: Hypervascular, normovascular, or hypovascular
  - Although the adrenal rests may surround testicular vessels, they neither narrow the vessel nor change their course

MR

- T1WI: Isointense or hyperintense relative to normal testicular parenchyma
- T2WI: Hypointense relative to normal testicular parenchyma
  - Halo of low signal intensity surrounding lesions has been described
- T1WI C+ FS: Diffuse enhancement

RELATED REFERENCES

1. Fitoz S et al: Testicular adrenal rests in a patient with congenital adrenal hyperplasia: US and MRI features. Comput Med Imaging Graph. 30(8):465-8, 2006
2. Nagamine WH et al: Testicular adrenal rest tumors in a patient with congenital adrenal hyperplasia: sonographic and magnetic resonance imaging findings. J Ultrasound Med. 24(12):1717-20, 2005

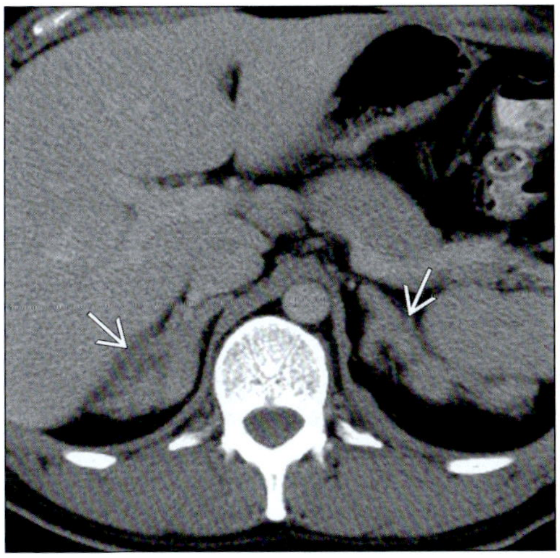

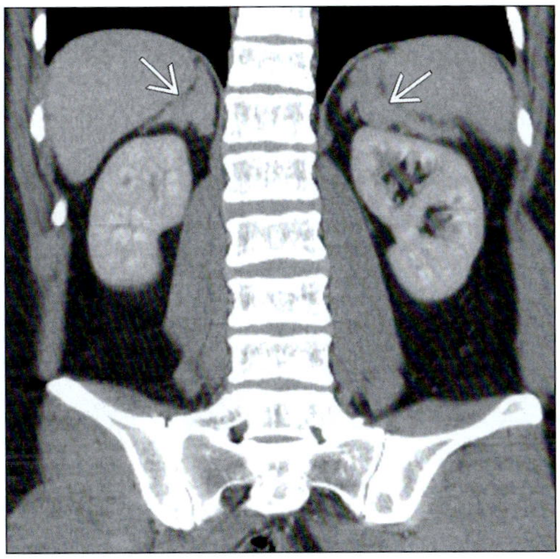

(Left) *Axial CECT in the same patient shows enlargement of both adrenal glands → with preservation of the normal adrenal shape.* ***(Right)*** *Coronal CECT in the same patient shows enlargement of both adrenal glands → with preservation of the normal adrenal shape.*

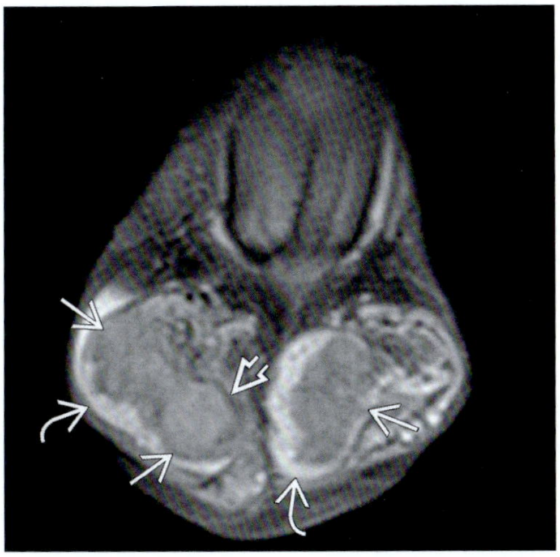

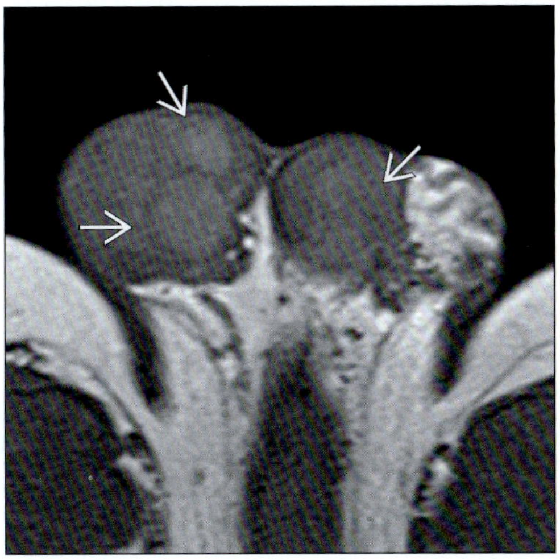

(Left) *Coronal T2WI in the same patient shows bilateral testicular masses →. The masses are hypointense relative to the normally bright testicular parenchyma ↷, stretched around the masses. A halo of low signal intensity ⇨ has been described around adrenal rests.* ***(Right)*** *Axial T1WI in the same patient shows bilateral testicular masses →. The masses are slightly hyperintense relative to the normally low signal intensity testicular parenchyma.*

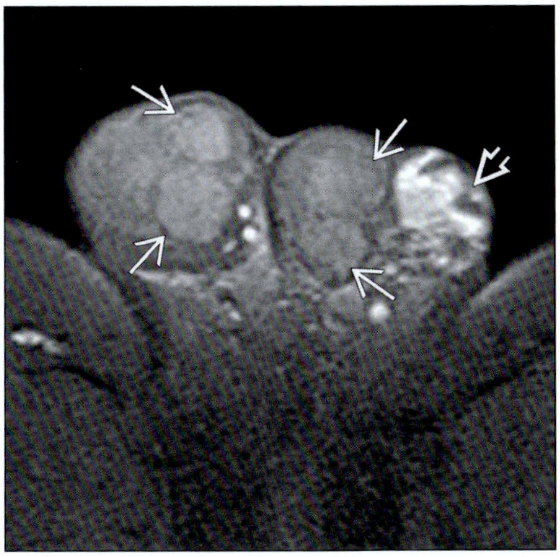

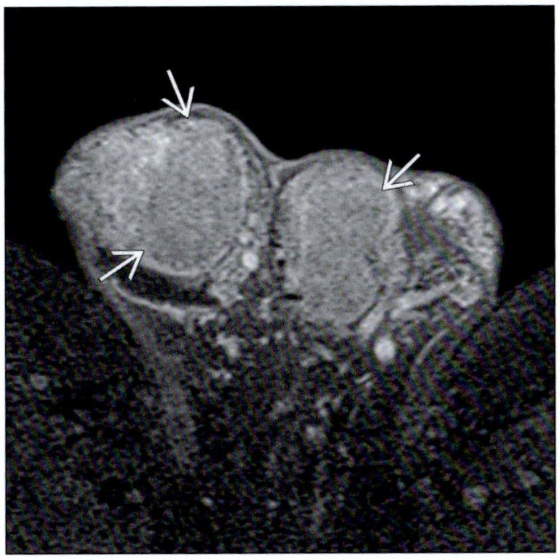

(Left) *Axial T1WI FS in the same patient shows multiple bilateral testicular masses → of slightly increased signal relative to the normally low signal intensity testicular parenchyma. The area of increased signal intensity ⇨ adjacent to the left testis represents fat due to incomplete fat suppression.* ***(Right)*** *Axial T1WI C+ FS in the same patient shows multiple bilateral testicular masses →. The masses show less enhancement relative to the normal testicular parenchyma.*

EPIDERMOID ONION RING SIGN

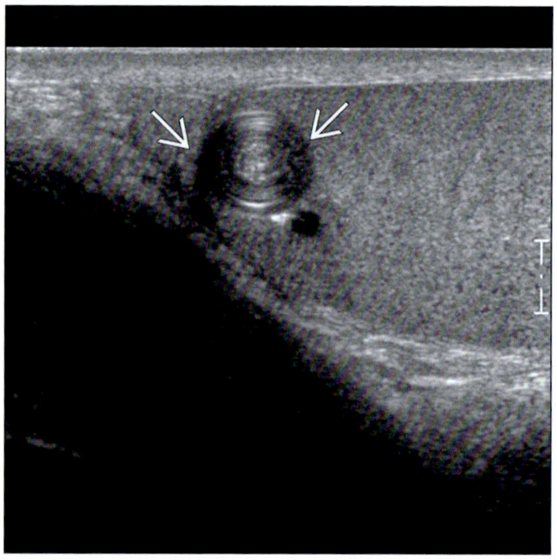

Longitudinal grayscale ultrasound examination of the scrotum demonstrates a well-circumscribed concentric laminated lesion, giving an onion ring appearance ➡ involving the upper pole of the left testicle.

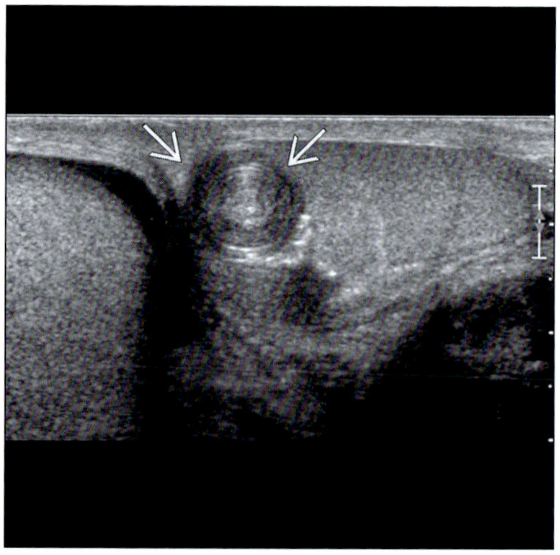

Transverse grayscale ultrasound examination of the scrotum shows the same lesion, giving an onion ring appearance ➡ involving the medial aspect of the left testicle.

CLINICAL SCENARIO

History

- 25-year-old man with nontender, palpable, firm left testicular mass
- No history of trauma

IMAGE INTERPRETATION

Appearance

- Onion ring sign is classic for testicular epidermoid cyst

BACKGROUND

General

- Benign lesion clinically indistinguishable from malignant testicular masses
- Typically present as smooth, firm, painless mass with mean diameter of 2-3 cm
- Normal surrounding testis

Epidemiology

- 1-2% of resected testicular tumors
- Most common benign testicular tumor
- Age: Most are in 2nd to 4th decades of life (range: 3-77 years)

Relevant Pathology

- Thick fibrous capsule filled with concentric rings of keratin debris
- Negative tumor markers (α-fetoprotein and β-human chorionic gonadotropin)
- Most acceptable current management is organ-preserving surgery (testis-sparing enucleation)

Relevant Embryology

- Metaplasia of seminiferous epithelium or rete testis is a suggested theory
- It has been reported that lesion represents monodermal development of a teratoma

IMAGING FEATURES

US

- Modality of choice for preoperative diagnosis
- Well-circumscribed intratesticular lesion with normal surrounding testis
- Usually surrounded by hypoechoic rim
- Typically, alternating hypoechoic and hyperechoic concentric rings (onion ring appearance) with echogenic peripheral rim
- Color Doppler US
  - Avascular

MR

- T1WI
  - Peripheral rim with low signal intensity
  - Alternating concentric rings of low and high signal intensity
- T2WI
  - Peripheral rim with low signal intensity
  - Alternating concentric rings of low and high signal intensity
- T1WI C+
  - No abnormal enhancement

RELATED REFERENCES

1. Arellano CM et al: Testicular epidermoid cysts in children: sonographic characteristics with pathological correlation. Pediatr Radiol. 41(6):683-9; quiz 796-7, 2011
2. Loya AG et al: Epidermoid cyst of the testis: radiologic-pathologic correlation. Radiographics. 24 Suppl 1:S243-6, 2004
3. Cho JH et al: Sonographic and MR imaging findings of testicular epidermoid cysts. AJR Am J Roentgenol. 178(3):743-8, 2002
4. Dogra VS et al: Testicular epidermoid cysts: sonographic features with histopathologic correlation. J Clin Ultrasound. 29(3):192-6, 2001
5. Langer JE et al: Epidermoid cysts of the testicle: sonographic and MR imaging features. AJR Am J Roentgenol. 173(5):1295-9, 1999

TUBULAR ECTASIA OF RETE TESTIS

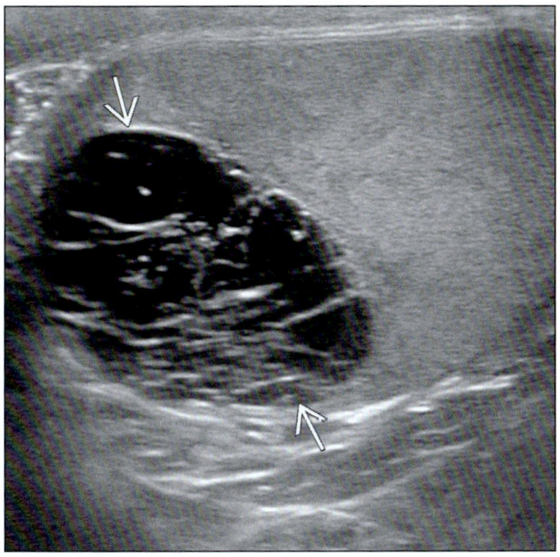

Scrotal ultrasound shows a multilocular cystic mass-like structure ➡ at the location of the mediastinum testis. A similar appearing lesion was present in the other testis.

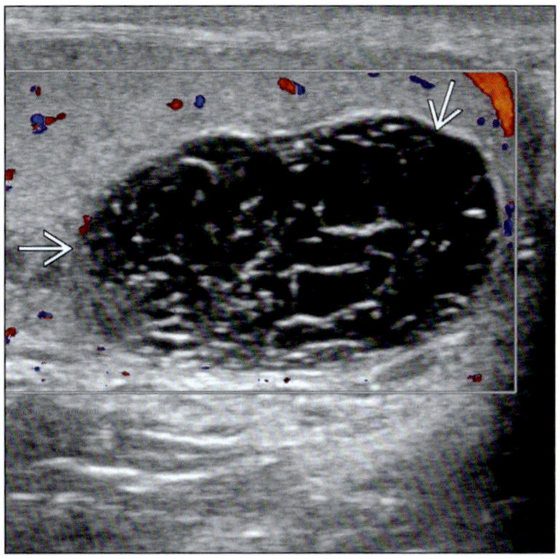

Scrotal color Doppler ultrasound shows a multilocular cystic mass ➡ without internal vascularity. Normal vascularity is seen in the surrounding testicular parenchyma.

CLINICAL SCENARIO

History
- 65-year-old man presenting with testicular discomfort

IMAGE INTERPRETATION

Pitfalls
- Can be misdiagnosed as cystic testicular neoplasm

Actual Diagnosis
- Tubular ectasia of rete testis

Clues to Correct Diagnosis
- Characteristic location
- Frequently bilateral
- Frequently accompanied with epididymal cysts

Key Teaching Point
- Should be recognized as benign entity and spare patient unnecessary orchiectomy

BACKGROUND

General
- Etiology
  - Results from conditions that cause epididymal or efferent duct obstruction
    - Vasectomy
    - Epididymal cysts or spermatoceles; testicular, epididymal or spermatic cord tumors
    - Longstanding epididymitis
    - Inguinal hernia repair

Epidemiology
- Usually in men > 55 years of age
- Bilateral in approximately 1/3 of cases; however, can be asymmetrical

Relevant Anatomy
- Rete testis is complex anastomosis of seminiferous tubules located in mediastinum testis
  - Drain via several efferent ductules, which open to form head of epididymis

Relevant Pathology
- Benign condition resulting from partial or complete obliteration of efferent ducts that cause ectasia of rete testis

IMAGING FEATURES

US
- Multilocular cystic and tubular structures in or adjacent to mediastinum testis
  - No internal flow on Doppler evaluation
- Individual cysts are usually small (< 3 mm) but can be large (> 7 mm)
- ± epididymal cysts

CT
- Focal area of decreased attenuation
- Difficult to discern internal architecture

MR
- Usually cystic and tubular structures of high signal intensity on T2WI and low signal intensity on T1WI
- May be difficult to identify on both T1- and T2WI because of similar signal intensity to that of normal testicular parenchyma
  - In this case, they are best appreciated on gadolinium-enhanced T1WI
    - Appear as tubular low signal intensity structures against background of enhancing testicular parenchyma

RELATED REFERENCES

1. Dieckmann KP et al: [Tubular ectasia of rete testis: a pitfall in ultrasonographic diagnostics of intratesticular cysts.] Urologe A. 50(1):57-63, 2011
2. Dogra VS et al: Sonography of the scrotum. Radiology. 227(1):18-36, 2003
3. Meyer DR et al: Pronounced cystic transformation of the Rete testis. MRI appearance. Invest Radiol. 34(9):600-3, 1999

SPERM GRANULOMA

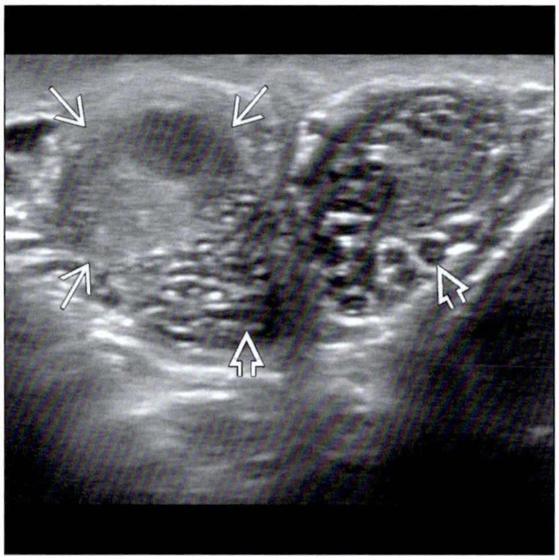

Scrotal ultrasound shows an epididymal head heterogeneous hypoechoic mass ➡. Note also the dilated tubular and cystic structures within the epididymal body ➡.

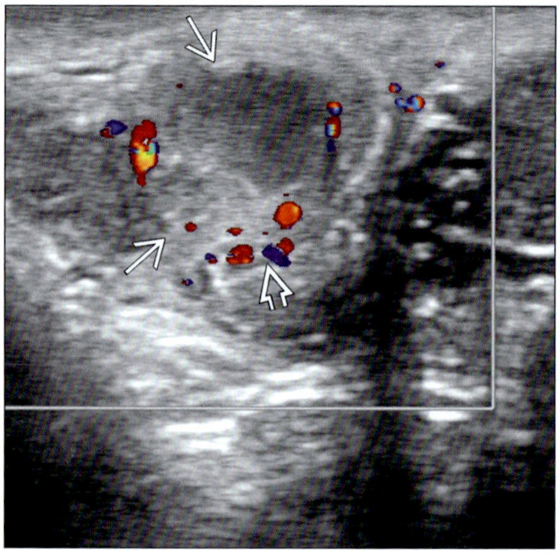

Scrotal color Doppler ultrasound shows an epididymal head heterogeneous hypoechoic mass ➡ with peripheral rim of increased vascularity ➡.

CLINICAL SCENARIO

History

- 45-year-old man with prior history of vasectomy presented with testicular discomfort

IMAGE INTERPRETATION

Pitfalls

- Epididymal lesion may be mistaken for neoplasm

Actual Diagnosis

- Sperm granuloma

Clues to Correct Diagnosis

- History of vasectomy
- May be bilateral and multiple
- May be associated with other sonographic features of vasectomy
- Since epididymal tumors are almost always benign, it is reasonable to follow-up epididymal lesion in postvasectomy patient

BACKGROUND

General

- ~ 50% of patients with spermatic granuloma after vasectomy are symptomatic, often with localized pain and scrotal mass
- Thought to represent chronic inflammatory response to extravasated sperm resulting from damaged tubules or obstructed vas deferens
  - Frequently seen within epididymis following vasectomy

Epidemiology

- Found in up to 42% of men who have undergone vasectomy and 2.5% of general population

Relevant Pathology

- Forms as foreign body giant cell reaction to extravasated sperm
- Histologically characterized by masses of sperm surrounded by epithelial cells and connective tissue
  - Lymphoid cells, lymphocytic debris, and granulomatous inflammation also are usually present
- Range in size from microscopic up to 4 cm, but most are < 1 cm

IMAGING FEATURES

US

- Well-circumscribed, hypoechoic, and heterogeneous lesions
- Can occur anywhere in ductal system
  - Most common at cut ends of vas deferens and can be multiple
- ± vascularity within mass on color Doppler images
- Other postvasectomy findings may be observed
  - Enlarged epididymides
  - Dilated tubular structures throughout epididymis
  - Punctate mobile echogenicities within dilated tubes (dancing filaria sign)
    - Occur in ~ 12% of men after vasectomy
    - May represent clumps of agglutinated sperm within dilated ducts

RELATED REFERENCES

1. Adejolu M et al: The "filarial dance" is not characteristic of filariasis: observations of "dancing megasperm" on high-resolution sonography in patients from nonendemic areas mimicking the filarial dance and a proposed mechanism for this phenomenon. J Ultrasound Med. 30(8):1145-50, 2011
2. Frates MC et al: Mobile echogenicities on scrotal sonography: is the finding associated with vasectomy? J Ultrasound Med. 30(10):1387-90, 2011
3. Woodward PJ et al: From the archives of the AFIP: extratesticular scrotal masses: radiologic-pathologic correlation. Radiographics. 23(1):215-40, 2003
4. Oh C et al: Sonographic demonstration, including color Doppler imaging, of recurrent sperm granuloma. J Ultrasound Med. 19(5):333-5, 2000

INTRATESTICULAR VARICOCELE

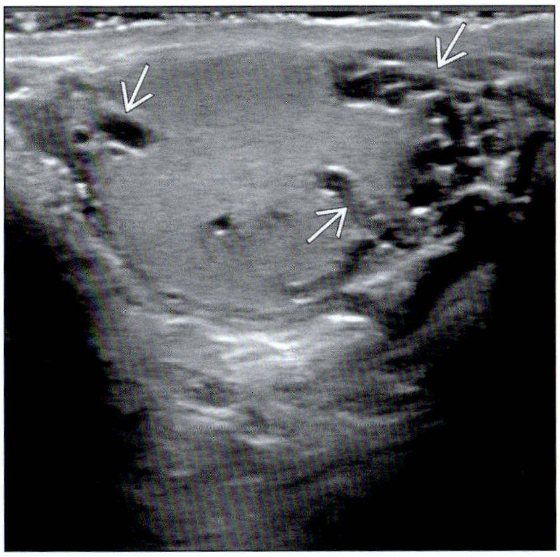

Longitudinal grayscale testicular ultrasound demonstrates anechoic subcapsular tubular and rounded structures ➔ *within the testis.*

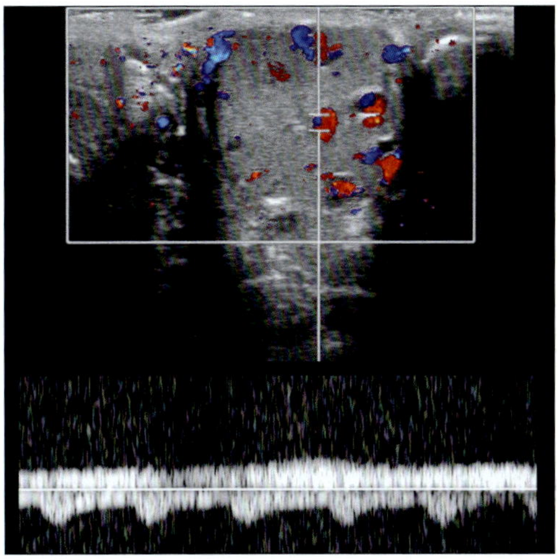

Longitudinal color Doppler testicular ultrasound shows the presence of tubular and rounded structures associated with a venous flow pattern. The amplitude increases with Valsalva maneuver.

CLINICAL SCENARIO

History

- 17-year-old boy presented with left testicular pain

IMAGE INTERPRETATION

Pitfalls

- Intratesticular varicoceles adjacent to mediastinum testis may mimic tubular ectasia of rete testis or cystic mass

Actual Diagnosis

- Intratesticular varicocele

Clues to Correct Diagnosis

- Color Doppler can confirm vascular nature of intratesticular varicocele and differentiate it from tubular ectasia

BACKGROUND

Epidemiology

- Rare and relatively new entity
- Reported in 0.9-2% of symptomatic men undergoing testicular sonography as opposed to extratesticular varicoceles, which are present in 15-20% of men
- Increased incidence in patients with prior orchiopexy

Relevant Anatomy

- Commonly unilateral
  - Most commonly left side
  - As with extratesticular varicocele, right-sided intratesticular varicocele should prompt evaluation for testicular venous obstruction
- Usually associated with extratesticular varicoceles
- Location may be subcapsular (under tunica albuginea) or adjacent to mediastinum testis

Relevant Physiology

- Patients with intratesticular component of varicocele have worsening asymmetry of testicular size and Doppler parameters, which ultimately requires surgical intervention
  - Presence of intratesticular component represents an unfavorable finding and can be regarded as indication for surgery
- Intratesticular component appears to be reversible following surgical treatment of varicocele

Clinical Features

- Testicular pain secondary to venous congestion → stretching of tunica albuginea
- Male infertility

IMAGING FEATURES

US

- Sonographic features of intratesticular varicoceles are similar to those of extratesticular varicoceles
- Grayscale sonography demonstrates tubular or serpentine structures > 2 mm in diameter with a positive Valsalva maneuver, confirming venous origin
- Involved testes may be smaller than contralateral side
- Color flow Doppler shows a characteristic venous spectral waveform
  - Retrograde blood flow, either spontaneously or during Valsalva maneuver
- Valsalva maneuver is very important as some vessels may not show spontaneous flow

RELATED REFERENCES

1. MacLachlan LS et al: Intratesticular varicoceles: are they significant? J Pediatr Urol. 9(6 Pt A):851-5, 2013
2. Bhatt S et al: Imaging of non-neoplastic intratesticular masses. Diagn Interv Radiol. 2011 Mar;17(1):52-63. Epub 2010 Jun 30. Review. Erratum in: Diagn Interv Radiol. 17(4):388, 2011
3. Bucci S et al: Intratesticular varicocele: evaluation using grey scale and color Doppler ultrasound. World J Urol. 26(1):87-9, 2008

BURNED-OUT TESTICULAR GERM CELL TUMOR

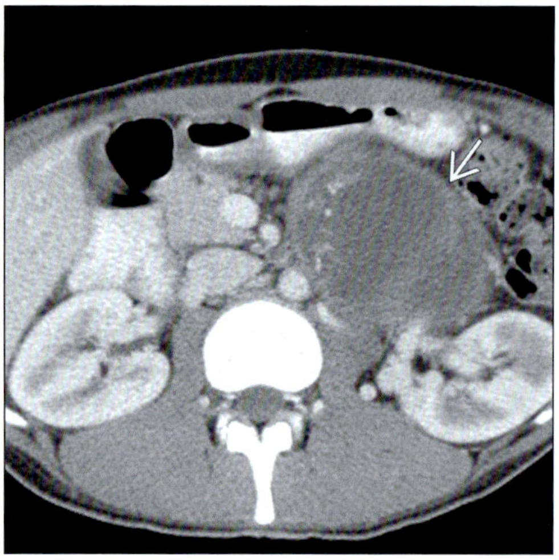

Axial CECT in a 24-year-old man shows a left paraaortic retroperitoneal mass ➔ containing calcifications. The mass was biopsied and showed yolk sac tumor.

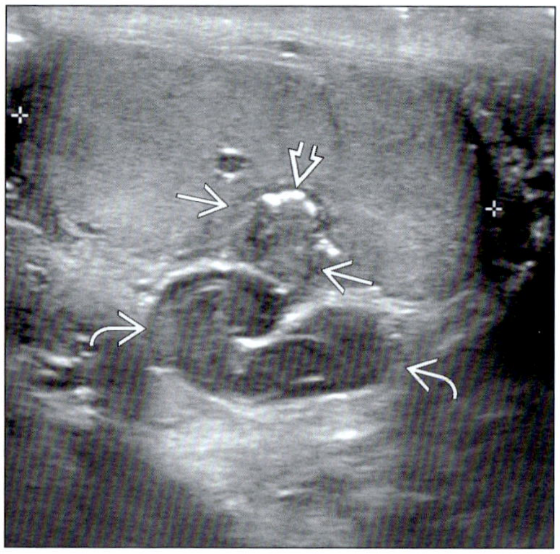

Sagittal testicular ultrasound shows a focal hypoechoic lesion ➔ with foci of ↑ echogenicity ⇨. Note also varicocele ↪ resulting from left testicular vein compression by the retroperitoneal mass.

CLINICAL SCENARIO

History

- 25-year-old man presenting with abdominal pain
- No palpable testicular mass on clinical examination

IMAGE INTERPRETATION

Pitfalls

- Presence of large retroperitoneal mass suggests presence of a primary retroperitoneal tumor
- Primary testicular tumor may be overlooked or dismissed because of its small, nonspecific appearance

Actual Diagnosis

- Burned-out testicular germ cell tumor (GCT) with retroperitoneal metastasis

Clues to Correct Diagnosis

- Primary extragonadal germ cell tumors are rare
- Biopsy-proven identification of a germ cell neoplasm in retroperitoneal, visceral, or mediastinal mass should prompt sonographic evaluation of testes in search of clinically unrecognized scar or mass

BACKGROUND

General

- Term burned-out tumor is used to describe a regressed testicular tumor that presents by its metastases
- Tumor is reduced to a fibrotic scar

Epidemiology

- ~ 2.5% of all testicular tumors
- May account for ~ 10% of "apparently" primary retroperitoneal germ cell tumors
- Mean age for discovery is 43 years, older than for testicular GCTs

Relevant Anatomy

- Metastatic sites include
  - Retroperitoneum, supraclavicular nodes, lungs, liver, and less commonly, bones

Relevant Pathology

- Macroscopic examination
  - Areas of testicular parenchymal scarring
- Microscopic examination
  - Intratubular germ cells or seminomatous foci
  - Sclerosis of seminiferous tubules and hyaline fibrosis in interstitium
  - Scar, which corresponds to a regressed GCT, has some features that distinguish it from the sequelae of trauma or infection
    - Hematoxyphilic bodies, hemosiderin pigmentation, and calcium phosphate deposits, indicating neoplasm and cell death

IMAGING FEATURES

US

- Sonographic features described include
  - Focal macrocalcification with posterior shadowing
  - Poorly circumscribed hypoechoic and hyperechoic areas
  - Microlithiasis in atrophic testis

MR

- Isointense to surrounding testicular parenchyma on unenhanced T1WI
- Hypointense band on T2WI
- Rapid and persistent enhancement on dynamic and delayed enhanced T1WI

RELATED REFERENCES

1. Patel MD et al: Sonographic and magnetic resonance imaging appearance of a burned-out testicular germ cell neoplasm. J Ultrasound Med. 26(1):143-6, 2007
2. Tasu JP et al: Imaging of burned-out testis tumor: five new cases and review of the literature. J Ultrasound Med. 22(5):515-21, 2003

SECTION 11
Female Pelvis

Technique-Related Pitfalls

Benign Conditions Simulating Malignancy

Benign Conditions Simulating Fibroid

Malignant Lesions Mimicking Benign Conditions

Treatment-Related Conditions Simulating Diseases

Vascular-Related Pitfalls

Cystic Lesions of Lower Female Urogenital Tract

Classic Signs and Appearances

PITFALLS OF SONOHYSTEROGRAPHY

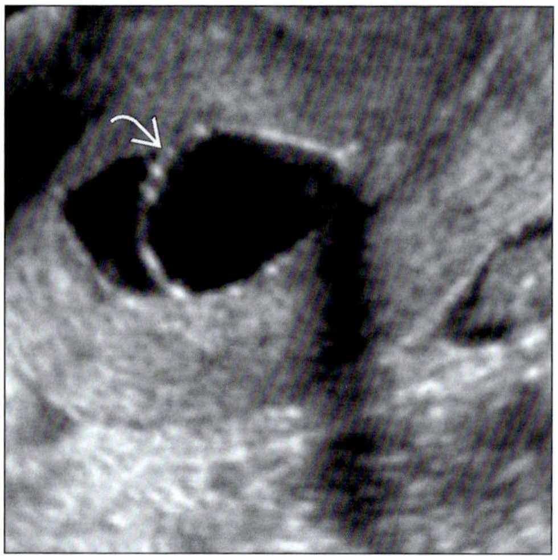

Longitudinal grayscale US shows hyperinflated balloon ➔ during sonohysterography. This is a common pitfall during sonohysterography, which may obscure underlying pathology.

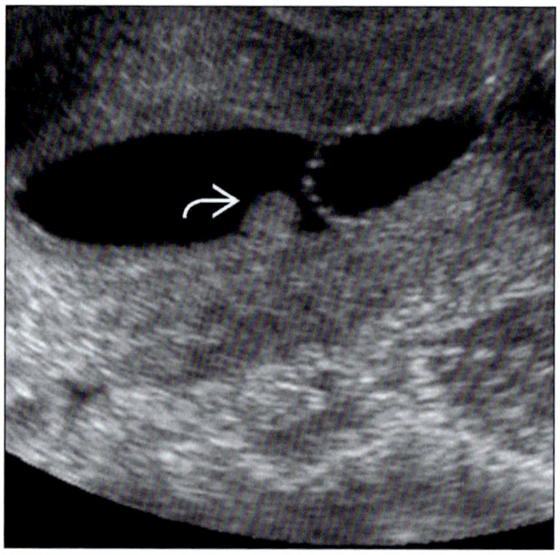

Longitudinal grayscale US shows a polyp ➔ that was initially obscured by balloon hyperinflation, subsequently revealed by deflating hyperinflated balloon to appropriate inflation level.

CLINICAL SCENARIO

History

- 40-year-old woman with irregular menstrual bleeding

IMAGE INTERPRETATION

Pitfalls

- Balloon hyperinflation is a common pitfall during sonohysterography (SHG), where it can obscure endometrial polyp

Clues to Correct Diagnosis

- Inflation of balloon to adequate level enables visualizing endometrial polyp

BACKGROUND

SHG

- Enables endometrial visualization by instilling saline into uterine cavity during transvaginal US

Indications of SHG

- Abnormal vaginal bleeding
  - In premenopausal women, SHG can differentiate anovulatory bleeding from anatomic lesion
  - In postmenopausal women, SHG can differentiate atrophy from anatomic lesions

TECHNIQUE

Technical Tips and Pitfalls

- SHG should be performed during follicular phase of cycle before day 10, when endometrium is thin
  - If performed during secretory phase, focal contour irregularities of endometrium may be mistaken for small polyps or focal areas of endometrial hyperplasia
- SHG catheter should be flushed with sterile saline prior to insertion to clear it of air
  - Air can cause echogenic artifact in uterine cavity
- Gently retract inflated balloon to occlude internal cervical os
  - If advanced too far into uterine cavity, → back flow of injected saline with nondistension of uterine cavity
- Catheter balloon tip is inflated 1-2 mL to help hold it in place
  - If balloon is hyperinflated, could obscure underlying pathology
- Proper visualization of endocervical canal often requires progressive collapse of balloon and fluid instillation into canal while catheter is slowly pulled back
  - If this step is not properly performed, underlying cervical pathology could be missed
- Other pitfalls can result from
  - Suboptimal visualization of endometrium due to improper distention of uterine cavity
  - Variable uterine position represents a common difficulty during procedure, making catheter insertion difficult
  - Cervical stenosis may require cervical dilatation or even use of guidewire
  - Blood clots can mimic endometrial masses
    - Blood products are usually mobile and may be displaced with brisk saline injection
  - Intrauterine synechiae may limit distention of uterine cavity

RELATED REFERENCES

1. Yang T et al: Sonohysterography: Principles, technique and role in diagnosis of endometrial pathology. World J Radiol. 5(3):81-7, 2013
2. Allison SJ et al: saline-infused sonohysterography: tips for achieving greater success. Radiographics. 31(7):1991-2004, 2011

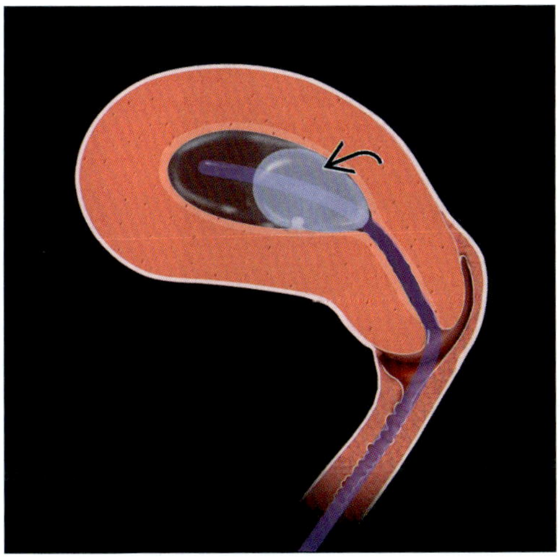

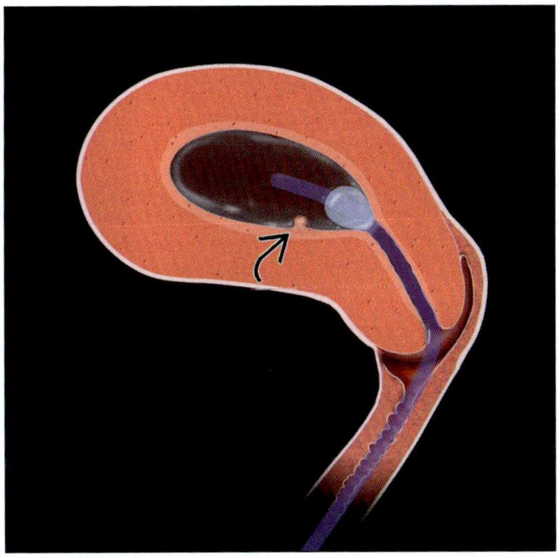

(Left) *Graphic shows balloon hyperinflation, which may obscure an underlying pathology. This could be overcome by correctly inflating the balloon to the appropriate level.* ***(Right)*** *Graphic shows a polyp that was initially obscured by balloon hyperinflation but is now revealed by deflating the hyperinflated balloon to appropriate inflation level.*

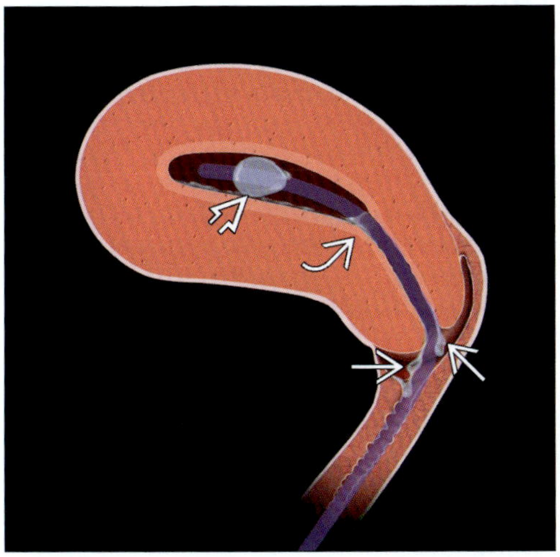

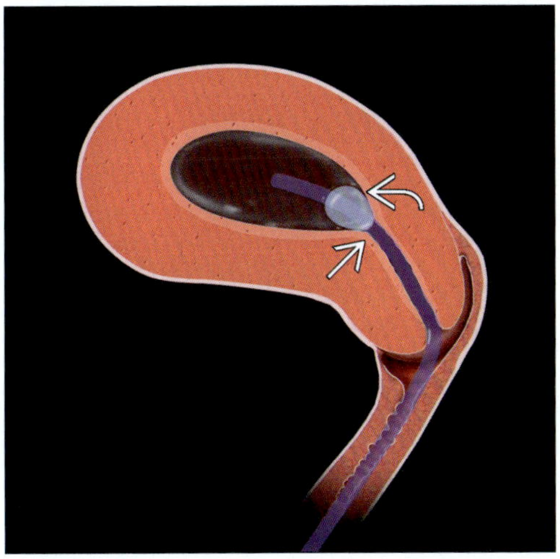

(Left) *Graphic shows backflow of saline. If the catheter is advanced too far into the uterine cavity, the balloon does not occlude the internal os. Fluid will leak out through the cervix with nondistension of the cavity.* ***(Right)*** *Graphic shows proper placement of the catheter balloon, which is gently retracted to occlude internal cervical os, allowing distension of the uterine cavity with the retained saline.*

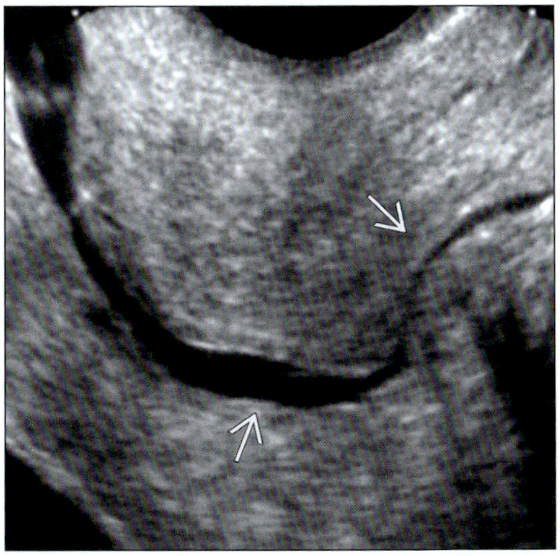

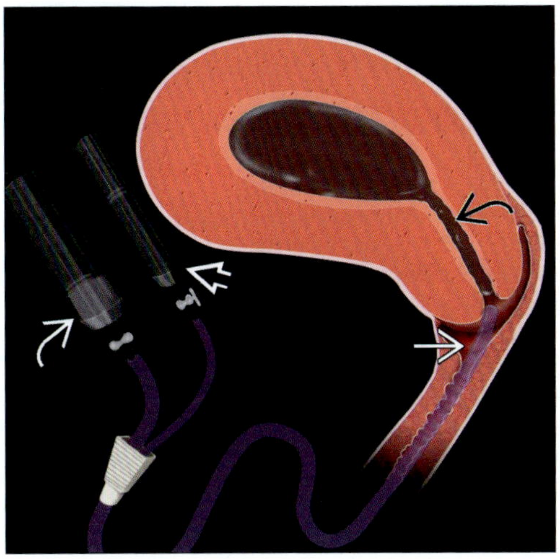

(Left) *Grayscale US during sonohysterography shows adequate distension of the endocervical canal. Inadequate distension of the canal may lead to missing pathology in this region.* ***(Right)*** *Graphic shows proper visualization of endocervical canal, which often requires progressive collapse of the balloon by slowly sucking air through the syringe and fluid instillation into the canal while the catheter is slowly pulled back.*

HSG: LARGE FIBROID MIMICKING UNICORNUATE UTERUS

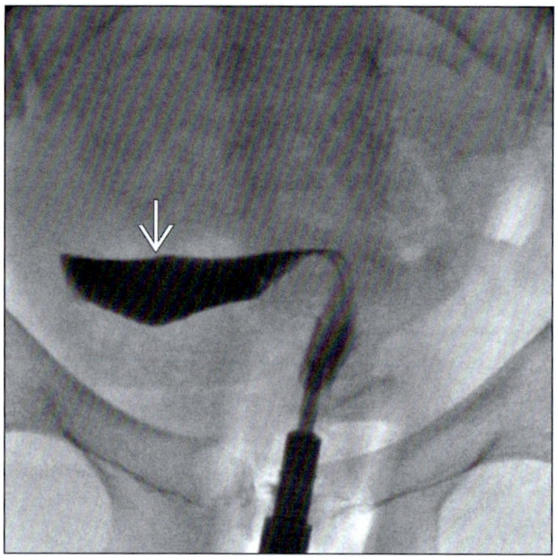

Hysterosalpingogram demonstrates deviation and flattening of the endometrial cavity to the right ➡ mimicking the appearance of a unicornuate uterus.

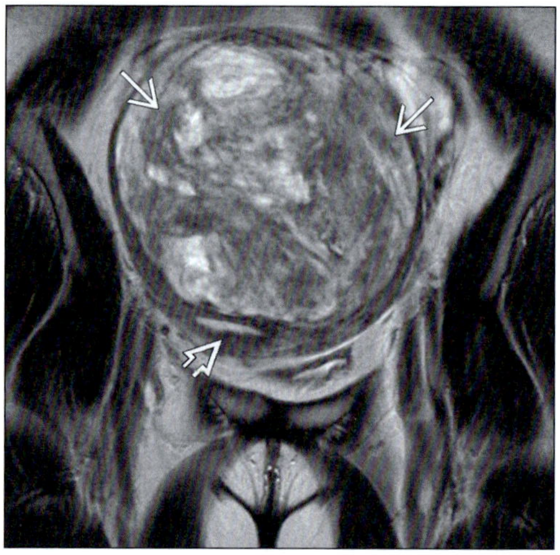

Coronal T2WI MR demonstrates a large mass ➡ with heterogeneous signal situated within the uterus exerting significant mass effect on the superior aspect of the endometrial cavity with flattened cavity ⇨.

CLINICAL SCENARIO

History

- 34-year-old woman with infertility

IMAGE INTERPRETATION

Pitfalls

- Mass effect from enlarged, degenerating fibroid can be misinterpreted as unicornuate uterus

Actual Diagnosis

- Large degenerating intramural fibroid blocking left fallopian tube

Clues to Correct Diagnosis

- Endometrial cavity does not taper at apex as with unicornuate uterus
- Mass effect seen on superior margin of endometrial cavity, giving somewhat flattened appearance

BACKGROUND

General

- Most common benign solid uterine neoplasm
- Can cause mass effect on endometrium and distort uterine contour
- Variable locations: Intramural, submucosal, subserosal, and pedunculated

Epidemiology

- Occurs in up to 25% of women of reproductive age
- Stimulated by estrogen exposure, enlarge during pregnancy, and involute at menopause

Relevant Pathophysiology

- Benign smooth muscle tumor
- Spindle-shaped smooth muscle cells
- Location often determines symptoms (e.g., submucosal most likely bleed and cause issues with fertility)
- May undergo hemorrhage, degeneration, atrophy, calcification, or fibrosis

IMAGING FEATURES

Hysterosalpingogram

- Submucosal fibroids → smooth filling defects in endometrial cavity (can mimic polyp)
- Large fibroids may distort and create mass effect on endometrial cavity

US

- Typically hypoechoic but can be iso- or hyperechoic
- Anechoic to mixed echogenic internal appearance in degenerating fibroids
- Calcified fibroids demonstrate echogenic appearance with shadowing

CT

- Usually difficult to differentiate from myometrium (isoattenuated) on noncontrast study
- Can cause contour abnormality of uterus or globular appearance
- Variable enhancement

MR

- T1WI: Intermediate to low signal compared to myometrium
- T2WI: Typically low signal to myometrium
  - Degenerating fibroids have variable but typically high signal (cystic degeneration → ↑ signal intensity and hyaline degeneration → ↓ signal)
- T1WI C+: Typically enhance, but degenerating fibroid exhibits less enhancement

RELATED REFERENCES

1. Nalaboff KM et al: Imaging the endometrium: disease and normal variants. Radiographics. 21(6):1409-24, 2001
2. Ueda H et al: Unusual appearances of uterine leiomyomas: MR imaging findings and their histopathologic backgrounds. Radiographics. 19 Spec No:S131-45, 1999
3. Weinreb JC et al: The value of MR imaging in distinguishing leiomyomas from other solid pelvic masses when sonography is indeterminate. AJR Am J Roentgenol. 154(2):295-9, 1990

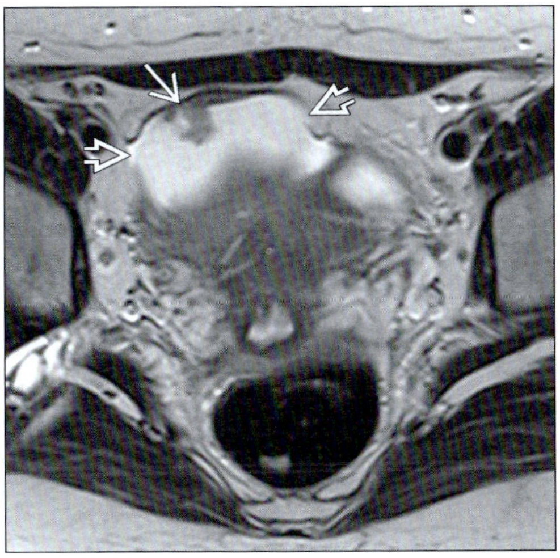

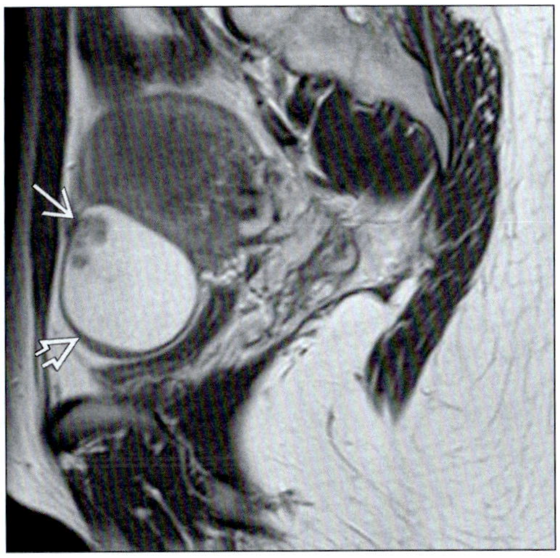

(Left) *Axial T2WI MR in the same patient obtained 4 weeks after delivery shows a right adnexal mass* ⇨ *of high signal intensity containing a small, slightly hyperintense (relative to pelvic skeletal muscles) lobular solid component* →. ***(Right)*** *Sagittal T2WI MR in the same patient shows a right adnexal mass* ⇨ *of high signal intensity containing a small, slightly hyperintense (relative to pelvic skeletal muscles) lobular solid component* →.

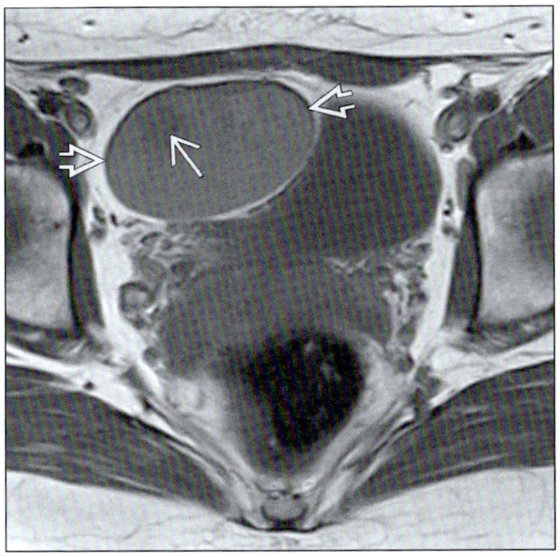

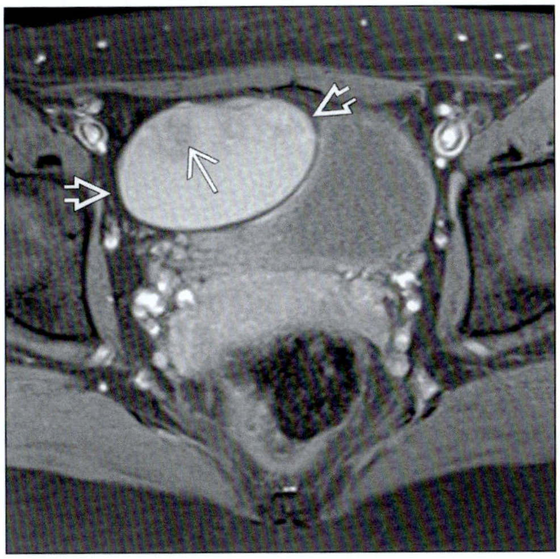

(Left) *Axial T1WI MR in the same patient shows a right adnexal mass* ⇨ *of slightly increased signal intensity containing a small isointense (relative to pelvic skeletal muscles) lobular solid component* →. ***(Right)*** *Axial T1WI FS MR in the same patient shows a right adnexal mass* ⇨ *of high signal intensity containing a small isointense (relative to pelvic skeletal muscles) lobular solid component* →.

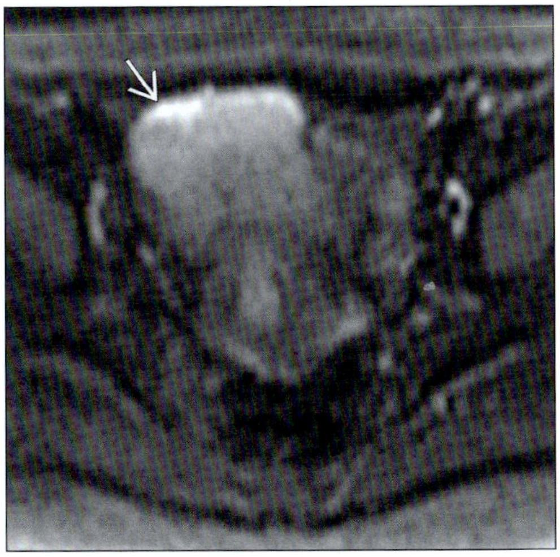

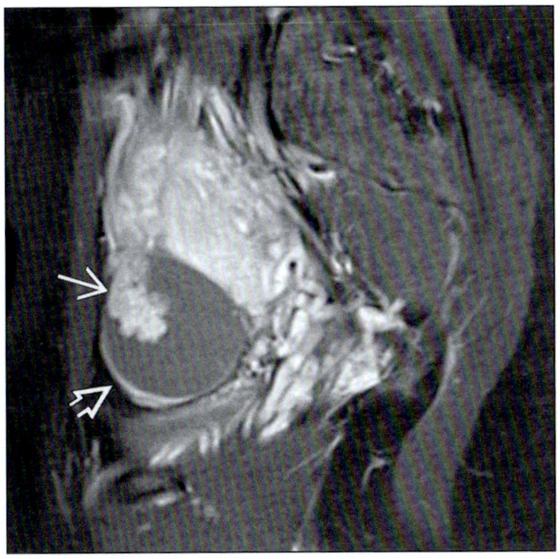

(Left) *Axial DWI b900 shows diffusion restriction of the focal solid component* → *within the cystic lesion.* ***(Right)*** *Sagittal T1WI C+ FS MR in the same patient shows a right adnexal mass* ⇨ *containing an enhancing lobular solid component* →. *Continuing follow-up revealed complete resolution of the solid component 3 months after delivery.*

APPENDICEAL MUCOCELE MIMICKING ADNEXAL MASS

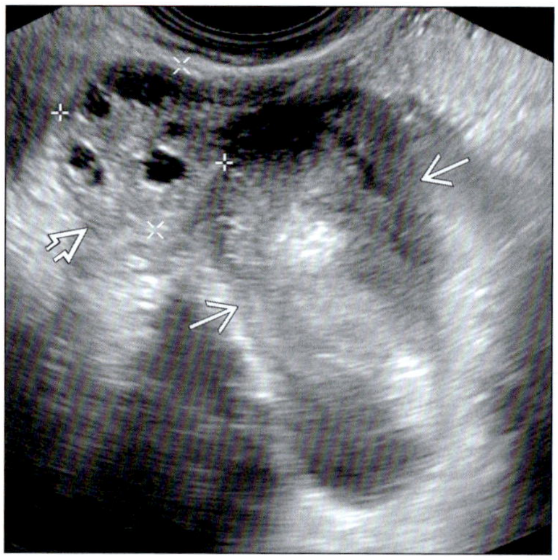

Axial transvaginal ultrasound shows a right adnexal heterogeneous lesion separate from the right ovary.

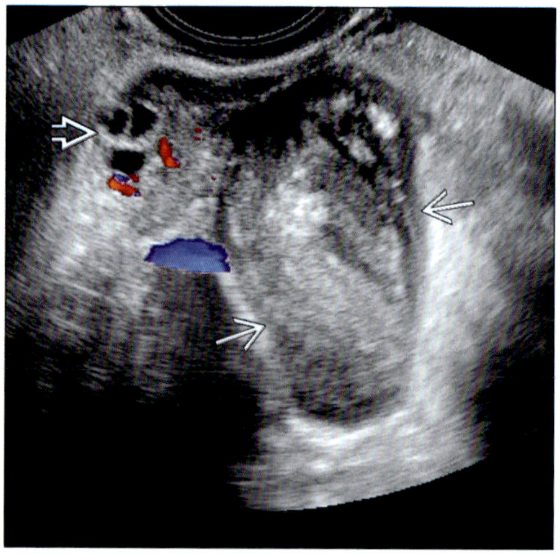

Axial transvaginal color Doppler ultrasound in the same patient shows a right adnexal lesion separate from the right ovary. There is no evidence of blood flow within the adnexal lesion.

CLINICAL SCENARIO

History

- 24-year-old woman presenting with pelvic pain

IMAGE INTERPRETATION

Pitfalls

- Elongated or tubular right adnexal structure may be mistaken for ovarian or tubal pathology

Actual Diagnosis

- Appendiceal mucocele

Clues to Correct Diagnosis

- Diagnosis may be difficult on ultrasound; however, should be considered whenever right adnexal tubular mass is found separate from ovary
- Can be differentiated from hydrosalpinx or pyosalpinx by absence of cog wheel sign
  - Cog wheel appearance of dilated fallopian tube when imaged in cross section is due to thickened longitudinal folds
- CT or MR can show tubular or funnel-shaped structure that can be traced to cecum

BACKGROUND

General

- Appendiceal dilatation due to abnormal mucus accumulation

Epidemiology

- 0.2-0.3% of all appendectomies
- Mean age is 54 years in benign conditions and 64 years in malignancy
- Female predominance (4:1-2:1)

Relevant Pathology

- Mucus is retained as a result of lumen obstruction or hyperproduction of mucus
- 4 different histologic subtypes of mucocele: Simple mucocele (18%), mucosal hyperplasia (20%), mucinous cystadenoma (52-84%), and mucinous cystadenocarcinoma (10-20%)

IMAGING FEATURES

Plain Radiography

- Curvilinear calcifications may be seen in right pelvis

US

- Echogenicity of mass depends on composition of mucus, thus leading to several sonographic patterns
  - Cyst with internal echoes and septa along with acoustic shadowing
  - Complex mass with acoustic enhancement
  - Cystic mass with layered walls and mural calcifications
  - Hypoechoic mass without posterior acoustic enhancement
    - Absence of posterior acoustic enhancement is due to attenuation of ultrasound beam by mucin
  - Onion skin sign
    - Layering mucin resulting from fluctuations in secretion and gelation of mucus in lumen

CT

- Tubular or spherical, well-circumscribed, thick-walled paracecal cystic mass ± mural calcification or internal septation

MR

- Cystic mass of low signal intensity on T1WI and high signal intensity on T2WI

RELATED REFERENCES

1. Papoutsis D et al: Mucocele of the vermiform appendix misdiagnosed as an adnexal mass on transvaginal sonography. J Clin Ultrasound. 40(8):522-5, 2012

APPENDICEAL MUCOCELE MIMICKING ADNEXAL MASS

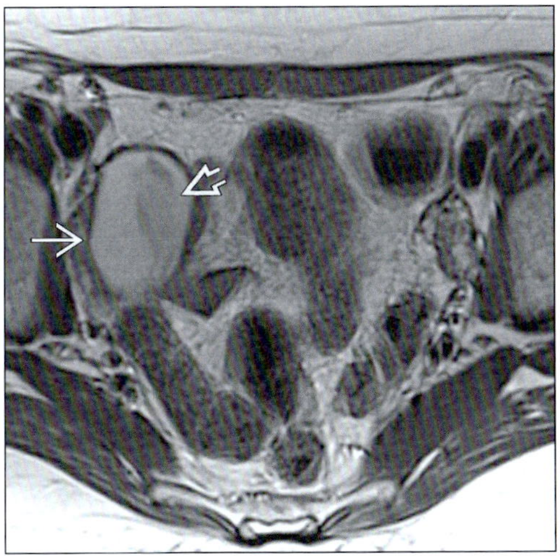

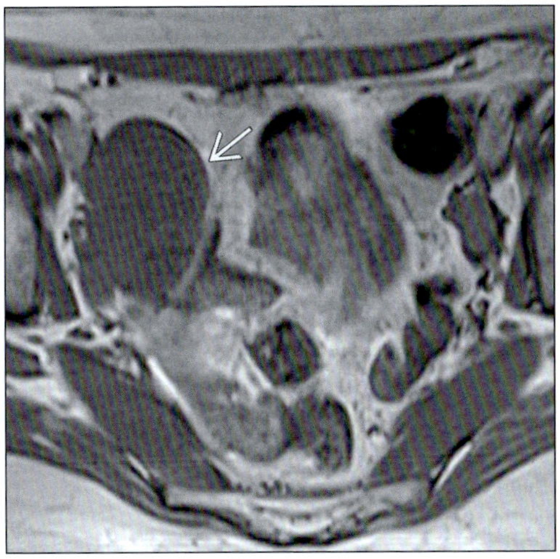

(Left) Axial T2WI MR in the same patient shows a right adnexal mass ➔ demonstrating predominantly high signal intensity. There is an area of heterogeneous signal intensity on the left side of the lesion ⇨. *(Right)* Axial T1WI MR in the same patient shows a right adnexal mass ➔ demonstrating signal intensity similar to pelvic skeletal muscles.

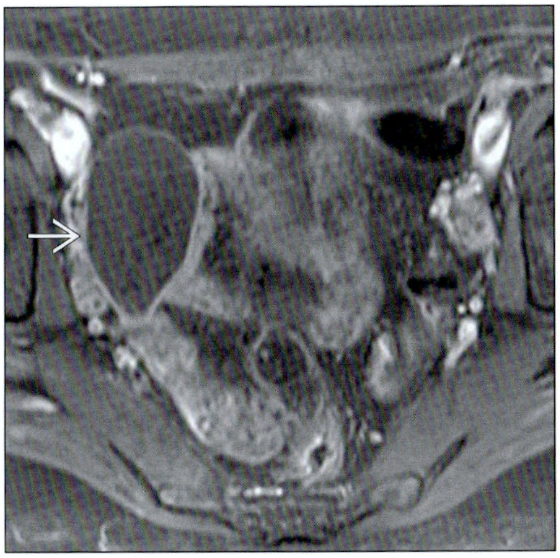

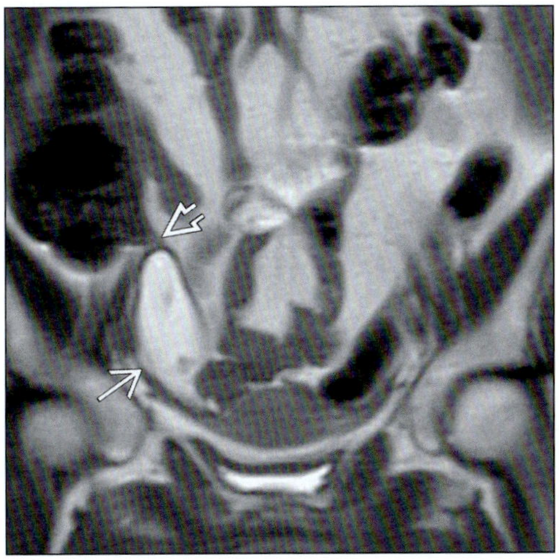

(Left) Axial T1WI C+ FS MR in the same patient shows a right adnexal mass ➔ demonstrating low signal intensity and uniform mild enhancement of the wall and no enhancement of the contents of the lesion. *(Right)* Coronal T2WI MR in the same patient shows a right adnexal mass ➔ demonstrating predominantly high signal intensity. The mass is attached to the cecum at the expected location of the appendix ⇨.

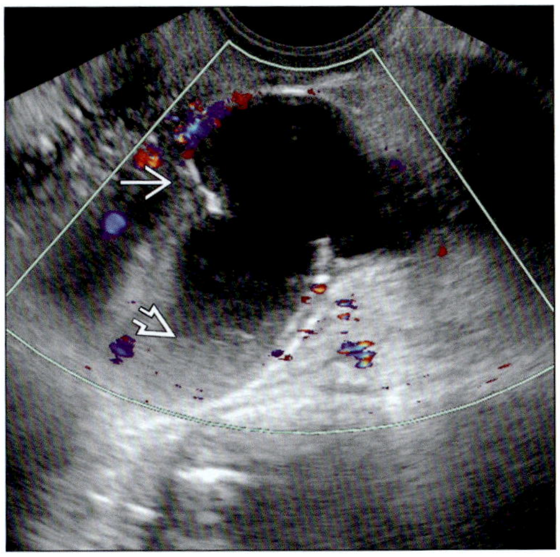

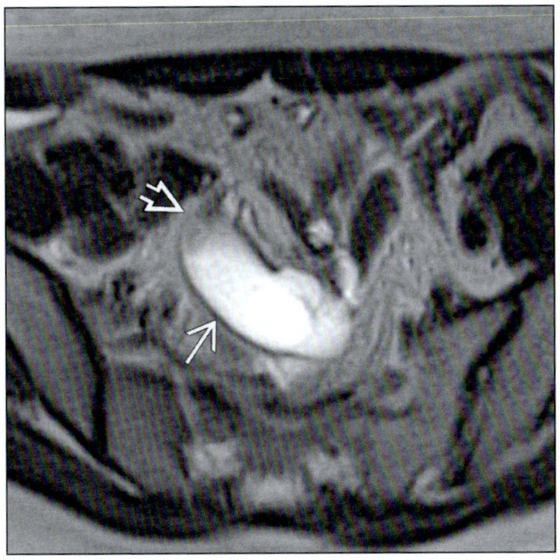

(Left) Axial transvaginal color Doppler ultrasound in a 33-year-old woman who presented with pelvic pain shows a midline pelvic lesion ➔ that is predominantly cystic with some layering debris ⇨. *(Right)* Axial T2WI MR in the same patient shows a midline pelvic tubular lesion ➔ demonstrating predominantly high signal intensity. The structure has a blunt tip ⇨ and is arising from the cecum, which is located deep within the pelvis.

ENDOMETRIOSIS MIMICKING CANCER

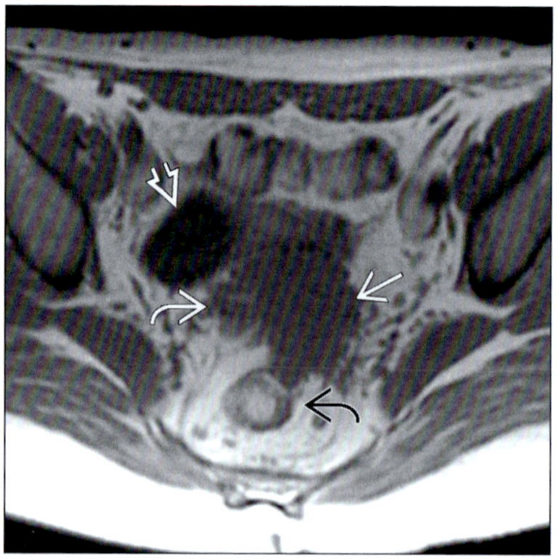

Axial T1WI MR shows an irregular low signal intensity mass ➔ in the left parametrium adjacent to the cervix ➔, abutting the rectum ➔ as well as the urinary bladder ➔.

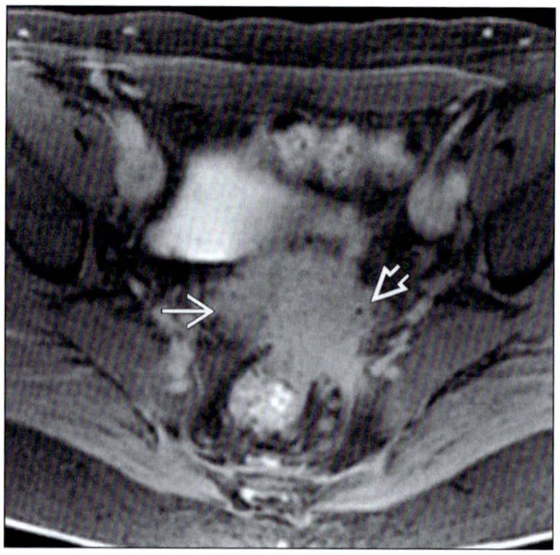

Axial T1WI C+ FS MR demonstrates homogeneous post-contrast enhancement of the irregular left parametrial mass ➔, which abuts the left aspect of the cervix ➔.

CLINICAL SCENARIO

History
- 48-year-old woman with history of metastatic thyroid cancer
- Left hydroureteronephrosis and pelvic mass on CT

Relevant Laboratory Tests
- CA125: 95.6 U/mL (normal: 0.0-35.0)

IMAGE INTERPRETATION

Pitfalls
- May be misdiagnosed as malignancy

Actual Diagnosis
- Endometriosis implant

Clues to Correct Diagnosis
- Characteristic location; CA125 may be elevated
- Fibrotic nature, possible tethering of adjacent bowel
- Occasional presence of high T2 signal intensity foci

BACKGROUND

General
- Ectopic endometrial glands and stroma outside uterus
- Benign (with < 1% risk of malignant transformation)
- Treatment: Surgical; medical: Hormonal and others

Epidemiology
- Prevalence: 5-10% of women (peak: 35-45 years old)

Relevant Anatomy
- Ovary most common site of endometriosis
- Other sites include uterine ligaments, serosal surfaces, fallopian tubes, rectosigmoid, and urinary bladder

Relevant Physiology
- Etiology uncertain; theories include retrograde menstruation vs. metaplasia of serosal epithelium
- CA125 may be elevated and can be followed

Relevant Pathology
- Gross
  - Translucent blebs; yellow-brown/red-blue staining
  - Thick fibrous capsule; chocolate-colored thick liquid
- Microscopic
  - Presence of endometrial epithelium, stroma, and glands with fibrous tissue, blood, and cysts
  - Extraovarian: Associated inflammatory cells

IMAGING FEATURES

US
- Hypoechoic nodule; thickening of adjacent tissue
- US sensitivity is low and varies with location

CT
- Nonspecific soft tissue with fibrous strands
- Cystic lesion with rim enhancement

MR
- T1WI: Typically low signal (due to fibrous component)
- T2WI: Hyperintense foci within hypointense fibrosis
- T1WI C+: Enhancement (2° to fibrosis)
- DWI: May show diffusion restriction

PET/CT
- Usually no/low FDG uptake, but increased uptake has been described likely due to cyclic changes or inflammation

Key Teaching Points
- Endometriosis could mimic pelvic mass
- CA125 may be elevated in endometriosis
- Characteristic appearance on T2WI can be seen

RELATED REFERENCES

1. Choudhary S et al: Unusual imaging appearances of endometriosis. AJR Am J Roentgenol. 192(6):1632-44, 2009
2. Kinkel K et al: Diagnosis of endometriosis with imaging: a review. Eur Radiol. 16(2):285-98, 2006

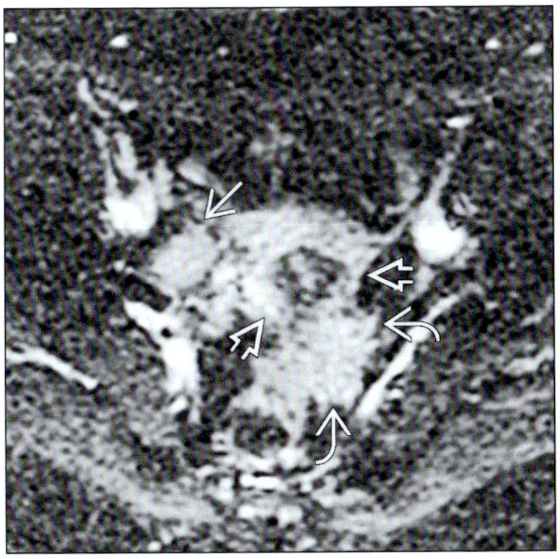

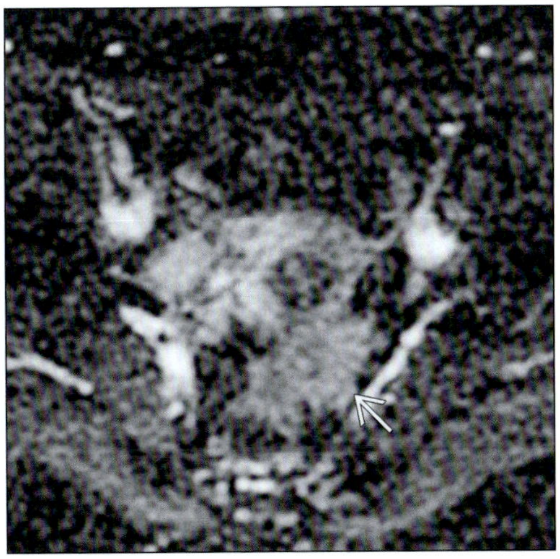

(Left) *Diffusion-weighted imaging (DWI) shows intermediate signal within the irregular parametrial lesion. There is high signal in the partially visible urinary bladder and uterus. Low signal of the cervix is seen.* ***(Right)*** *Apparent diffusion coefficient (ADC) map shows low to intermediate signal within the lesion, indicative of mild diffusion restriction.*

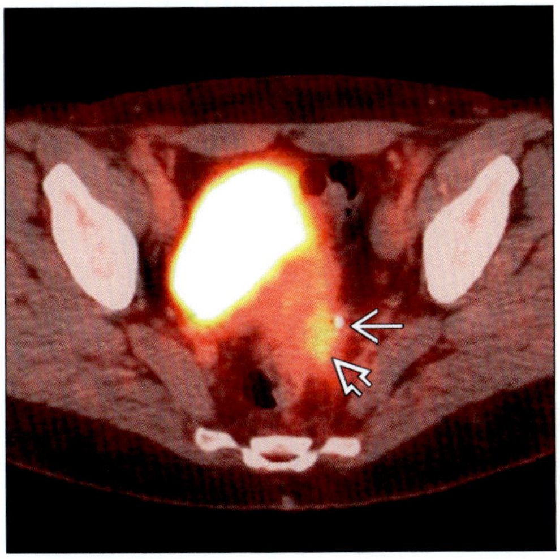

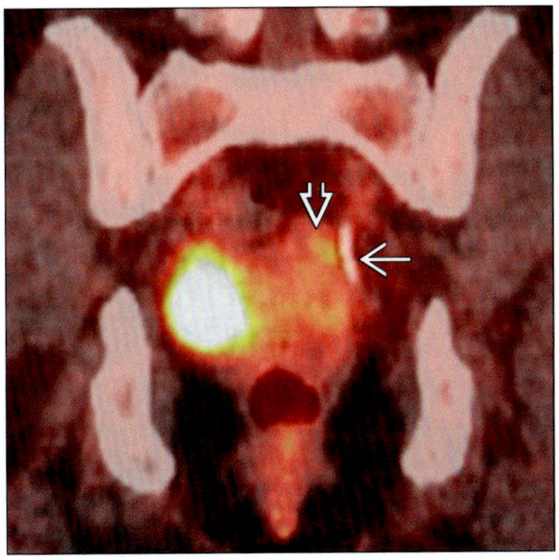

(Left) *Axial PET/CT shows mild uptake in the bulk of the left parametrial mass. There is a small focus of moderate uptake in the superolateral aspect of the lesion adjacent to the ureter stent (which was placed for hydronephrosis caused by the mass).* ***(Right)*** *Coronal PET/CT shows mild uptake in the bulk of the left parametrial mass, adjacent to the ureter stent.*

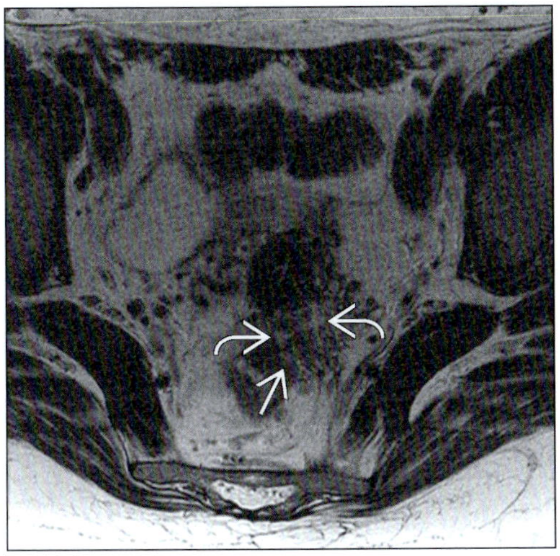

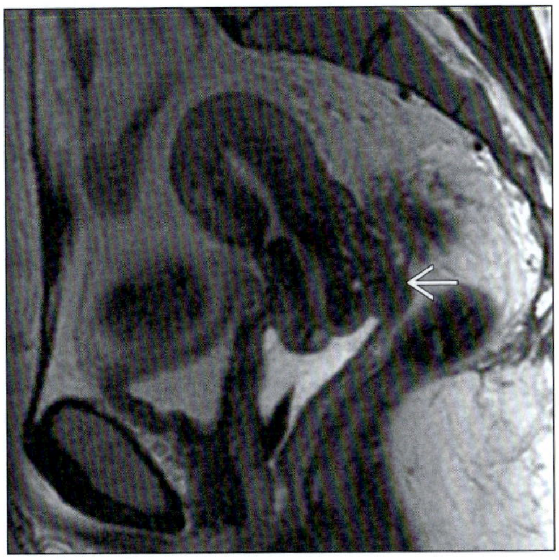

(Left) *Oblique coronal T2WI MR through the pelvis shows numerous high signal foci throughout the irregular left parametrial lesion, with a surrounding low signal intensity indicating fibrosis.* ***(Right)*** *Sagittal T2WI MR through the pelvis shows the irregular mass to abut the posterior wall of the cervix.*

PARASITIC LEIOMYOMA

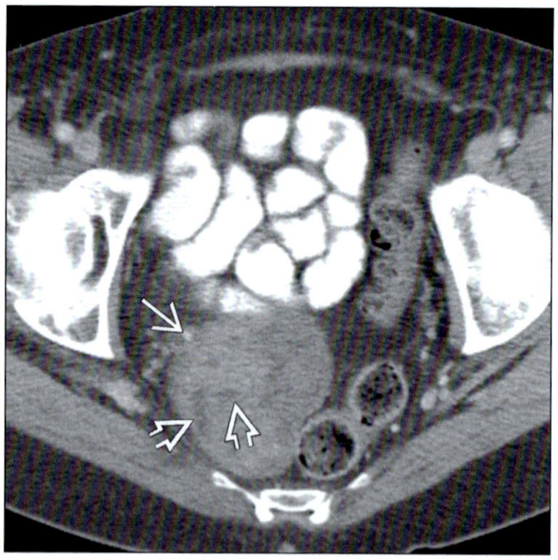

Axial CECT shows a right-side enhancing solid pelvic mass ➡. The mass shows areas of lower attenuation ➪ likely due to cystic changes.

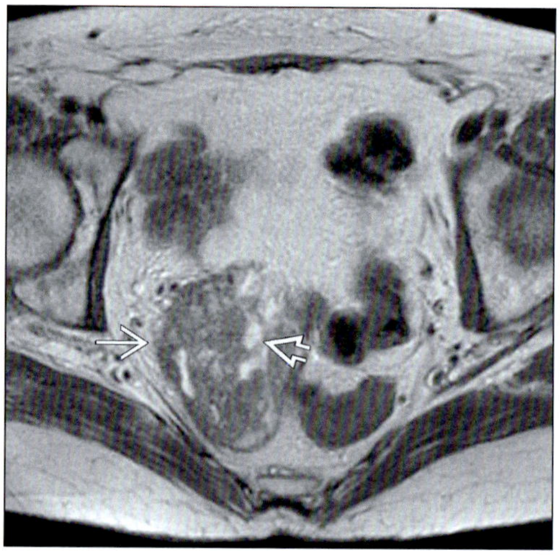

Axial T2WI MR shows a right pelvic mass ➡. The mass is predominantly solid and hyperintense relative to pelvic skeletal muscles, with areas of very high signal intensity ➪ representing cystic changes.

CLINICAL SCENARIO

History

- 62-year-old woman who underwent laparoscopic hysterectomy and bilateral oophorectomy and was recently diagnosed with colon cancer

IMAGE INTERPRETATION

Pitfalls

- May be misdiagnosed as peritoneal metastasis

Actual Diagnosis

- Parasitic leiomyoma

Clues to Correct Diagnosis

- History of laparoscopic myomectomies or hysterectomies with use of electric tissue morcellator
- Imaging features are similar to typical uterine leiomyomas
- Aberrant supplying vessels may be seen on CTA or MRA

BACKGROUND

General

- Leiomyomas that become adherent to surrounding structures develop an auxiliary blood supply and lose their original attachment to uterus, thus becoming parasitic
  - Primary parasitic leiomyomas are extremely rare
    - Likely arise from pedunculated subserosal myomas that have completely separated from uterus and have acquired blood supply
  - Iatrogenic origin
    - Develop after laparoscopic myomectomies or hysterectomies with use of electric tissue morcellator
    - Small fragments may implant in abdominopelvic cavity and subsequently develop into large fibroid

Epidemiology

- Prevalence of iatrogenic parasitic leiomyoma ranges from 0.12-0.9% after morcellation procedures

Clinical Presentation

- May be asymptomatic
- Pelvic pain
  - Pressure on adjacent organs (e.g., urethra, bladder neck, ureter, rectum)
- Can be associated with pleural effusion, ascites (pseudo-Meigs syndrome)

IMAGING FEATURES

US

- Whorled appearance and variable echogenicity depending on extent of degeneration, fibrosis, and calcification

CT

- Usually uniform, solid soft tissue attenuation
- Calcifications can be seen in 3-10% of all leiomyomas

MR

- T1WI: Isointense to normal myometrium
- T2WI: Hypointense to normal myometrium
  - Degenerative changes are also identical to uterine leiomyomas
- T1WI C+ FS: Heterogeneously enhancing

PET/CT

- Mild or moderate uptake of FDG-18 may be seen and declines with age

RELATED REFERENCES

1. Leren V et al: Parasitic leiomyomas after laparoscopic surgery with morcellation. Acta Obstet Gynecol Scand. 91(10):1233-6, 2012
2. Fasih N et al: Leiomyomas beyond the uterus: unusual locations, rare manifestations. Radiographics. 28(7):1931-48, 2008

PARASITIC LEIOMYOMA

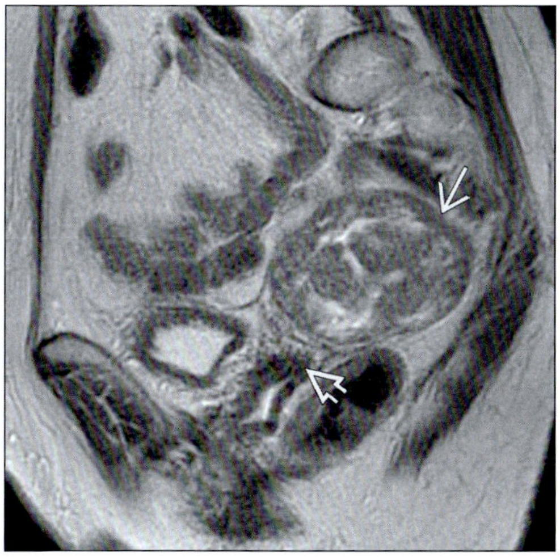

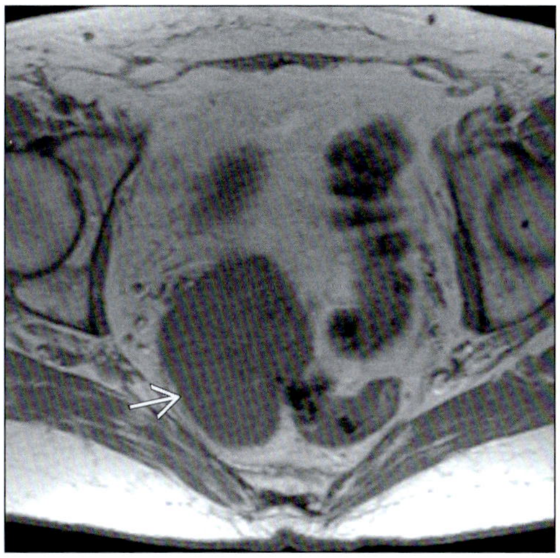

(Left) *Sagittal T2WI MR in the same patient shows a pelvic mass just superior to and separate from the vaginal cuff.* ***(Right)*** *Axial T1WI MR in the same patient shows a right pelvic adnexal mass demonstrating homogeneous signal intensity similar to or slightly lower compared to pelvic skeletal muscles.*

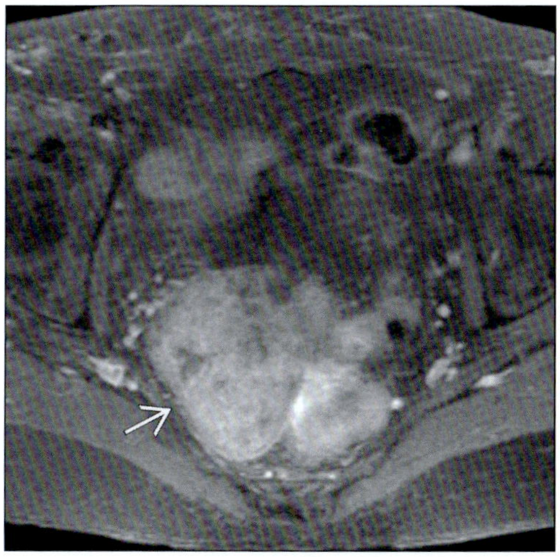

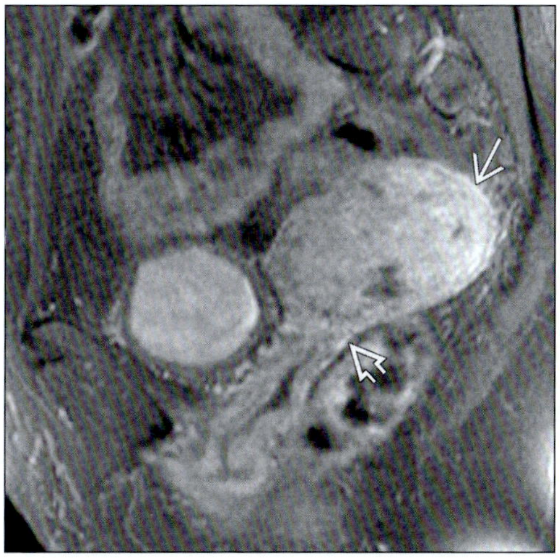

(Left) *Axial T1WI C+ FS MR in the same patient shows a right pelvic mass demonstrating heterogeneous intense enhancement. The appearance of the mass is similar to a typical leiomyoma.* ***(Right)*** *Coronal T1WI C+ FS MR in the same patient shows a pelvic mass above the vaginal cuff demonstrating heterogeneous intense enhancement. Biopsy revealed spindle cells consistent with parasitic leiomyoma.*

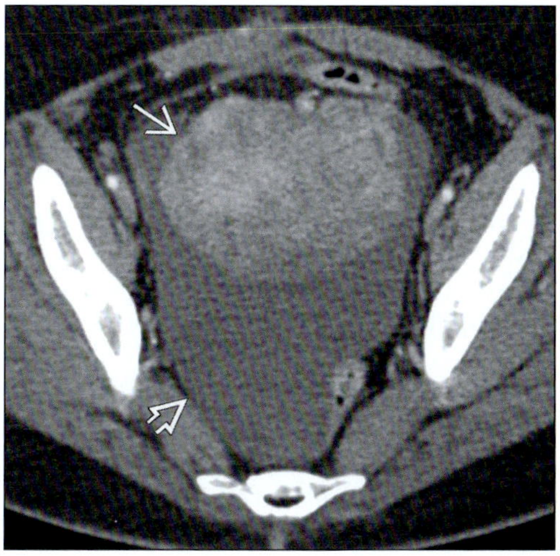

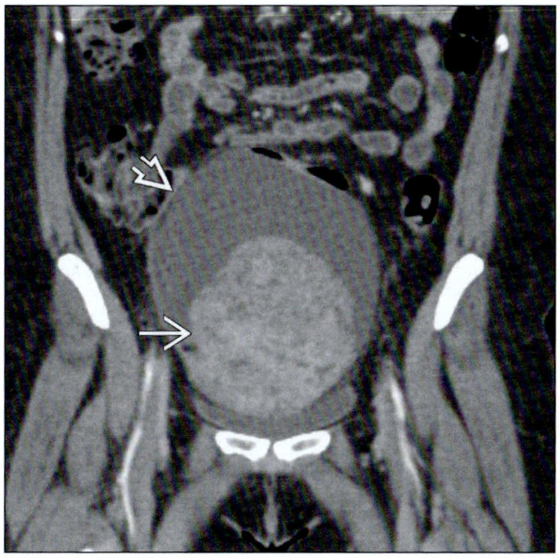

(Left) *Axial CECT in a 55-year-old woman who underwent hysterectomy for diffuse leiomyomatosis 3 years ago and recently presented with hydrothorax shows a heterogeneous midline pelvic mass and pelvic ascites.* ***(Right)*** *Coronal CECT in the same patient shows a heterogeneous pelvic mass and localized ascites. This is an example of pseudo-Meigs syndrome, which consists of pleural effusion, ascites, and benign pelvic tumors (other than ovarian fibromas).*

HIGH-POSITIONED OVARY

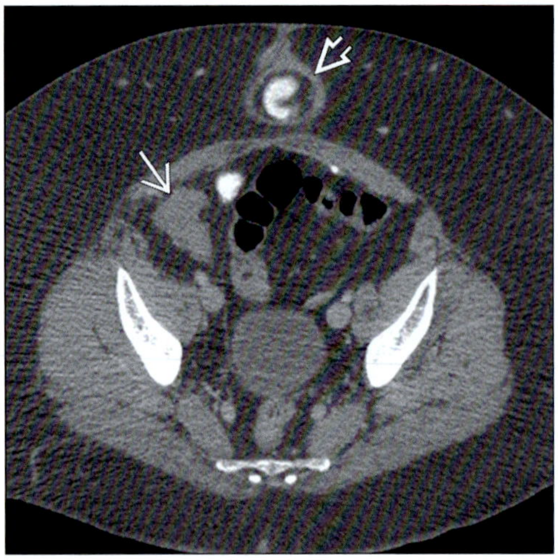

Axial CECT reveals a lobulated soft tissue attenuation lesion (isoattenuating to the skeletal muscles) ➡ within the right side of the pelvis. An incidental ventral hernia is noted ➡.

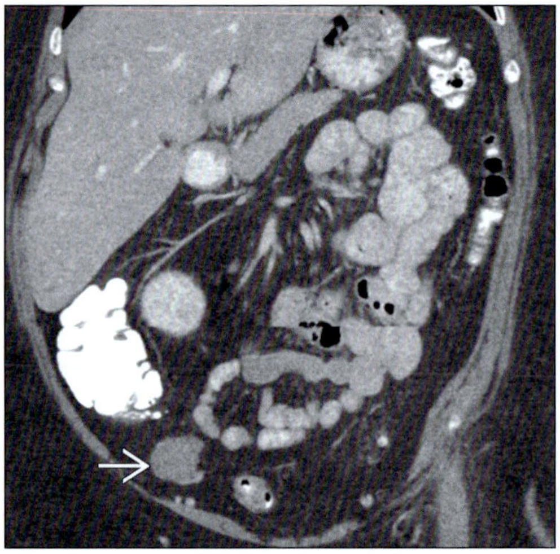

Coronal reformatted CECT shows a homogeneous soft tissue attenuation lesion ➡ in the right side of the pelvis.

CLINICAL SCENARIO

History

- 54-year-old woman post right hemicolectomy for colon cancer and hysterectomy for endometriosis

IMAGE INTERPRETATION

Pitfalls

- Can be mistaken for lymphadenopathy, recurrence, or peritoneal metastasis in light of patient's history

Actual Diagnosis

- High-positioned normal right ovary

Clues to Correct Diagnosis

- Morphology and location
- Tracking ovarian vein, draining to IVC on right and to left renal vein on left (both usually course anterior to psoas muscle)
- Suspensory or utero-ovarian ligament leads to ovary
- Ovaries are usually located anterior to ureter
- Ovarian mass displaces ureter posteriorly and laterally
  - Conversely, lymph node displaces ureter anteriorly and medially
- Ovaries lie posterior to broad ligament

BACKGROUND

General

- Uterus aids in identifying ovaries; when absent, ovaries can be mistaken for pathology
- Lymph nodes can be misinterpreted for normal ovaries

Relevant Anatomy of Ovaries

- Located in fossa of Waldeyer or ovarian fossa
- Posteriorly: Ureter; laterally: Pelvic wall
- Superior border: External iliac vein

IMAGING FEATURES

US

- Homogeneous texture with anechoic follicles
- Central iso- to hyperechoic medulla
- Size varies with hormonal status and menstrual cycle
- Color Doppler: Minimal vascularity as opposed to highly vascular metastasis

CT

- Ovoid low-attenuation structures in adnexa
  - Measures ~ 1.5-3 cm
- Attached by mesovarium to broad ligament, by suspensory ligament to pelvic wall, and by utero-ovarian ligament to uterus

MR

- T1WI: Hypointense to isointense
- T2WI: Hyperintense medulla, isointense cortex (relative to skeletal muscles)
- Post-contrast T1WI: Mild enhancement
- DWI: Varies with cycle

PET/CT

- Varies with menstrual cycle; can be high with benign processes such as physiological cysts or infection

Key Teaching Points

- If present in high position, normal ovaries can be misinterpreted for other pathologies including pelvic lymphadenopathy

RELATED REFERENCES

1. Laing FC et al: US of the ovary and adnexa: to worry or not to worry? Radiographics. 32(6):1621-39; discussion 1640-2, 2012
2. Saksouk FA et al: Recognition of the ovaries and ovarian origin of pelvic masses with CT. Radiographics. 24 Suppl 1:S133-46, 2004
3. Langer JE et al: High-resolution computed tomography of the female pelvis: spectrum of normal appearances. Semin Roentgenol. 31(4):267-78, 1996

HIGH-POSITIONED OVARY

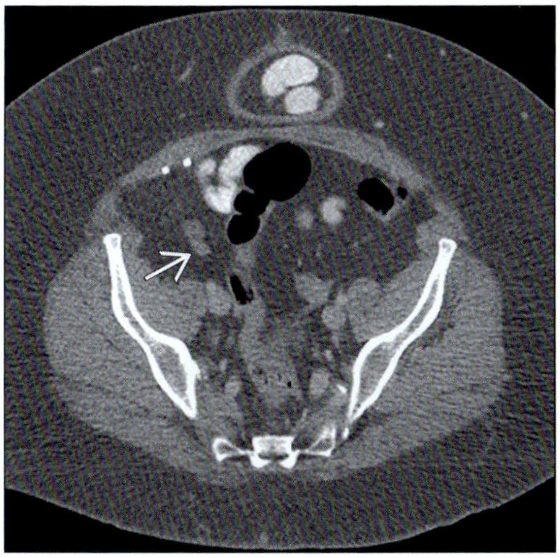

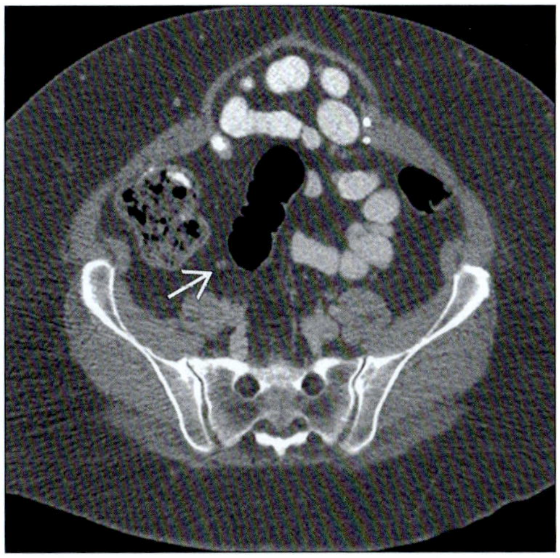

(Left) *Axial CECT reveals the right ovarian vein* ➔ *with a normal course, originating from the right pelvic mass and tracking anteriorly to the right psoas muscle.* ***(Right)*** *Axial CECT reveals the right ovarian vein* ➔ *with a normal course, originating from the right pelvic mass and tracking anteriorly to the right psoas. The right ovarian vein was found to drain to the IVC (not shown).*

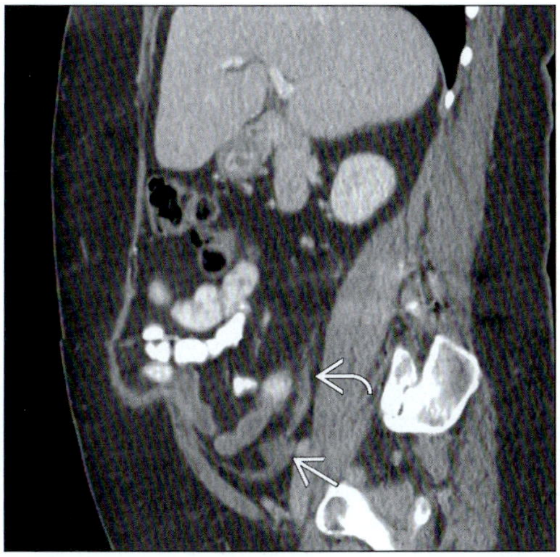

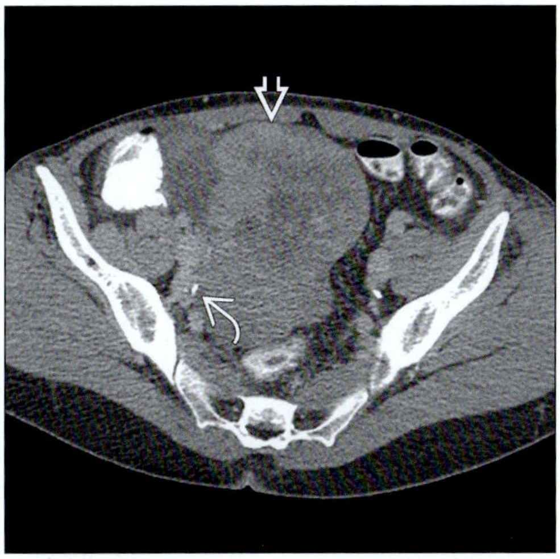

(Left) *Sagittal reconstruction reformatted CECT depicts the right ovarian vein* ↪ *tracking toward the right ovary* ➔*.* ***(Right)*** *Axial CECT in delayed phase demonstrates that the right ureter is opacified with contrast* ↪ *and displaced laterally by the pelvic mass* ⇨ *in a different patient (47-year-old woman with a right pelvic mass, surgically proven to be ovarian serous carcinoma).*

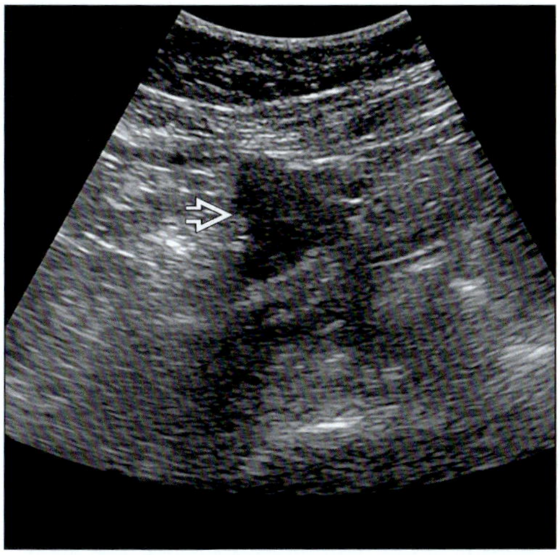

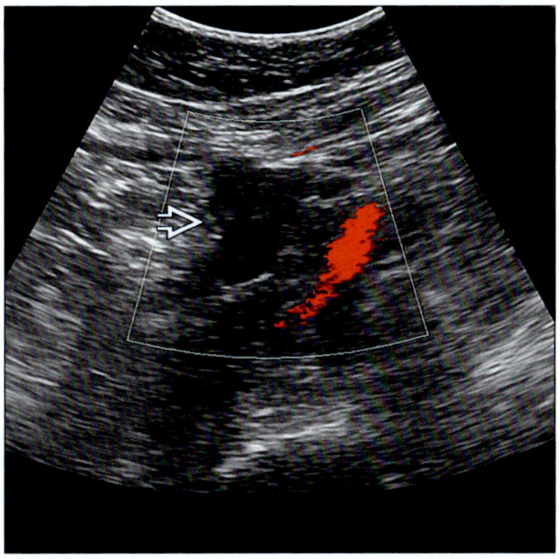

(Left) *Longitudinal grayscale ultrasound demonstrates a lobulated hypoechoic right ovary* ⇨ *with heterogeneous echo texture.* ***(Right)*** *Longitudinal color Doppler ultrasound demonstrates no evidence of abnormal vascularity in the right ovary* ⇨*. A metastatic lymph node or implant would be expected to demonstrate increased vascularity.*

ACTINOMYCOSIS

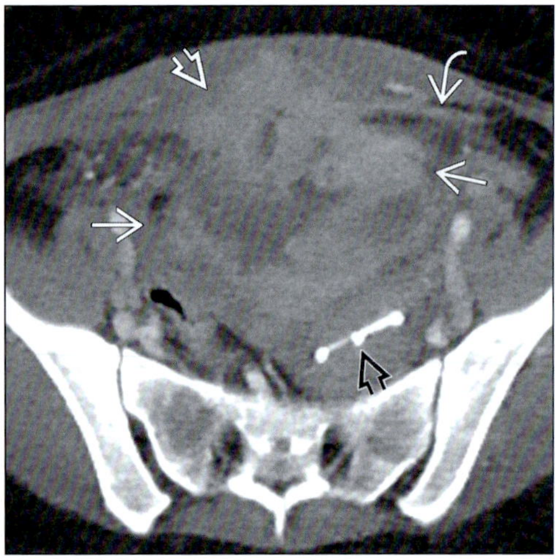

Axial CECT shows an aggressive soft tissue mass ➡ with invasion of the abdominal wall ➡ and thickening of the pelvic peritoneum ➡. An IUCD ➡ is present within the uterus.

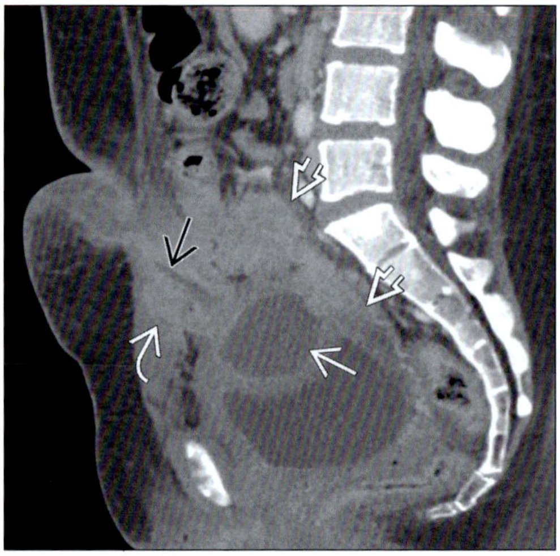

Sagittal CECT in the same patient shows a fluid collection ➡, a thick irregular rim of enhancing soft tissue ➡, invasion of the abdominal wall ➡, and a thick-walled sinus tract ➡.

CLINICAL SCENARIO

History

- 37-year-old woman presenting with draining anterior abdominal wall sinus

IMAGE INTERPRETATION

Pitfalls

- Aggressive soft tissue mass with extensive local invasion can be mistaken for pelvic malignancy

Actual Diagnosis

- Pelvic actinomycosis

Clues to Correct Diagnosis

- Presence of intrauterine contraceptive device (IUCD)
- Extension across tissue planes, fistula formation + IUCD are highly suggestive of diagnosis

BACKGROUND

General

- Slowly progressing chronic granulomatous infectious disease
- Associated with prolonged use of IUCDs
  - May occur months or years after IUCD removal

Relevant Microbiology

- Gram-positive anaerobic bacteria genera *Actinomyces*, most frequently *Actinomyces israelii*
  - Opportunistic pathogens, normal inhabitants of oropharynx, bowel, and female genital tract
    - Organism is found on cultures in 3-4% of normal women
    - ~ 25% of IUCDs eventually become colonized by *Actinomyces*
- Definitive diagnosis requires positive anaerobic culture or identification of *Actinomyces* granules
  - Organism isolation achieved in < 50% of cases
- Most actinomycotic infections are polymicrobial
  - Mix of other microorganisms is frequently found at infection associated with *Actinomyces* species
- Penicillin G is drug of choice regardless of disease extent or severity

Relevant Pathology

- Most commonly involve ovaries and fallopian tubes
  - Can involve uterus, urinary bladder, rectum, and abdominal wall
- Organisms produce proteolytic enzymes, which facilitate spread through normal anatomic barriers
  - Result in abscesses, sinus tracts, and fistulas surrounded by indurated firm fibrotic tissue

IMAGING FEATURES

General Features

- Can present as fistula, sinus tract, inflammatory solid pseudotumor, or abscess
- Strong enhancement of solid component
- Small rim-enhancing abscesses within solid lesions
- Tubo-ovarian actinomycosis usually appears to be more solid than typical tubo-ovarian abscess

US

- Nonspecific solid and cystic pelvic mass(es)

CT

- Abscess cavity with thick irregular wall or solid mass
- Thickening and enhancement of fascial planes

MR

- Intermediate to low signal intensity of solid component on T2WI due to prominent fibrotic tissue

RELATED REFERENCES

1. Heo SH et al: Imaging of actinomycosis in various organs: a comprehensive review. Radiographics. 34(1):19-33, 2014
2. Rezvani M et al: Fallopian tube disease in the nonpregnant patient. Radiographics. 31(2):527-48, 2011
3. Lely RJ et al: Case 85: pelvic actinomycosis in association with an intrauterine device. Radiology. 236(2):492-4, 2005

FOCAL ADENOMYOMA

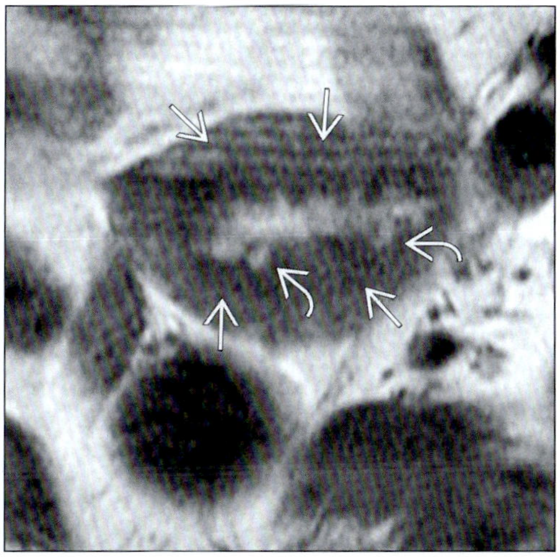

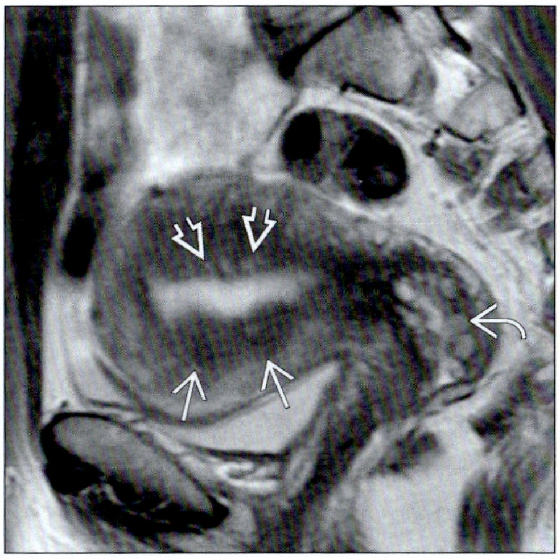

(Left) *Axial T2WI MR demonstrates thickening of the junctional zone →. Multiple small, round, T2-hyperintense foci → are seen deep to the endometrium-myometrial junction.* ***(Right)*** *Sagittal T2WI MR demonstrates thickening of the junctional zone → with multiple small, round, T2-hyperintense subendometrial foci →. Nabothian cysts → are noted at the cervix.*

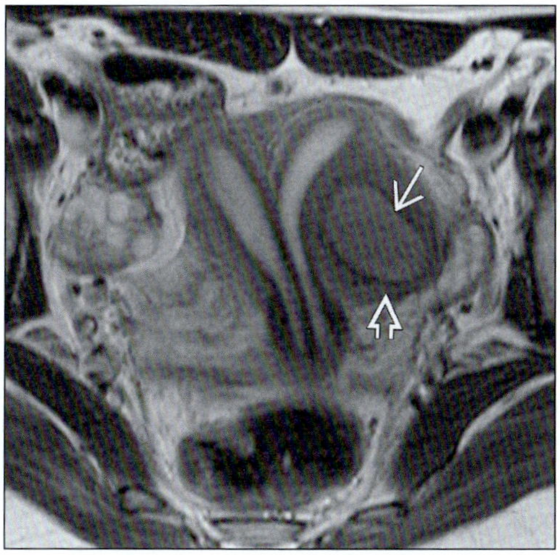

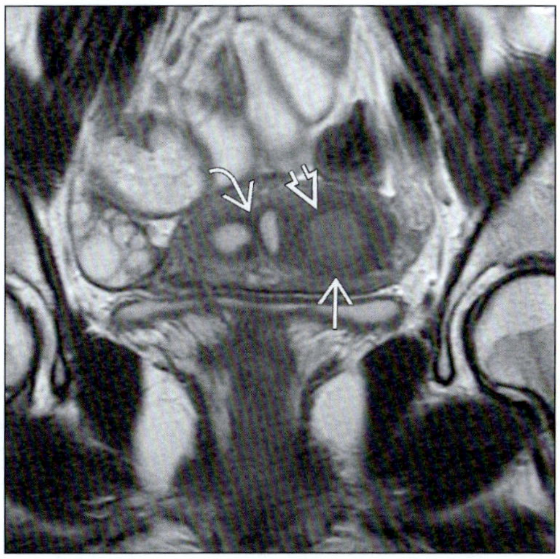

(Left) *Axial T2WI MR demonstrates a well-circumscribed lesion → with mildly increased signal due to the presence of blood products, surrounded by low-signal rim → representing an adenomyotic cyst. A septate uterus is present.* ***(Right)*** *Coronal T2WI MR shows a well-circumscribed lesion → with intermediate signal (representing blood products) with surrounding low-signal rim → compatible with an adenomyotic cyst. A fibrous uterine septum is noted →.*

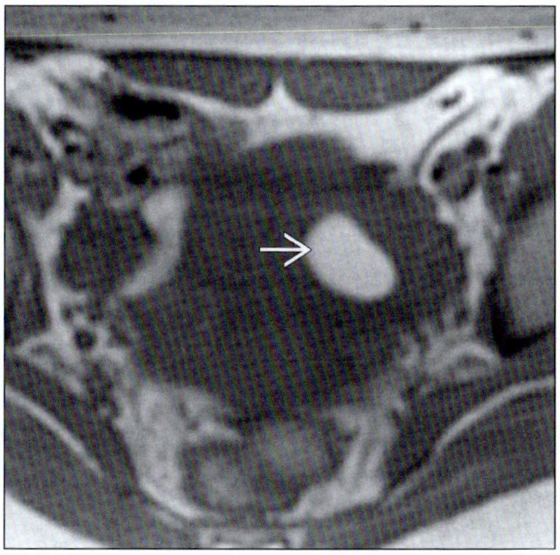

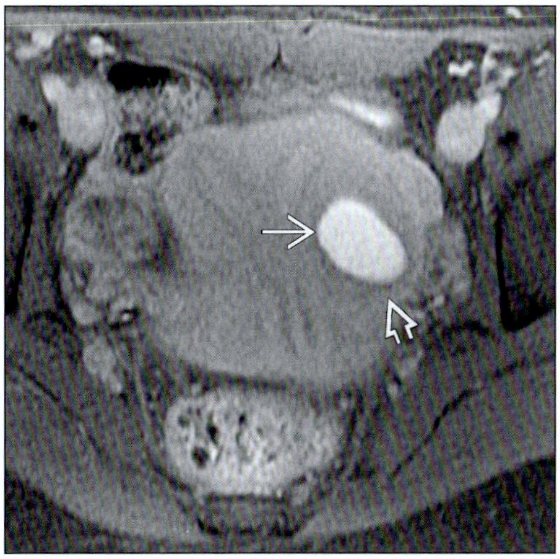

(Left) *Axial T1WI MR shows a well-circumscribed myometrial lesion → demonstrating high signal compatible with hemorrhage within an adenomyotic cyst.* ***(Right)*** *Axial T1WI C+ FS MR shows a hemorrhagic adenomyotic cyst → surrounded by a low-signal rim → with no appreciable enhancement.*

UTERINE LEIOMYOSARCOMA

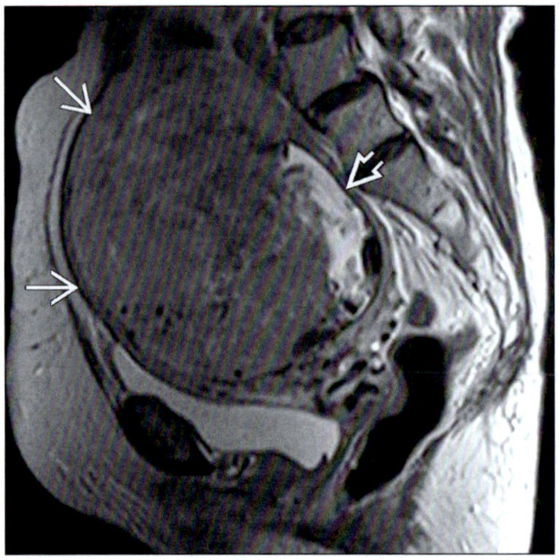

Sagittal T2WI MR demonstrates a large mass involving the uterus with heterogeneous increased signal intensity with an area of markedly increased signal posteriorly.

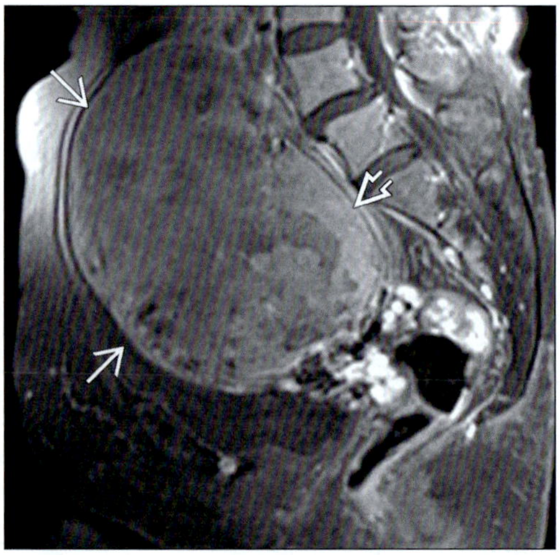

Sagittal T1WI C+ MR demonstrates heterogeneous enhancement of the mass, with more confluent enhancement involving the posterior area corresponding to the area of T2 hyperintensity.

CLINICAL SCENARIO

History

- 28-year-old woman with anemia and heavy menstrual bleeding

IMAGE INTERPRETATION

Pitfalls

- May be mistaken for large uterine fibroid

Actual Diagnosis

- Uterine leiomyosarcoma

Clues to Correct Diagnosis

- Very large size (nonspecific)
- Lack of calcifications (calcifications are more common in fibroids)
- Moderately high signal intensity on T2WI with post-contrast enhancement
  - Fibroids are usually low signal on T2WI
  - Cystic degeneration in fibroids: Areas of high signal on T2WI that do not enhance
  - Myxoid degeneration in fibroids: Very high signal on T2WI with minimal enhancement

BACKGROUND

General

- May present with palpable mass, pain, and bleeding
- Aggressive tumor with high recurrence rate

Epidemiology

- Rare: 3-7 per 100,000 in USA; peak age: 40-69 years
- 2x more common in African Americans than Caucasians
- Risk factors include increasing age, postmenopausal status, long-term tamoxifen use, and pelvic radiation

Relevant Pathology

- Gross: Usually infiltrative, large fleshy tumor
- Microscopic: Hypercellular with spindle cells, pleomorphism; areas of hemorrhage and necrosis

IMAGING FEATURES

US

- Large mass with mixed echogenicity
- Often hypoechoic areas compatible with necrosis
- Color Doppler (nonspecific): Irregular vessel distribution, low impedance to flow, and high peak systolic velocity

CT

- Large mass
- Shows contrast enhancement
- Low-attenuation areas of hemorrhage and necrosis
- Calcifications less common compared to fibroids

MR

- Large mass with irregular margins
- T1WI: Isointense to myometrium; areas of hemorrhage may have high signal on T1
- T2WI: Moderately high signal intensity
- T1WI C+: Moderate contrast enhancement

PET/CT

- Usually, moderate to intense FDG uptake (rarely, mild)

KEY TEACHING POINTS

Large Fibroid vs. Leiomyosarcoma

- Differentiation is challenging and often not possible
- Consider sarcoma if large mass with areas of moderately increased T2 signal and contrast enhancement
- Atypical uterine fibroids are still much more common

RELATED REFERENCES

1. Kitajima K et al: Spectrum of FDG PET/CT findings of uterine tumors. AJR Am J Roentgenol. 195(3):737-43, 2010

UTERINE LEIOMYOSARCOMA

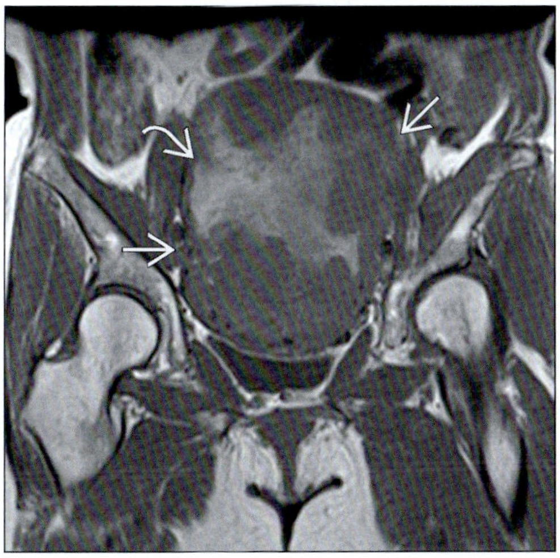

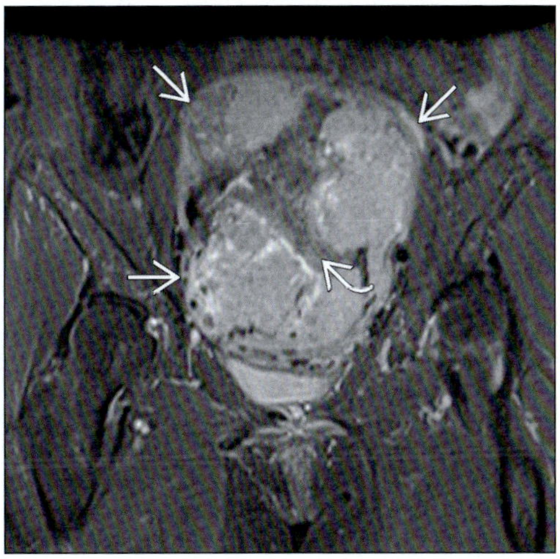

(Left) *Coronal T1WI MR demonstrates a large, lobulated, heterogeneous, exophytic uterine mass with a large central hyperintense area representing hemorrhage.* ***(Right)*** *Coronal T1WI C+ MR demonstrates significant heterogeneous enhancement, which is predominantly peripheral, with a central nonenhancing area representing hemorrhage.*

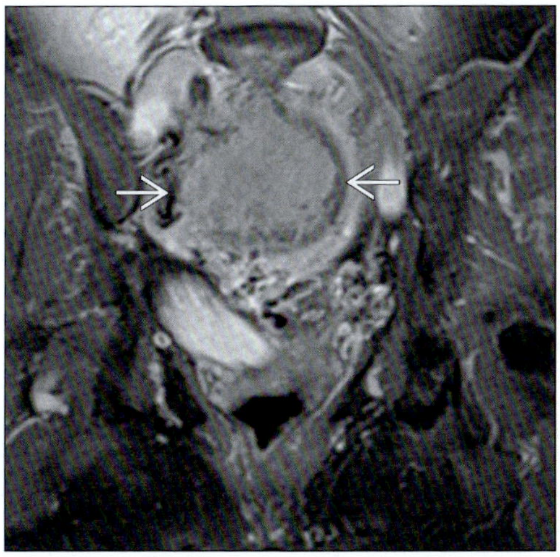

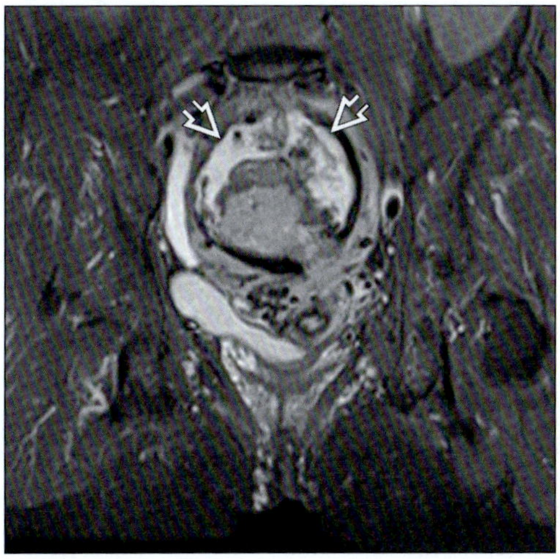

(Left) *A more posterior coronal T1WI C+ MR in the same patient shows an area of significant enhancement.* ***(Right)*** *Coronal T2WI MR in the same area shows that the mass is very heterogeneous with internal hyperintense areas. When a mass is this heterogeneous and avidly enhancing, leiomyosarcoma should always be considered and the patient must go to surgery.*

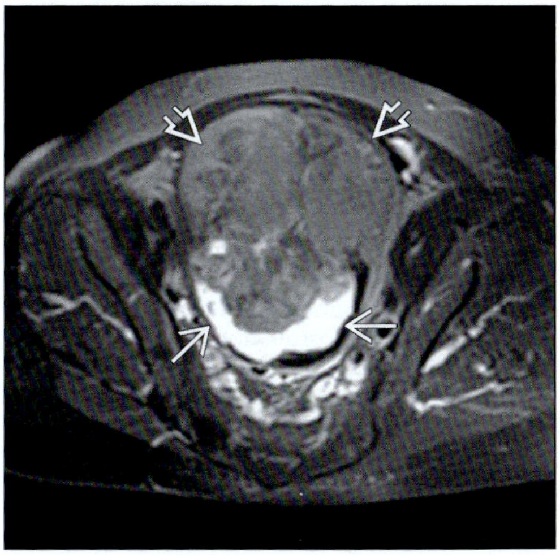

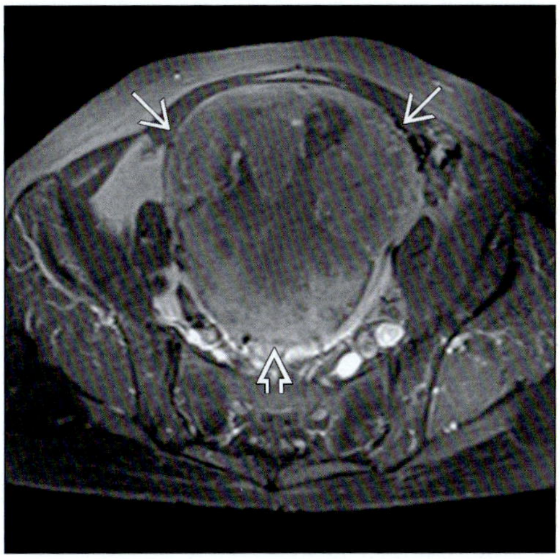

(Left) *Axial T2WI MR demonstrates a large heterogeneous mass lesion that is predominantly hyperintense, with a markedly hyperintense posterior area.* ***(Right)*** *Axial T1WI C+ MR demonstrates significant, predominantly peripheral enhancement with a notable enhancement of the posterior aspect.*

GRANULOSA CELL TUMOR

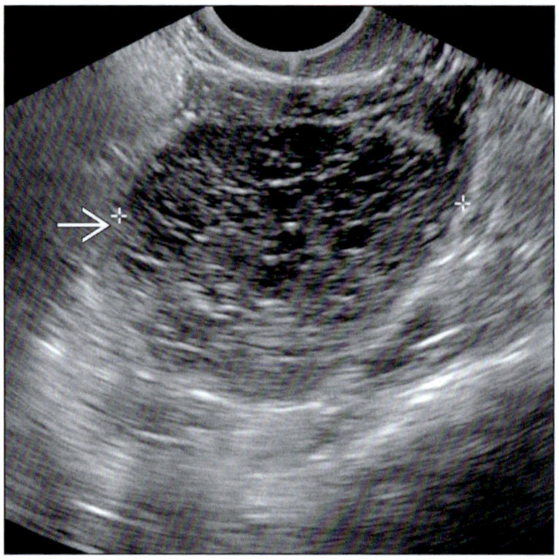

Sagittal transvaginal ultrasound shows an ovarian mass ➔ composed of numerous small cystic spaces separated by thin septa, giving the lesion a fishnet appearance.

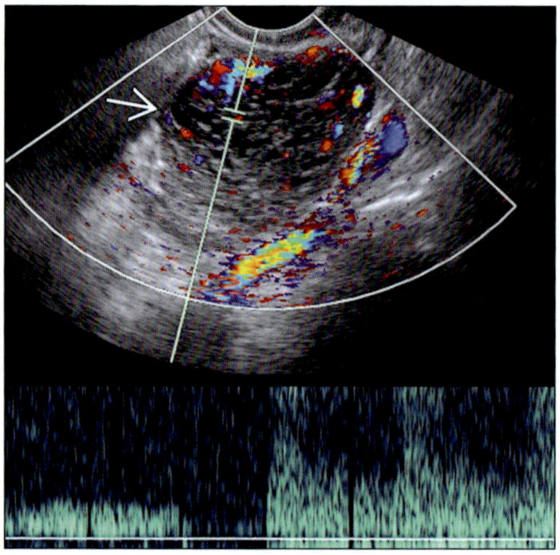

Sagittal transvaginal duplex Doppler ultrasound in the same patient shows the ovarian mass ➔ with definite blood flow within the septa separating the small cystic spaces.

CLINICAL SCENARIO

History

- 36-year-old woman presenting with pelvic pain

IMAGE INTERPRETATION

Pitfalls

- Lesion resembles fishnet pattern characteristic of hemorrhagic cyst

Actual Diagnosis

- Granulosa cell tumor (GCT)

Clues to Correct Diagnosis

- Presence of vascular flow within lesion
  - Hemorrhagic cysts are avascular on Doppler studies
- GCT may be associated with estrogenic manifestations, including endometrial hyperplasia and carcinoma
  - Resulting in endometrial thickening

BACKGROUND

General

- Classified as sex cord-stromal tumor
- Believed to arise from cells surrounding germinal cells in ovarian follicles
- 2 subtypes
  - Adult: ~ 95% of all GCTs
  - Juvenile: ~ 5% of all GCTs

Epidemiology

- Incidence: 0.5-1.5 per 100,000 women per year
  - ~ 3-5% of all malignant ovarian tumors
  - Most common sex cord-stromal tumor after fibromas and fibrothecomas
  - Most common malignant sex cord-stromal tumor
- Wide age range (newborn to postmenopausal)
  - ~ 5% in prepubertal period
  - ~ 35% in premenopausal women
  - ~ 60% in postmenopausal women

IMAGING FEATURES

General

- Different patterns have been described
  - Multilocular cystic lesions with solid components
  - Solid masses
  - Solid with sponge-like appearance resembling Swiss cheese or fishnet
  - Completely cystic tumors with thick rind of soft tissue
- Enlarged uterus with endometrial thickening

CT

- Solid, enhancing mass with variable cystic or hemorrhagic/necrotic areas of low attenuation

MR

- T1WI
  - Cysts may have increased signal intensity due to hemorrhage
- T2WI
  - Solid mass with internal cysts (Swiss cheese appearance)
  - Low signal on T2WI or fluid-fluid levels with intracystic hemorrhage
  - Septations may have low signal intensity
- T1WI C+
  - Septa enhance

PET/CT

- Usually very low FDG avidity

RELATED REFERENCES

1. Kim JA et al: High-resolution sonographic findings of ovarian granulosa cell tumors: correlation with pathologic findings. J Ultrasound Med. 29(2):187-93, 2010
2. Van Holsbeke C et al: Imaging of gynecological disease (3): clinical and ultrasound characteristics of granulosa cell tumors of the ovary. Ultrasound Obstet Gynecol. 31(4):450-6, 2008

HEMOPERITONEUM DUE TO RUPTURED OVARIAN CYST

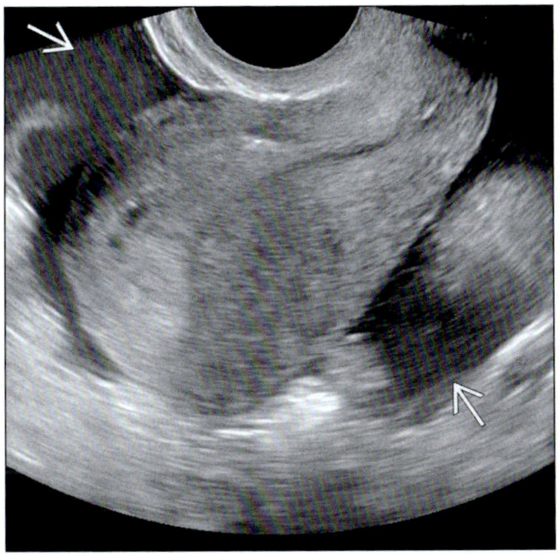

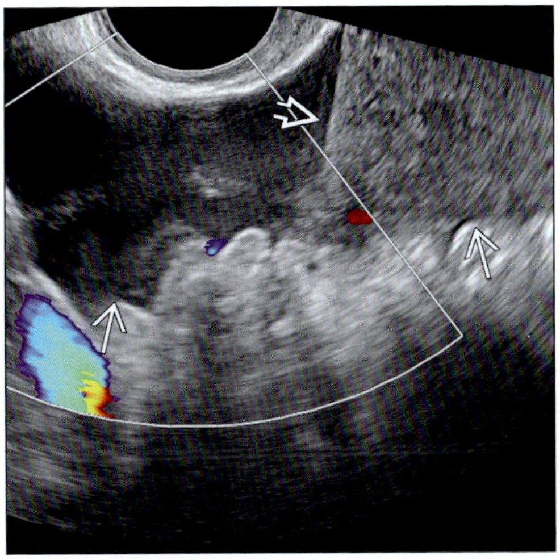

(Left) *Sagittal transvaginal ultrasound in a 24-year-old woman who presented with sudden severe pelvic pain and had a negative pregnancy test shows a large amount of free pelvic fluid with low-level echoes.* ***(Right)*** *Sagittal transvaginal color Doppler ultrasound in the same patient shows a large amount of free pelvic fluid. A fluid-fluid level is present due to layering of blood components.*

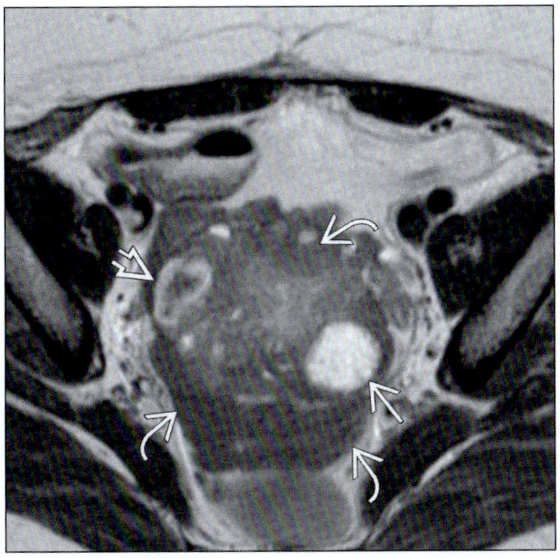

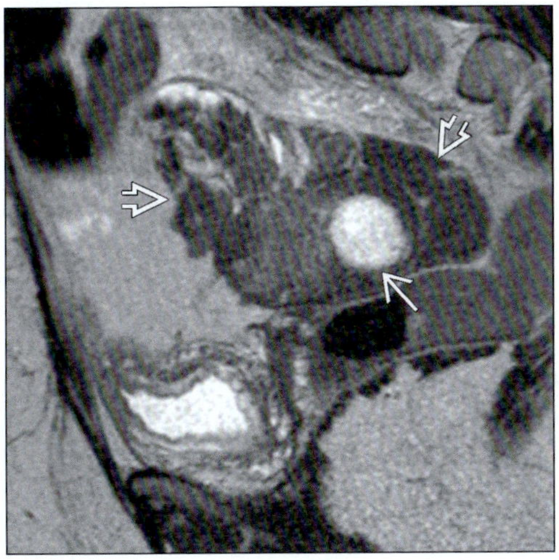

(Left) *Axial T2WI MR in a 34-year-old woman who had a hysterectomy and presented with severe abdominal pain shows a left ovarian hemorrhagic cyst, a right ovarian corpus luteum, and a moderate amount of pelvic heterogeneous fluid.* ***(Right)*** *Sagittal T2WI MR in the same patient shows the left ovarian hemorrhagic cyst bathed in a moderate amount of heterogeneous blood.*

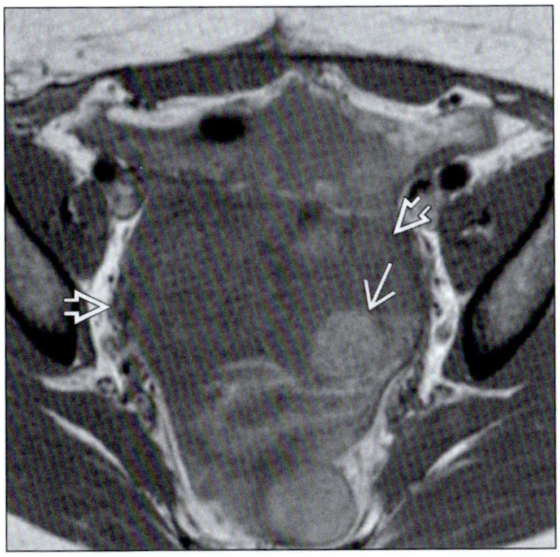

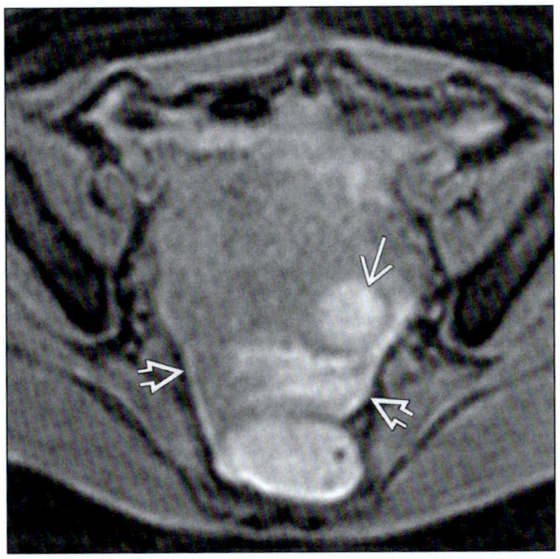

(Left) *Axial T1WI MR in the same patient shows the high signal intensity left ovarian hemorrhagic cyst and a moderate amount of pelvic heterogeneous fluid showing layers of high and low signal intensity.* ***(Right)*** *Axial T1WI FS MR in the same patient shows the high signal intensity left ovarian hemorrhagic cyst and a moderate amount of pelvic heterogeneous fluid. Fat-suppressed T1 sequences are important to differentiate a ruptured hemorrhagic cyst from a ruptured dermoid cyst.*

SKENE GLAND CYST

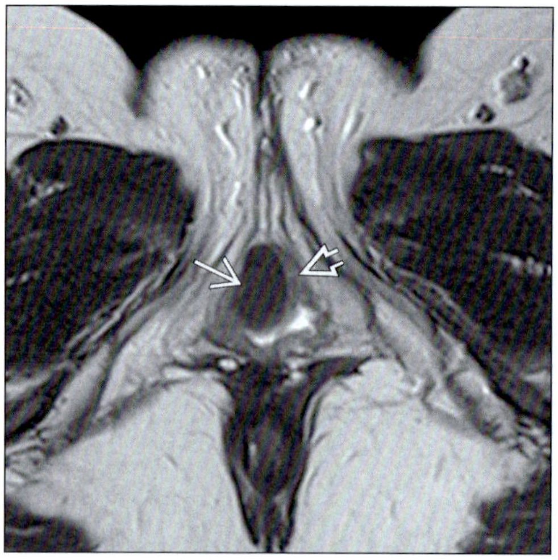

Axial T2WI MR shows an ovoid, hypointense structure located to the right of the distal urethra, which is flattened and stretched over the lesion.

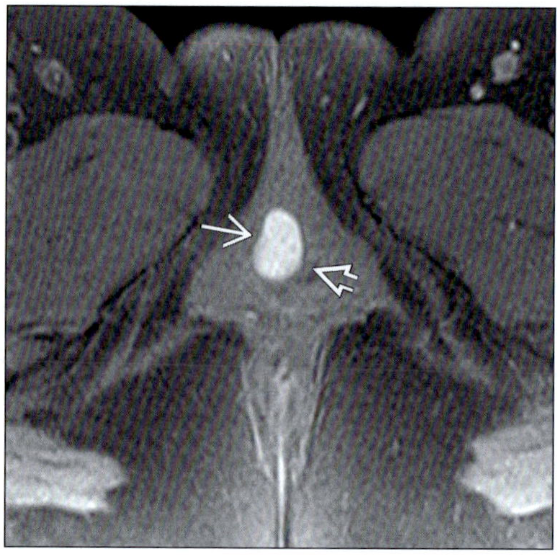

Axial T1WI FS MR in the same patient shows an ovoid, hyperintense structure located to the right of the distal urethra.

CLINICAL SCENARIO

History

- Incidentally discovered lesion on pelvic MR

IMAGE INTERPRETATION

Pitfalls

- May be mistaken for other cysts of female lower genital tract

Actual Diagnosis

- Skene gland cyst

Clues to Correct Diagnosis

- Rounded or ovoid lesions at or lateral to external urethral orifice inferior to pubic symphysis and perineal membrane
- Periurethral and originating at anterior aspect of superficial perineal pouch

BACKGROUND

Relevant Anatomy

- Skene glands are also known as periurethral glands
- Paired glands at 3- and 9-o'clock positions along distal urethra
- Function to lubricate distal urethra
- Considered female analogue to male prostate gland

Etiology

- Results from ductal obstruction from prior infection, inflammation, or trauma

Clinical Features

- Often asymptomatic and incidentally identified
- Complications
  - May become infected (skenitis)
  - Can cause urethral obstruction when large
  - May rarely undergo malignant degeneration into adenocarcinoma
    - Elevated prostate-specific antigen (PSA) levels

Management

- Asymptomatic cysts may not require treatment
- Symptomatic cysts (abscesses or sterile cysts) may require antibiotic therapy, excision, or marsupialization

IMAGING FEATURES

US

- Anechoic cyst when uncomplicated
- Low-level echoes in presence of hemorrhage or infection

CT

- Fluid attenuation with thin, nonenhancing wall when uncomplicated
- High attenuation in presence of proteinaceous debris or hemorrhage
- Thickening of wall and stranding of surrounding fat if infected

MR

- Fluid signal intensity with thin, nonenhancing wall when uncomplicated
- Variable T1 and T2 signal intensity in presence of proteinaceous debris or hemorrhage
- If infected, heterogeneous cyst content with varied signal intensity and thickened, irregular, enhancing wall

RELATED REFERENCES

1. Tubay M et al: Resident and fellow education feature: what is that cyst? Common cystic lesions of the female lower genitourinary tract. Radiographics. 34(2):427-8, 2014
2. Surabhi VR et al: Magnetic resonance imaging of female urethral and periurethral disorders. Radiol Clin North Am. 51(6):941-53, 2013

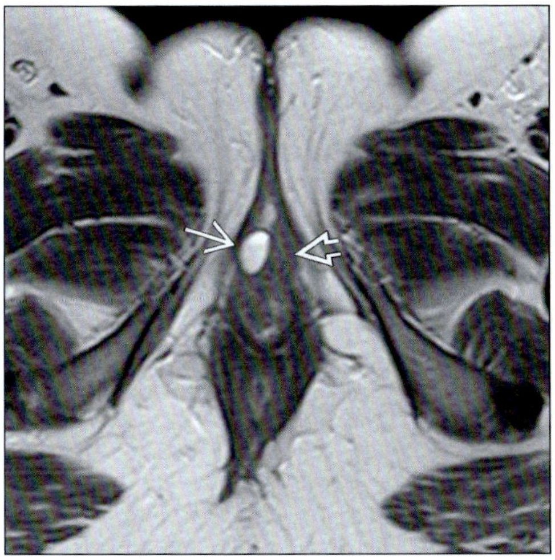

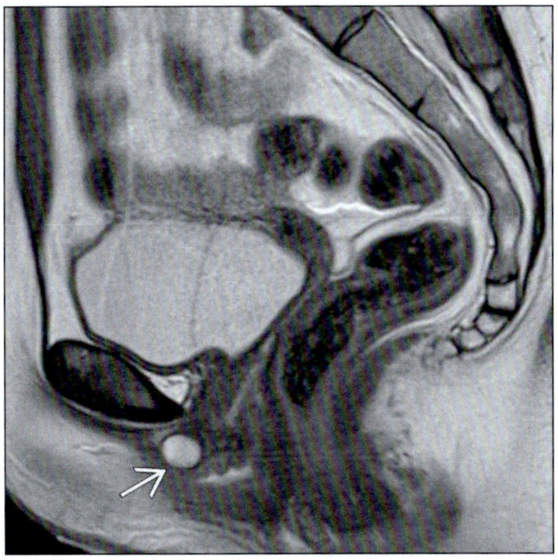

*(**Left**) Axial T2WI MR shows an ovoid, hyperintense structure ➡ located to the right of the distal urethra ➡. Skene gland cysts usually contain fluid of high signal intensity, when uncomplicated. (**Right**) Sagittal T2WI MR in the same patient shows an ovoid, hyperintense structure ➡ positioned at the anterior vaginal vestibule, inferior to the level of the pubic symphysis and perineal membrane.*

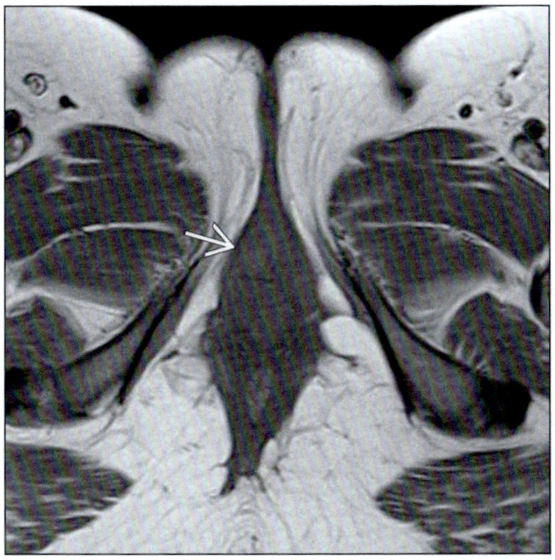

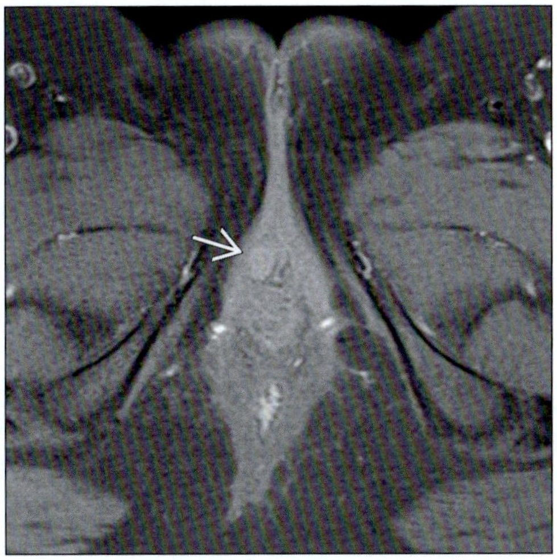

*(**Left**) Axial T1WI MR in the same patient shows an ovoid structure ➡ located at the vaginal introitus. It demonstrates signal intensity that is more or less similar to pelvic skeletal muscles. (**Right**) Axial T1WI FS MR in the same patient shows an ovoid structure ➡ located at the vaginal introitus. The uncomplicated cyst may be difficult to visualize on T1WI because its signal intensity is similar to surrounding structures.*

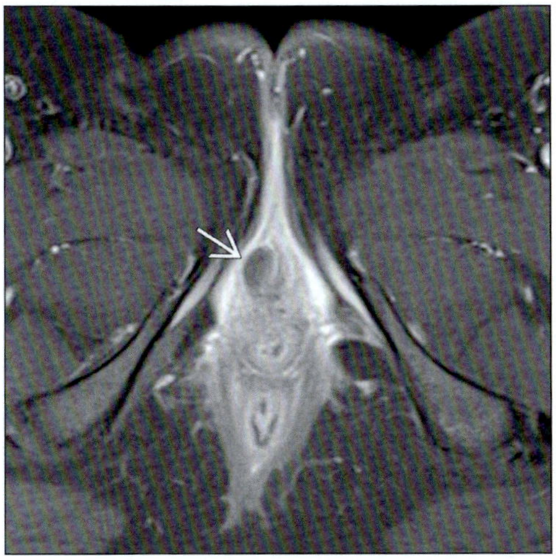

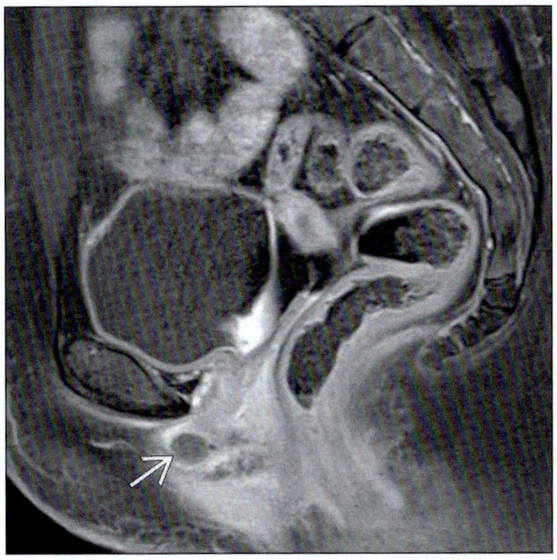

*(**Left**) Axial T1WI C+ FS MR in the same patient shows an ovoid structure ➡ located at the vaginal introitus. The thin cyst wall demonstrates mild enhancement after gadolinium administration. The cyst is much better seen because of intense enhancement of the surrounding tissues. (**Right**) Sagittal T1WI C+ FS MR in the same patient shows an ovoid structure ➡ with a thin, uniform, enhancing wall, located inferior to the level of the pubic symphysis and perineal membrane.*

GARTNER DUCT CYST

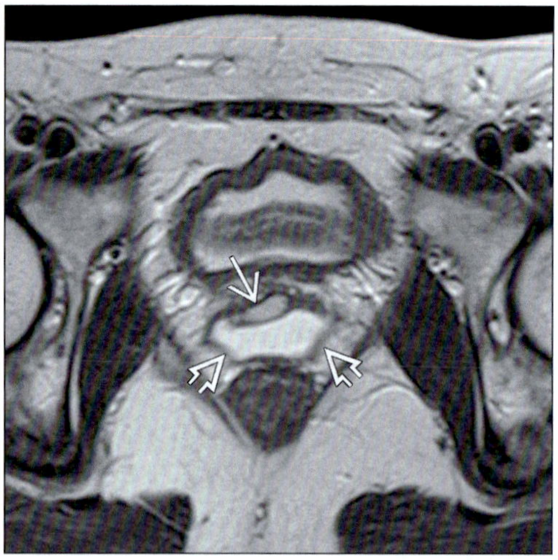

Axial T2WI MR shows an ovoid, hyperintense structure ➡ located at the right anterolateral aspect of the gel-filled vagina ⇨. The signal intensity is less than that of simple fluid due to hemorrhage.

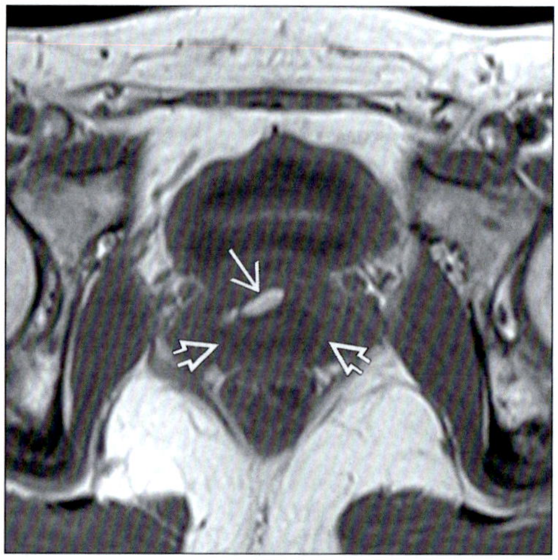

Axial T1WI MR shows an ovoid, hyperintense structure ➡ located at the right anterolateral aspect of the gel-filled vagina ⇨. The high signal intensity is due to intracystic hemorrhage.

CLINICAL SCENARIO

History

- 25-year-old woman with incidental finding on pelvic MR

IMAGE INTERPRETATION

Pitfalls

- May be mistaken for other other cysts of female lower genital tract

Actual Diagnosis

- Gartner duct cyst

Clues to Correct Diagnosis

- Cystic structure usually arising from anterolateral wall of upper vagina
- Above level of perineal membrane and pubic symphysis

BACKGROUND

General

- Typically solitary, < 2 cm in size

Epidemiology

- Most common benign cyst of vagina
  - Seen in up to 1% of women

Relevant Embryology

- Arises from remnants of distal mesonephric (wolffian) ducts
- May be associated with other congenital urogenital abnormalities, such as ectopic ureteral insertion and unilateral renal agenesis or hypoplasia

Relevant Pathology

- Retention-type cysts lined by non-mucin-secreting cells

Clinical Features

- Usually asymptomatic
- Commonly manifests as palpable anterior vaginal mass
- Complications
  - Infection
  - Hemorrhage
  - Malignant transformation
  - If large and inferiorly located, may have mass effect on urethra

Management

- Small cysts may be treated with aspiration
- Large, symptomatic cysts are typically treated with excision, sclerotherapy, or marsupialization

IMAGING FEATURES

US

- Anechoic cyst when uncomplicated
- Low-level echoes in presence of hemorrhage or infection

CT

- Fluid attenuation with thin, nonenhancing wall when uncomplicated
- High attenuation in presence of proteinaceous debris or hemorrhage

MR

- Fluid signal intensity with thin, nonenhancing wall when uncomplicated
- Variable T1 and T2 signal intensity in presence of proteinaceous debris or hemorrhage

RELATED REFERENCES

1. Tubay M et al: Resident and fellow education feature: what is that cyst? Common cystic lesions of the female lower genitourinary tract. Radiographics. 34(2):427-8, 2014
2. Walker DK et al: Overlooked diseases of the vagina: a directed anatomic-pathologic approach for imaging assessment. Radiographics. 31(6):1583-98, 2011

T2 SHADING OF OVARY

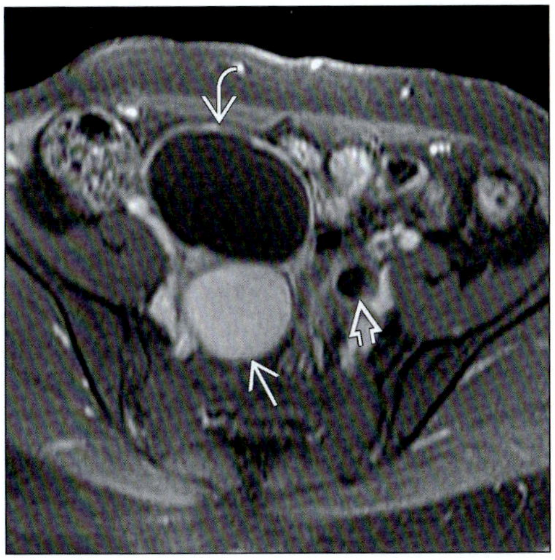

Axial T1WI C+ FS MR shows a well-circumscribed ovoid lesion ➔ within the right adnexa posterior to urinary bladder ➔. Normal left ovarian follicle ➔ demonstrating ↓ signal intensity is noted.

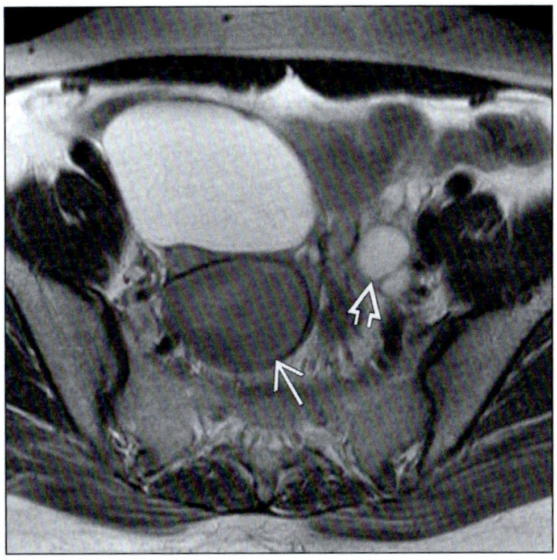

Axial T2WI MR demonstrates low signal intensity of the right adnexal mass T2 shading ➔ and high signal intensity of the left ovarian follicular cyst ➔.

CLINICAL SCENARIO

History

- 29-year-old woman with chronic cyclical pelvic pain

IMAGE INTERPRETATION

Appearance

- T2 shading sign is classic for endometrioma

BACKGROUND

General

- High protein content is due to repetitive cyclical hemorrhage, causing degenerated blood products to accumulate in hemosiderin-laden macrophages
- T2 shading indicates chronicity as it takes multiple cycles for blood products (proteins) to reflect on MR

Related Pathology

- Endometriosis is ectopic growth of functional endometrial cells outside endometrial cavity (most accepted theory is retrograde menstruation)
- Influenced by cyclical hormonal changes
- Can vary from microscopic foci to grossly visible cysts
- Repeated cyclical hemorrhage in deep peritoneal implants over surface of ovary → endometriotic cyst (a.k.a. endometrioma/chocolate cyst)
- Typically in women during reproductive years (25-30)
- Clinically: Infertility (2° to fibrosis), dysmenorrhea, dyspareunia, dysfunctional bleeding, & acute abdomen
- Associated with adenomyosis in 20% of cases
- Can → clear cell or endometrioid carcinoma
    - 2.5% of cases, ↑ when > 15 cm
    - Enhancing mural nodule on MR
    - Better prognosis than with no endometriosis due to lower grade & discovery at earlier stage
- In pregnancy, enhancing mural nodule can develop 2° to ↑ progesterone (not to be confused for cancer)

IMAGING FEATURES

US

- Well-circumscribed complex cystic mass that is homogeneously hypoechoic with low-level echoes & posterior acoustic enhancement
- Occasional fluid-fluid levels (different ages of blood or peripheral echogenic nodules due to blood clots)
- Color Doppler: No internal blood flow, so abnormal vascularity suggests malignant transformation

CT

- Nonspecific: Nonenhancing complex cystic mass

MR

- Highly specific due to ability to detect blood products of different ages
- T1WI: Hyperintense (no drop on FS)
- T2WI: Variable according to stage of blood product
- T2 shading (↑ SI on T1WI & ↓ SI on T2WI) is 90-98% specific, reflects T1 & T2 shortening 2° to high protein content & viscosity
- Multiplicity ↑ specificity for endometriomas
- T1WI C+: No enhancement
    - If enhances, suspect malignant transformation
- Endometriomas can show restricted diffusion

PET/CT

- Mostly low uptake on FDG PET scans (photopenic)
    - Normal increased uptake can be seen in menstrual & ovulatory phases of menstrual cycle

RELATED REFERENCES

1. Siegelman ES et al: MR imaging of endometriosis: ten imaging pearls. Radiographics. 32(6):1675-91, 2012
2. Chamié LP et al: Findings of pelvic endometriosis at transvaginal US, MR imaging, and laparoscopy. Radiographics. 31(4):E77-100, 2011
3. Lerman H et al: Normal and abnormal 18F-FDG endometrial and ovarian uptake in pre- and postmenopausal patients: assessment by PET/CT. J Nucl Med. 45(2):266-71, 2004

T2 DARK SPOT SIGN OF ENDOMETRIOMA

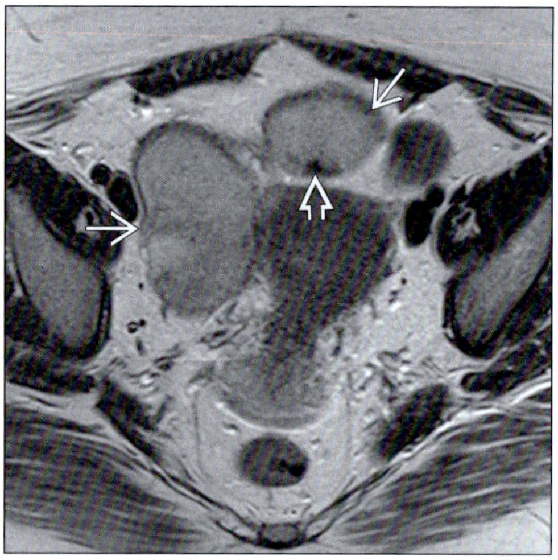

Axial T2WI MR shows bilateral ovarian hyperintense lesions ➡. Both lesions showed increased signal intensity on T1WI. There is a focal area of very low signal intensity ➪ within the left ovarian lesion.

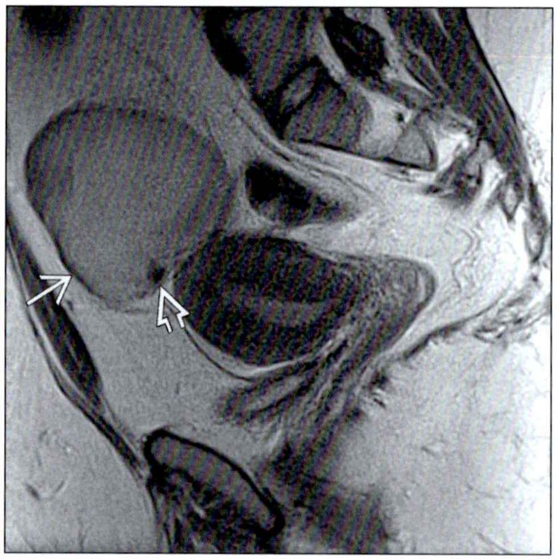

Sagittal T2WI MR shows the left ovarian hyperintense lesions ➡ with a focal area of very low signal intensity ➪.

IMAGING FEATURES

Appearance

- Small (mean: 6.3 mm) foci of very low T2 signal intensity within cystic lesion
  - Can be seen within cyst, often against cyst wall, but not within cyst wall itself

Clinical Significance

- T2 dark spot sign is highly specific for chronically hemorrhagic lesions (such as endometriomas)
- Can be used to differentiate ovarian endometriomas from functional hemorrhagic cysts
  - Sensitivity: 36%
  - Specificity: 93%
    - Not seen in hemorrhagic cysts
    - May be seen in hemorrhagic neoplasms
  - Positive predictive value: 89%
  - Negative predictive value: 48%
- May correspond to mural echogenic foci described in endometriomas at US

Other Imaging Findings

- Endometriomas characteristically have high signal intensity on T1WI
  - Hemorrhagic cysts and hemorrhagic neoplasms also have high signal intensity on T1WI
- T2 shading
  - Classic MR feature of endometrioma
    - Defined as cystic lesion with high signal intensity on T1WI that demonstrates T2 shortening resulting in signal intensity that is lower than simple fluid on T2WI
    - Likely secondary to high concentration of protein and degraded blood products that result from repeated hemorrhage
  - Performance of T2 shading in differentiating ovarian endometriomas from functional hemorrhagic cysts
    - Sensitivity: 93%
    - Specificity: 45%
    - Positive predictive value: 72%
    - Negative predictive value: 81%
- Presence of multiple hyperintense lesions on T1WI is specific for diagnosis of endometriomas
- Benign endometriomas show restricted diffusion

BACKGROUND

Explanation

- Exact cause is unclear
  - No pathologic correlate was found
- May represent chronic retracted blood clots that contain high concentration of protein &/or hemosiderin
  - Chronically retracted clots may become concentrated with protein and hemoglobin products to exhibit T2 shortening seen with T2 dark spots
- Because of rapid resolution of hemorrhagic cysts, retracted clots within hemorrhagic cysts may not have sufficient time to lose free water or progress to hemosiderin to cause marked T2 shortening

Pathology

- Endometriosis is defined as presence of endometrial tissue outside of uterine cavity
  - Estimated prevalence of 5-10% of women per year
- Endometriomas results from repeated hemorrhage with formation cystic lesions, commonly on ovaries

RELATED REFERENCES

1. Corwin MT et al: Differentiation of ovarian endometriomas from hemorrhagic cysts at MR imaging: utility of the T2 dark spot sign. Radiology. 271(1):126-32, 2014
2. Siegelman ES et al: MR imaging of endometriosis: ten imaging pearls. Radiographics. 32(6):1675-91, 2012
3. Glastonbury CM: The shading sign. Radiology. 224(1):199-201, 2002
4. Woodward PJ et al: Endometriosis: radiologic-pathologic correlation. Radiographics. 21(1):193-216; questionnaire 288-94, 2001

RING OF FIRE

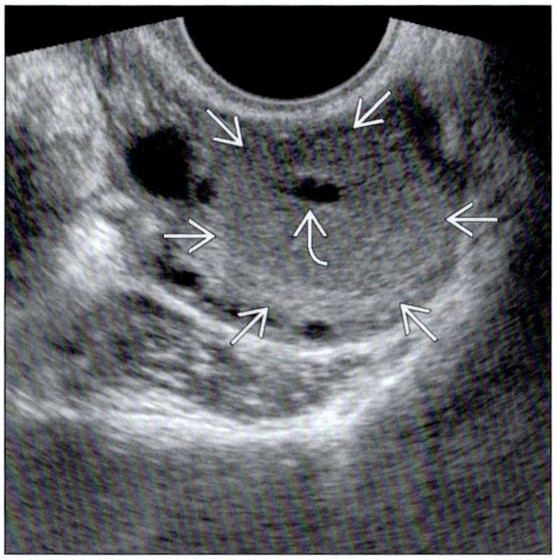

Transverse transvaginal grayscale ultrasound demonstrates a left adnexal mass with a small central cystic area with an echogenic periphery.

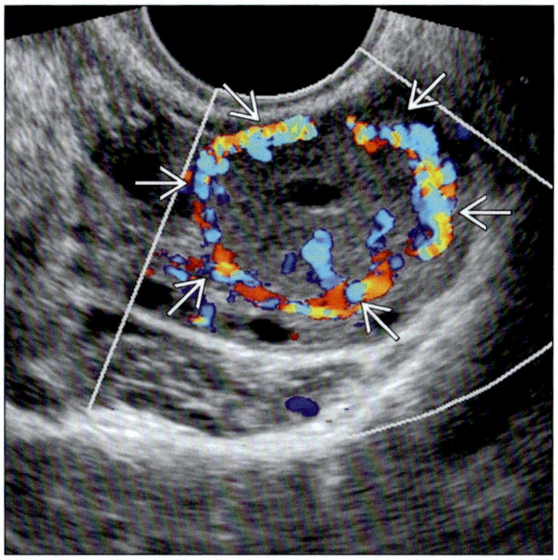

Transverse transvaginal color Doppler ultrasound demonstrates increased vascularity surrounding the cystic mass (ring of fire).

CLINICAL SCENARIO

History

- 25-year-old pregnant woman with pelvic pain and vaginal bleeding
- History of pelvic inflammatory disease
- Quantitative urine β-hCG is positive, indicating early pregnancy

IMAGE INTERPRETATION

Classic Sign

- Ring of fire represents peripheral hypervascularity of adnexal cyst (possibly extrauterine gestational sac)
  - Consistent with ectopic pregnancy in presence of proper clinical and laboratory settings

Differential Diagnosis

- Nonspecific sign; can be seen surrounding normal maturing follicle or corpus luteal cyst

BACKGROUND

Epidemiology

- Incidence: 2% of pregnancies
- 9-14% mortality rate

Relevant Pathology

- Ectopic pregnancy occurs with implantation of blastocyst outside of endometrium
- Risk factors: History of ectopic pregnancy, tubal surgery, pelvic inflammatory disease, and use of intrauterine device
- Locations
  - Fallopian tube is most common, accounting for ~ 95% of cases
  - Less common locations include interstitial, cornual, ovarian, cervical, scar, intraabdominal, and heterotopic
- Risk of rupture increases when ectopic pregnancy enlarges

IMAGING FEATURES

US

- No intrauterine pregnancy; no gestational sac, no yolk sac, and no fetal pole in endometrium
- Pseudosac (10%) can be occasionally seen; fluid centrally located in endometrial cavity with absent double decidual reaction, which is most often irregular in shape or flat
- Complex lesion in adnexa (most common location), which has echogenic ring that may demonstrate increased vascularity (ring of fire)
- Complex free fluid with debris suggesting hemorrhage
- When neither intrauterine pregnancy nor specific findings of ectopic pregnancy can be documented in patient with subthreshold β-hCG level
  - Patient should be closely monitored with serial US, and β-hCG levels should be continually tested until either ectopic or intrauterine pregnancy is identified

CT

- NECT: Complex-looking cystic lesion with internal high attenuation
- Peripheral enhancement correlating to ring of fire

MR

- T1WI: High signal intensity intracystic content
- T2WI: Low signal intensity internal content with high signal intensity wall
- T1WI C+: Peripheral enhancement 2° to wall hypervascularity

RELATED REFERENCES

1. Kao LY et al: Beyond ultrasound: CT and MRI of ectopic pregnancy. AJR Am J Roentgenol. 202(4):904-11, 2014
2. Lin EP et al: Diagnostic clues to ectopic pregnancy. Radiographics. 28(6):1661-71, 2008
3. Pellerito JS et al: Ectopic pregnancy: evaluation with endovaginal color flow imaging. Radiology. 183(2):407-11, 1992

COG WHEEL SIGN

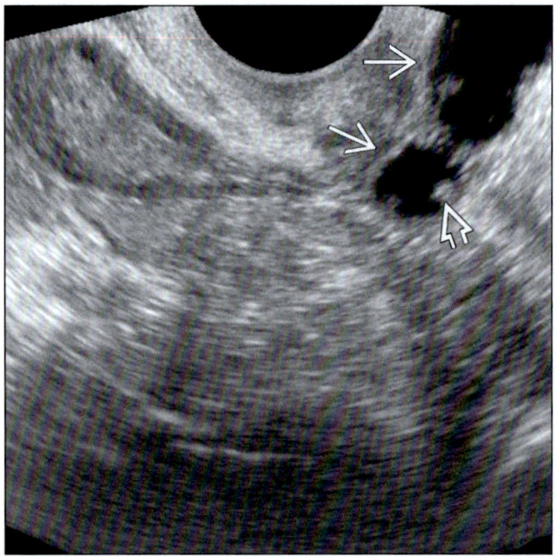

Longitudinal transvaginal grayscale ultrasound of the right adnexal region demonstrates a tubular structure ➡ with peripheral nodularities ➡ due to endosalpingeal folds thickening.

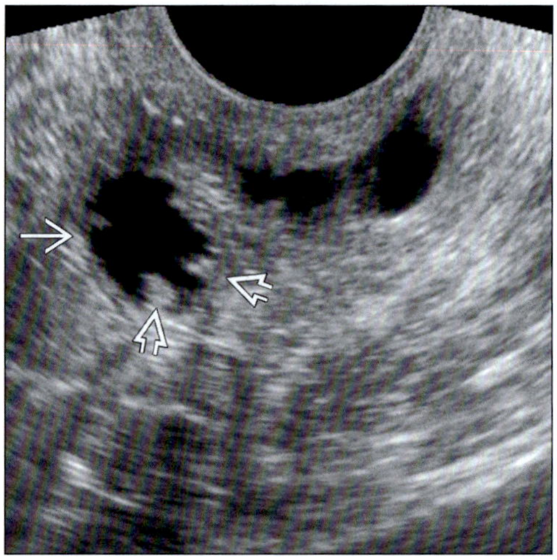

Transverse transvaginal grayscale US of right adnexa shows dilated tube in cross section ➡ with peripheral nodularities ➡ due to endosalpingeal folds thickening, resulting in cog wheel appearance.

CLINICAL SCENARIO

History

- 37-year-old woman with severe right lower quadrant pain & fever

IMAGE INTERPRETATION

Findings

- US shows markedly thickened endosalpingeal folds (cog wheel), wall thickening, and internal debris

Diagnosis

- Hydrosalpinx
- Presence of cog wheel appearance indicates that cystic adnexal structure represents dilated fluid-filled fallopian tube
  - Useful sign to differentiate ovarian cystic lesions from dilated fallopian tubes

BACKGROUND

General

- Hydrosalpinx is a chronic manifestation of pelvic inflammatory disease
- Usually starts with salpingitis → tubal and peritubal adhesions → obstruction of fimbrial end → fluid accumulation → hydrosalpinx

Epidemiology

- > 1 million cases of acute salpingitis reported annually in USA
- For women 16-25 years, salpingitis is most common serious infection (11% of females of reproductive age)
- ↑ incidence in low socioeconomic and young females (earlier sex, multiple partners, poor health care)
- 3x increase of PID with use of IUCD
- Also occurs via childbirth, abortion, endometrial biopsy, IUCD insertion, miscarriage

Relevant Pathology

- Commonest organisms: *Neisseria gonorrhoeae* and *Chlamydia*
- Marked neutrophilic infiltrate, congestion, and edema
- Mucosal ulceration and reactive epithelial change

IMAGING FEATURES

US (Transvaginal)

- Serpentine dilated, ovoid or pear-shaped fallopian tube with echogenic material
- Usually unilateral, but as disease progresses, infection could spread to other fallopian tube
- Thickened endosalpingeal folds → cog wheel sign
- Incomplete septa: Distended tortuous tubes with prominent folds
- Gain needs to be adjusted to visualize internal echoes
- Color Doppler: Increased vascularity in thickened walls
- Findings resolve promptly after adequate treatment

CECT

- Findings may be very subtle, particularly early
- Dilated fallopian tubes, which may show post-contrast enhancement
- Fat stranding with enhancing bands if infected

MR

- T1WI: Variable due to variable protein content (usually hypointense to intermediate signal intensity)
- T2WI: Intermediate to high signal intensity
- T1WI C+: Enhancing thickened/dilated fallopian tubes, surrounded by stranding of peritoneal fat

RELATED REFERENCES

1. Rezvani M et al: Fallopian tube disease in the nonpregnant patient. Radiographics. 31(2):527-48, 2011
2. Horrow MM: Ultrasound of pelvic inflammatory disease. Ultrasound Q. 20(4):171-9, 2004
3. Tukeva TA et al: MR imaging in pelvic inflammatory disease: comparison with laparoscopy and US. Radiology. 210(1):209-16, 1999

SNOWSTORM SIGN: MOLAR PREGNANCY

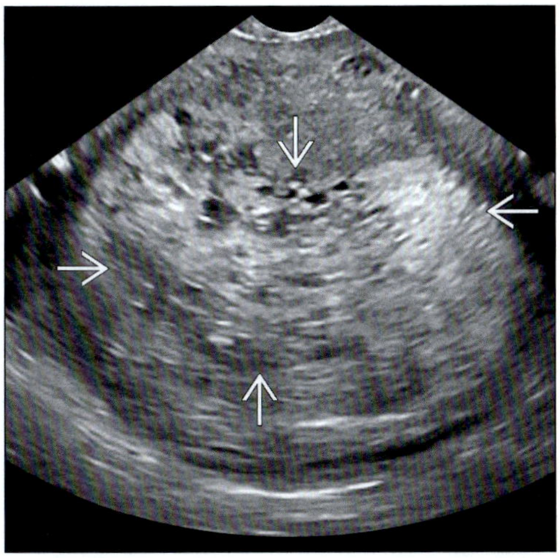

Transverse transvaginal ultrasound demonstrates a large mass ➡ distending the uterine cavity with multiple cystic and solid areas giving snowstorm appearance with absence of fetal parts.

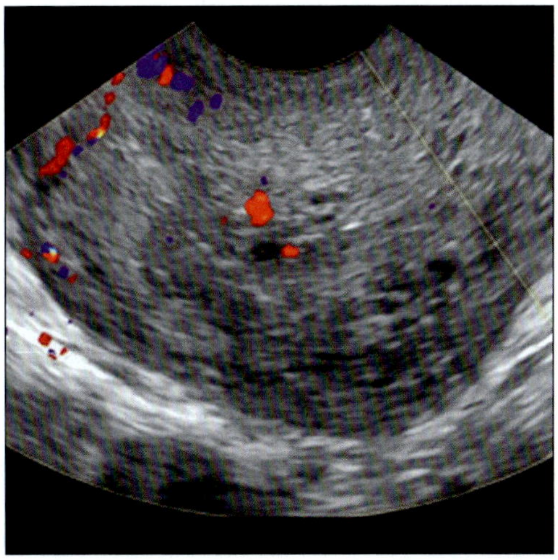

Color Doppler examination in the same patient demonstrates some increased blood flow within the mass.

CLINICAL SCENARIO

History

- 19-year-old woman with vaginal bleeding and morning sickness

IMAGE INTERPRETATION

Classic Sign

- Alternation of cystic and solid areas gives snowstorm appearance within uterine cavity and is consistent with hydatiform mole in proper clinical and laboratory setting

BACKGROUND

General

- Hydatiform mole is most common gestational trophoblastic disease (GTD)
- GTD is a manifestation of an aberrant fertilization event that leads to proliferative process
- Spectrum of GTD: Hydatididiform moles (complete and partial), invasive mole, choriocarcinoma, and placental site trophoblastic disease (rare)
- 90% of complete moles have 46,XX diploid chromosomes (paternal origin, suggesting fertilization of single ovum that has lost its chromosomes by 2 sperms)
- Partial mole has a triploid (69,XXY) karyotype and results from fertilization of a normal egg by 2 sperms; one is 23X chromosomes, other a 23Y chromosomal pattern
- Rarely coexists with normal pregnancy
- Marked increase in β-HCG production causing hyperemesis gravidarum and theca lutein cysts

Epidemiology

- Incidence: 1:1,000-2,000 pregnancies and as high as 1:41 miscarriages
- Age: Teens and adults between 40-50 years old, but can occur in any age group
- History of molar pregnancy increases risk of similar subsequent lesion
- More prevalent in Asia and Latin America than in North American and Europe
- 20% of complete moles are followed by malignant sequelae of invasive mole or choriocarcinoma

Relevant Pathology

- Cystic dilatation of chorionic villi producing cluster of grapes appearance
- Noninvasive mole does not invade myometrium
- Invasive mole in 20% after complete mole

IMAGING FEATURES

US

- Uterine cavity filled with multiple sonolucent areas of varying size and shape (alternation of cystic and solid areas gives snowstorm appearance), with no fetal parts (complete mole) or with fetal parts (partial mole)
- 1st trimester moles may have sonographic appearance simulating that of incomplete abortion
- Ovarian theca lutein cysts: Up to 50%
- Color Doppler: Highly vascular

CT

- Limited role in evaluation
- CECT demonstrates heterogeneously enhancing endometrial mass with occasional reticular pattern

MR

- T1WI: Uterine mass isointense to myometrium (areas of hemorrhage are hyperintense)
- T2WI: Markedly hyperintense mass distending endometrial cavity
- T1WI C+: Enhancing mass ± numerous small cysts

RELATED REFERENCES

1. Elsayes KM et al: Imaging of the placenta: a multimodality pictorial review. Radiographics. 29(5):1371-91, 2009

TIP OF ICEBERG: OVARIAN DERMOID

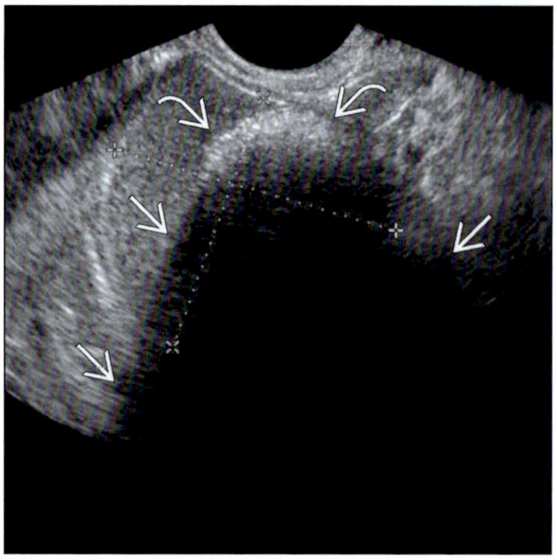

Longitudinal grayscale ultrasound demonstrates a curvilinear echogenic structure ➔ with posterior acoustic shadowing ➔ obscuring the borders of the mass giving tip of iceberg appearance.

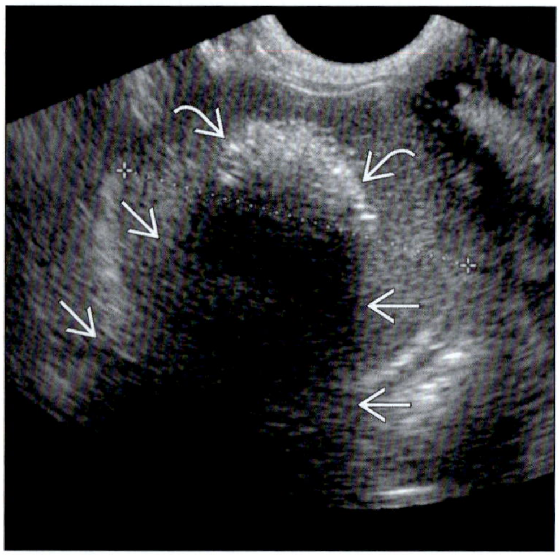

Transverse grayscale ultrasound demonstrates and confirms the findings in a different plane, with echogenic structure ➔ and posterior acoustic shadowing ➔ obscuring the mass.

CLINICAL SCENARIO

History

- 33-year-old woman with palpable right adnexal mass

IMAGE INTERPRETATION

Classic Sign

- Tip of iceberg sign is classic for ovarian dermoid

BACKGROUND

Explanation of Sign

- Due to hyperechogenicity of structures (hair and sebaceous material) inside cyst that may be diffuse, with shadowing often obscuring lesion
- Acoustic shadowing could be seen 2° to calcification
- Posterior shadowing should be differentiated from bowel gas with reverberation artifacts

General

- a.k.a. benign cystic teratoma
- Present from birth but usually not detected until 2nd or 3rd decade of life because of slow growth
- Usually incidental or palpated on physical exam
- Large dermoid cysts are usually removed as they may torse or rupture, presenting with acute abdominal pain

Epidemiology

- Most common ovarian neoplasm in women (< 45 years) and most common germ cell neoplasm
- Account for 10-20% of ovarian neoplasms
- Bilateral in 10-20% of cases

Relevant Pathology

- Composed of mature cells of all 3 germ cell layers with predominance of ectodermal elements, including hair, skin, teeth, and desquamated epithelium
- Cyst wall is made of stratified squamous epithelium & is filled with sebaceous material
- Rokitansky nodule arises from wall and contains bone, teeth, and hair follicles from which hair arises
- Malignant transformation in 1-2% of dermoid cysts, most commonly squamous cell carcinoma

IMAGING FEATURES

US

- Variable appearances depending on epithelial contents
- Diffuse or focal echogenic areas & posterior shadowing
- Classic sonographic findings
  - Tip of iceberg sign
  - Dermoid plug (a.k.a. Rokitansky nodule): Mural nodule containing hair follicles &/or other solid elements, echogenic with posterior shadowing; may be single or multiple
  - Dermoid mesh: Multiple linear & punctate echoes, corresponding with interweaving strands of hair
- Fat-fluid level and focal calcification (tooth)

CT

- Fat attenuation (both adipose-containing dermoid plug and lipid-laden sebaceous cystic material)
- May or may not see calcifications within wall
- Hairball or fat-fluid level are sometimes seen

MR

- Various components including fat and calcification
- T1WI: Hyperintense (similar to fat)
- T2WI: Moderate signal (similar to fat)
- Signal loss on fat-saturated T1 and T2WI

RELATED REFERENCES

1. Wasnik AP et al: Multimodality imaging of ovarian cystic lesions: Review with an imaging based algorithmic approach. World J Radiol. 5(3):113-25, 2013
2. Jung SE et al: CT and MR imaging of ovarian tumors with emphasis on differential diagnosis. Radiographics. 22(6):1305-25, 2002
3. Beller MJ: The "tip of the iceberg" sign. Radiology. 209(2):395-6, 1998

FISHNET SIGN: OVARIAN HEMORRHAGIC CYST

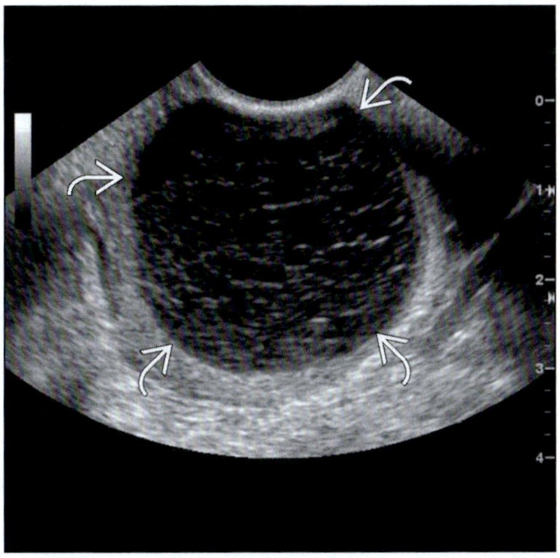

Grayscale transvaginal ultrasound of the left ovary demonstrates a complex cystic lesion exhibiting a fine reticular pattern giving appearance of fishnet with posterior acoustic enhancement.

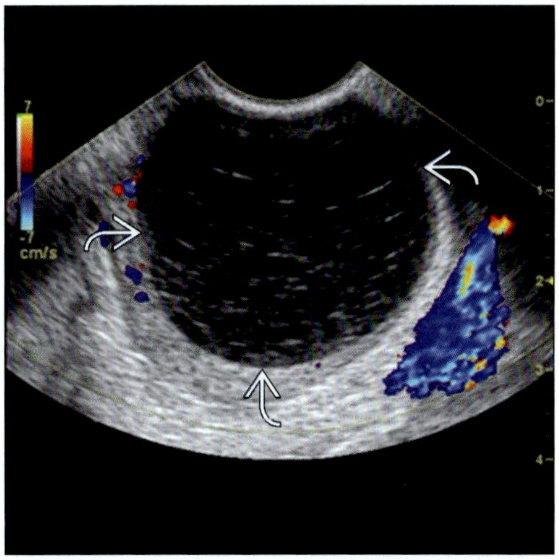

Color Doppler interrogation of transvaginal ultrasound examination of the left ovary demonstrates no definite evidence of abnormal internal vascularity of the lesion.

CLINICAL SCENARIO

History

- 32-year-old woman with left lower quadrant pain

IMAGE INTERPRETATION

Classic Sign

- Fine reticular echoes in fishnet pattern in ovarian cyst without internal vascularity is classic for hemorrhagic ovarian cyst

BACKGROUND

General

- Hemorrhage within corpus luteum cyst
- Benign without malignant potential
- Typically resolves within 2 menstrual cycles
- May be present with pain or may be asymptomatic

Epidemiology

- Women of reproductive age

Relevant Physiology

- Granulosa cell layer is avascular until ovulation
- After release of an egg, granulosa cell layer becomes highly vascularized
- Blood vessels in granulosa cell layer are fragile and prone to rupture, which leads to hemorrhage within corpus luteum cyst

Relevant Pathology

- Gross: Typically 3-8 cm, thin-walled and unilocular cyst with internal hemorrhage
- Microscopic: Luteinized granulosa cells, fibroblasts, hemosiderin-laden macrophages, and abundant fibrin

IMAGING FEATURES

US

- Preferred modality
- Thin-walled cyst
- Typical size is about 3 cm
- Fishnet sign of fine reticular echoes within hemorrhagic cyst representing fibrin strands
- Retracting clot within a hemorrhagic cyst may appear as a triangular or curvilinear clump of echoes
- No internal color Doppler signal

MR

- Well-circumscribed cystic lesion
- Internal signal characteristics are variable depending on age of hemorrhage
- Most common pattern is T1-hyperintense signal and T2-heterogeneous or hyperintense signal
- No internal contrast enhancement on gadolinium-enhanced images

CT

- Ovarian mass with internal contents measuring > 10 HU

PET/CT

- Variable, but increased FDG uptake has been reported

Key Teaching Points

- Describes fine reticular echoes representing fibrin strands within hemorrhagic cyst
- Classic for ovarian hemorrhagic cyst

RELATED REFERENCES

1. Kanso HN et al: Variable MR findings in ovarian functional hemorrhagic cysts. J Magn Reson Imaging. 24(2):356-61, 2006
2. Patel MD et al: The likelihood ratio of sonographic findings for the diagnosis of hemorrhagic ovarian cysts. J Ultrasound Med. 24(5):607-14; quiz 615, 2005
3. Jain KA: Sonographic spectrum of hemorrhagic ovarian cysts. J Ultrasound Med. 21(8):879-86, 2002

ENTRAPPED OVARY SIGN

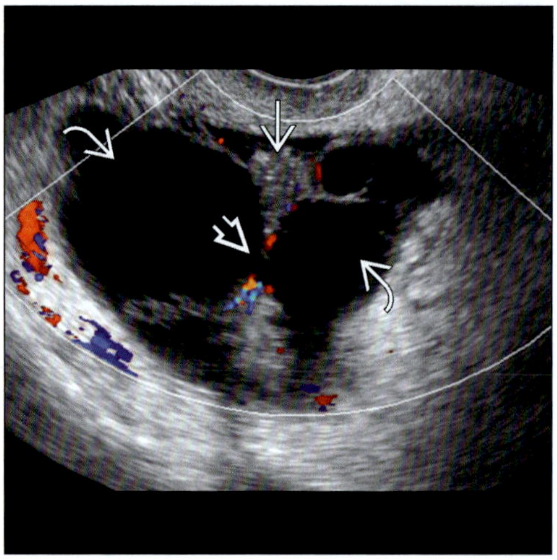

Color Doppler transvaginal ultrasound shows a well-defined multiloculated cystic lesion ➡ seen surrounding the right ovary ➡ with mildly vascularized septations ➡.

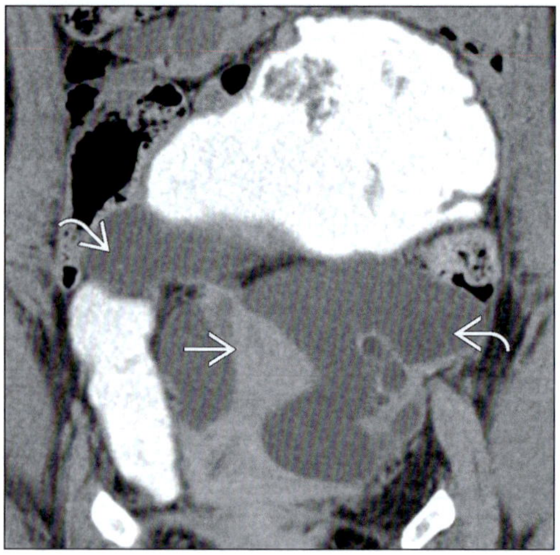

Coronal reformatted CECT shows a well-circumscribed lobulated multiloculated cystic collection ➡ seen surrounding the ovary ➡, showing the entrapped ovary sign.

IMAGE INTERPRETATION

Appearance and Explanation

- Classic appearance of peritoneal inclusion cyst
- Results from accumulation of ovarian fluid that is not absorbed by peritoneum

Pitfalls

- Peritoneal inclusion cyst can be misinterpreted as paraovarian cyst, hydrosalpinx, pyosalpinx, multicystic mesothelioma, and malignant cystic ovarian neoplasm

BACKGROUND

Clinical Presentation

- Most patients present with pelvic pain or pelvic mass

Epidemiology

- Occurs almost exclusively in premenopausal women

Relevant Pathology

- Development of peritoneal inclusion cyst depends on presence of active ovary and peritoneal adhesions
  - Peritoneal adhesions result from abdominal or pelvic surgery, trauma, pelvic inflammatory disease, or endometriosis
    - Nonneoplastic, reactive mesothelial proliferation → ↓ absorptive capacity of peritoneum → accumulation of fluid around ovary
- Varies in size from several mm to large masses that may occupy the whole pelvis and abdomen
- Primarily occurs in pelvis and rarely in other intraperitoneal locations

IMAGING FEATURES

General

- Loculated septated fluid collection within pelvis with normal ovary in middle or at edge of fluid collection
  - Entrapped ovary appears like spider in web of linear peritoneal adhesions and may be mistaken for solid nodular portion of tumor with surrounding septations
- Insinuating pattern of expansion between pelvic structures without considerable mass effect
  - This pattern helps distinguish peritoneal inclusion cysts from other cystic pelvic lesions

US

- Cyst content is usually anechoic with fine septations and thin wall
- Rarely low-resistance flow from vascularized septations

CT

- Cyst content is usually fluid attenuation

MR

- Fluid-signal intensity, low on T1WI, high on T2WI, and no enhancement of cyst walls
- The location of ovary in relation to cysts is clearly displayed

Key Teaching Points

- Entrapped ovary sign is typical for peritoneal inclusion cyst
- Peritoneal inclusion cyst can be misinterpreted for other pathologies, including malignant cystic ovarian neoplasm

RELATED REFERENCES

1. Brown DL et al: Adnexal masses: US characterization and reporting. Radiology. 254(2):342-54, 2010
2. Jeong YJ et al: Neoplastic and nonneoplastic conditions of serosal membrane origin: CT findings. Radiographics. 28(3):801-17; discussion 817-8; quiz 912, 2008
3. Jeong JY et al: Sclerotherapy of peritoneal inclusion cysts: preliminary results in seven patients. Korean J Radiol. 2(3):164-70, 2001

FDG UPTAKE WITHIN THROMBUS

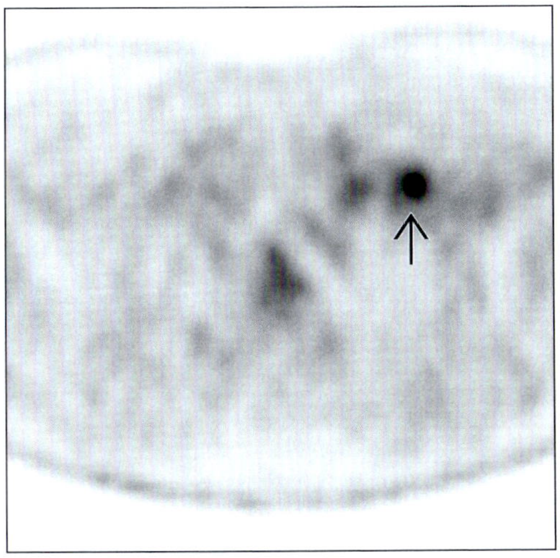

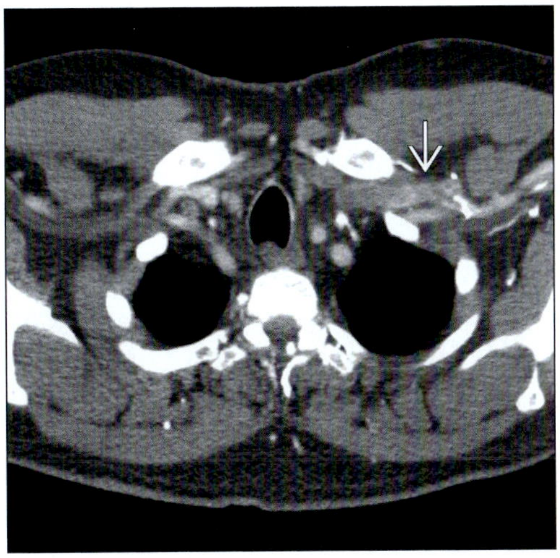

(Left) *Axial PET demonstrates increased radiotracer uptake* → *corresponding to left subclavian vein intraluminal filling defect seen on the contrast-enhanced CT, consistent with FDG uptake within a thrombus.* ***(Right)*** *Axial contrast-enhanced CT from the same patient demonstrates left subclavian vein intraluminal filling defect* ➡*.*

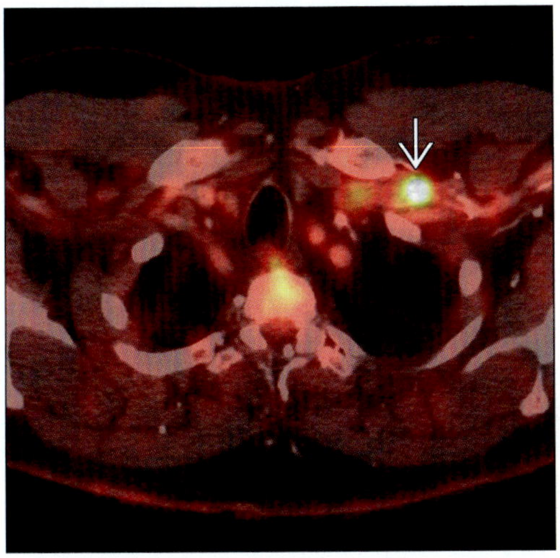

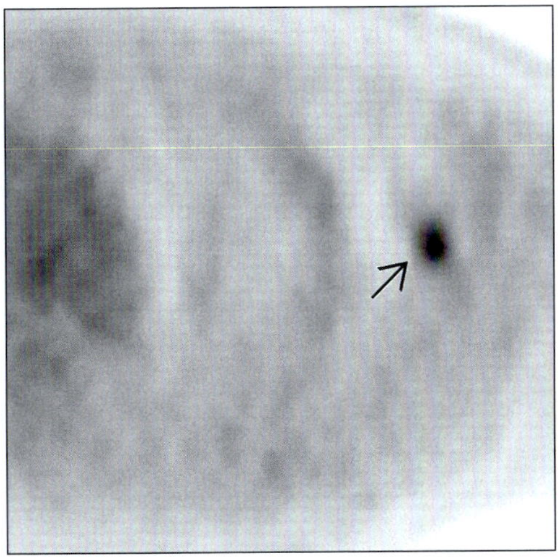

(Left) *Axial fused PET/CT from the same patient demonstrates increased radiotracer uptake* ➡ *corresponding to left subclavian vein intraluminal filling defect seen on the contrast-enhanced CT, consistent with FDG uptake within a thrombus.* ***(Right)*** *Axial PET in a different patient demonstrates increased radiotracer activity* → *corresponding to an intravascular filling defect on contrast-enhanced CT, consistent with thrombus or embolus.*

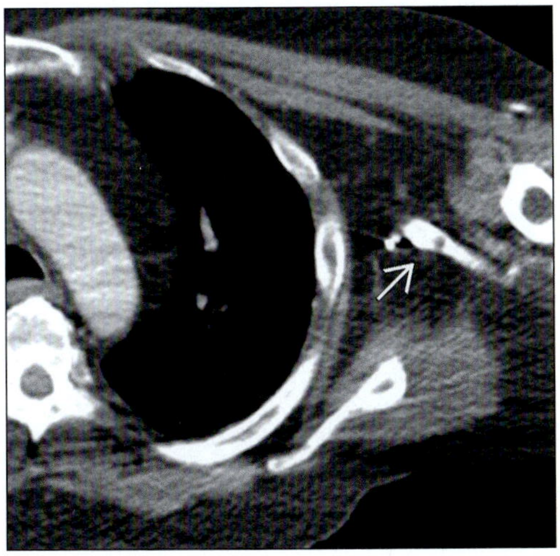

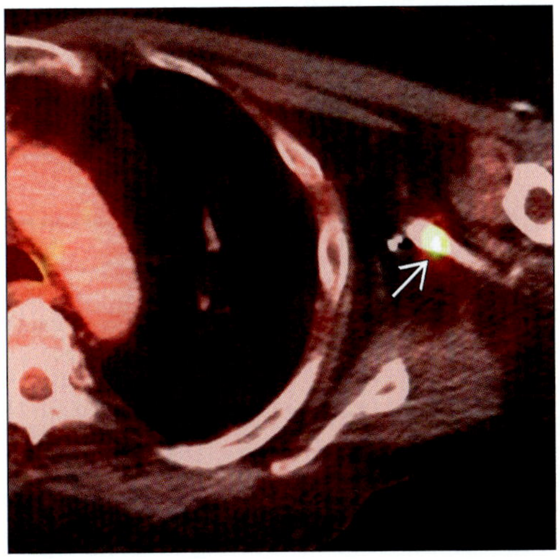

(Left) *Axial CT from the same patient demonstrates an intravascular filling defect* ➡ *on contrast-enhanced CT, consistent with thrombus or embolus.* ***(Right)*** *Axial fused PET/CT from the same patient demonstrates increased radiotracer activity* ➡ *corresponding to an intravascular filling defect on contrast-enhanced CT, consistent with thrombus or embolus.*

POSTPROCEDURAL FDG UPTAKE

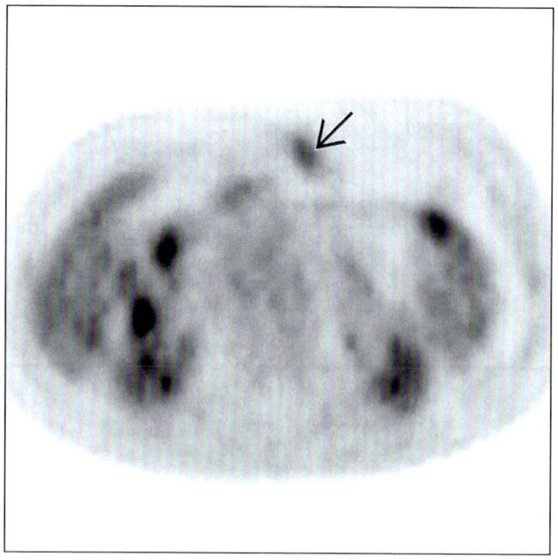

Axial PET demonstrates a linear focus of increased radiotracer activity at a gastrostomy tube insertion site ➔.

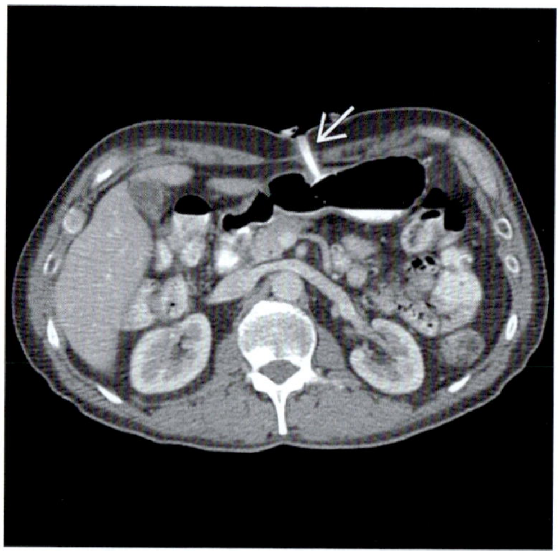

Axial NECT demonstrates gastrostomy tube ➔ traversing through the skin and subcutaneous tissue toward the gastric lumen.

CLINICAL SCENARIO

History

- 63 year old with lung adenocarcinoma and lymphatic metastasis undergoing chemotherapy/radiation
- Percutaneous endoscopic gastrostomy (PEG) tube placed 5 months prior to PET/CT examination

IMAGE INTERPRETATION

Pitfalls

- Postoperative hypermetabolic uptake surrounding PEG insertion site may be misinterpreted for malignancy or infection

Actual Diagnosis

- Normal FDG uptake surrounding PEG insertion site

Clues to Correct Diagnosis

- Correlate with additional imaging (CT)
  - Nodularity may represent metastasis or infection
    - Infection more frequently demonstrates adjacent inflammatory changes (e.g., fat stranding)
- Obtaining clinical history of patient symptoms and physical examination for evidence of infection

BACKGROUND

General

- Postoperative FDG uptake can be seen with a variety of iatrogenic procedures including gastrostomy tube, implanted port, and hernia repair with mesh
- Gastrostomy tube placement can be performed endoscopically or fluoroscopically
- Many patients undergoing PEG placement have known malignancy, particularly head and neck cancer
  - Though rare, abdominal wall metastases can occur
    - Metastasis along PEG insertion site often presents late, PET/CT may provide early detection

Epidemiology

- Patients with underlying squamous cell carcinoma of pharynx or esophagus are more likely to develop seeding at PEG site
  - Risk factors for development of seeding in this setting include PEG placement with untreated or advanced stage squamous cell carcinoma or PEG placement with endoscopic pull string gastrostomy

IMAGING FEATURES

CT

- No nodularity or fluid collection if uncomplicated PEG
  - Mild soft tissue stranding if recently placed PEG
- Soft tissue nodularity ± enhancement suspicious for metastatic disease
- Hypoattenuating complex fluid collection with peripheral enhancement suggestive of abscess

PET/CT

- Mild increased metabolic activity may be physiologic or secondary to granulation tissue
- Intensely increased FDG uptake with associated abnormal finding on CT is more concerning for metastatic disease
  - Small nodules may represent metastasis or infection/abscess
- Correlation for secondary signs of inflammation or infection such as fat stranding should be performed

RELATED REFERENCES

1. de Monès E et al: Diagnosis of squamous cell carcinoma metastasis with 18F-FDG PET/CT in stoma after percutaneous endoscopic gastrostomy: a rare and poorly known iatrogenic cause of spread of head and neck cancer. Clin Nucl Med. 39(6):544-6, 2014
2. Purandare NC et al: Percutaneous endoscopic gastrostomy site metastases in head and neck cancer: use of FDG PET-CT. Diagn Interv Radiol. 14(2):88-93, 2008

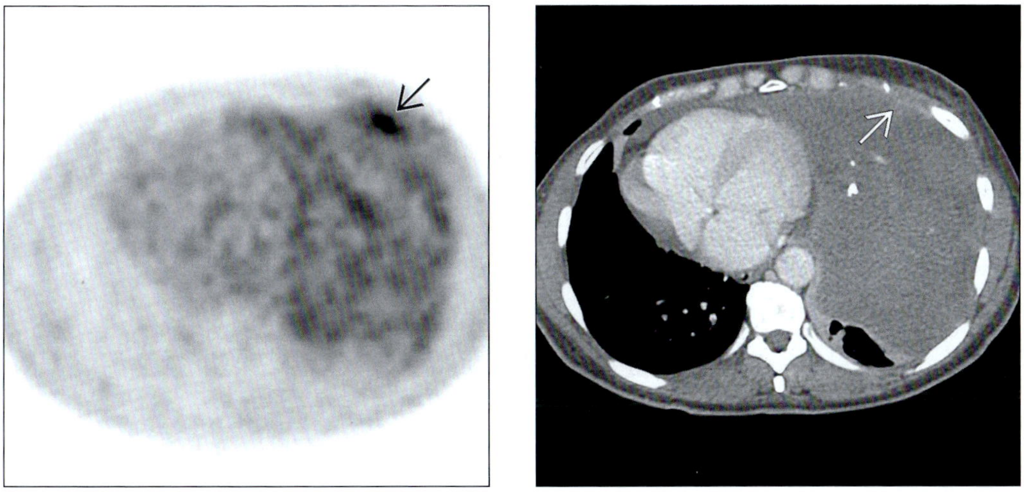

(Left) *Axial PET in a 50-year-old woman with nodular sclerosing Hodgkin lymphoma demonstrates a linear area of increased FDG-18 activity → (SUVmax: 4.2) in the left chest wall.* ***(Right)*** *Axial CECT demonstrates no definite abnormality within the intercostal space at the site of increased activity →.*

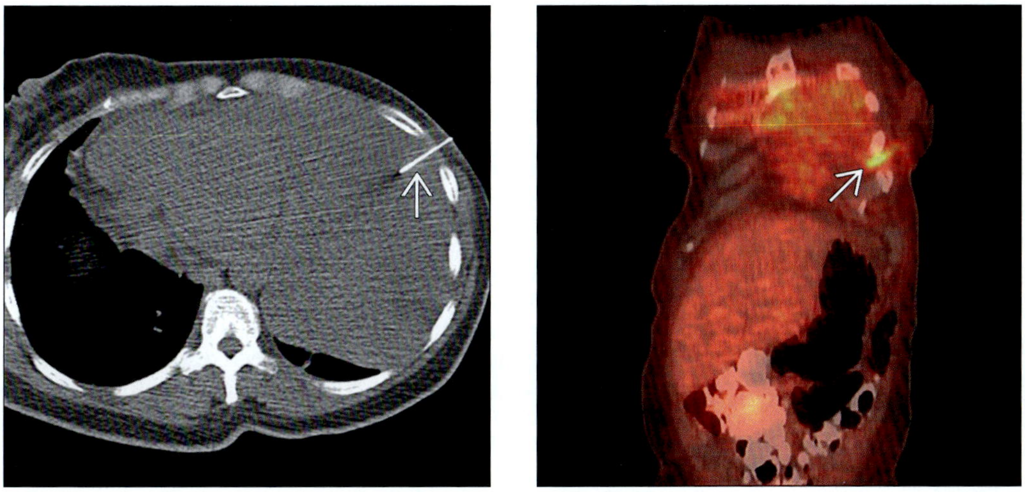

(Left) *Axial NECT demonstrates a biopsy needle → traversing through the same location during a previous needle biopsy procedure.* ***(Right)*** *Coronal fused PET/CT demonstrates a linear area of increased FDG-18 activity → (SUVmax: 4.2) within the intercostal space between the 6th and 7th ribs from recent needle biopsy.*

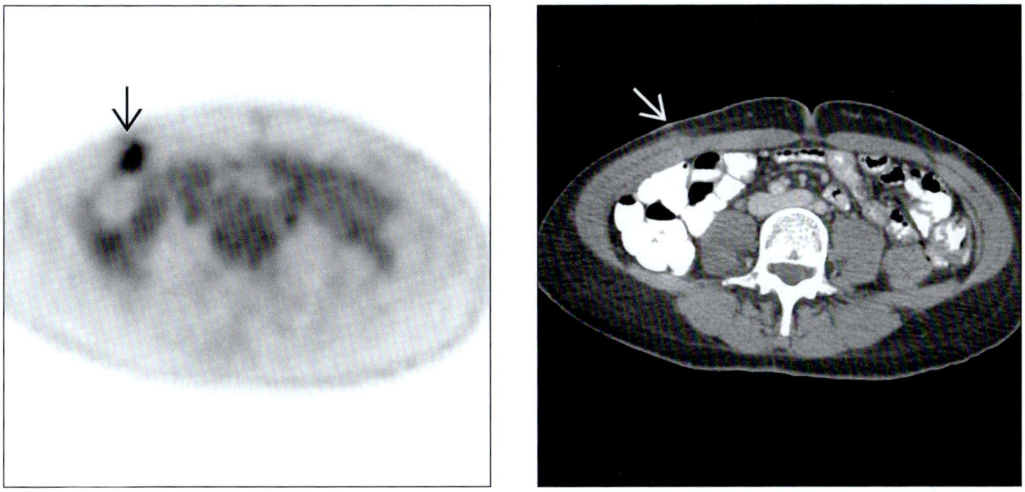

(Left) *Axial PET demonstrates a focus of increased radiotracer activity → in the right lower anterior abdominal wall.* ***(Right)*** *Axial CT demonstrates a soft tissue stranding →, corresponding to a laparoscopic port insertion site.*

PHYSIOLOGIC ACTIVITY IN FEMALE REPRODUCTIVE ORGANS

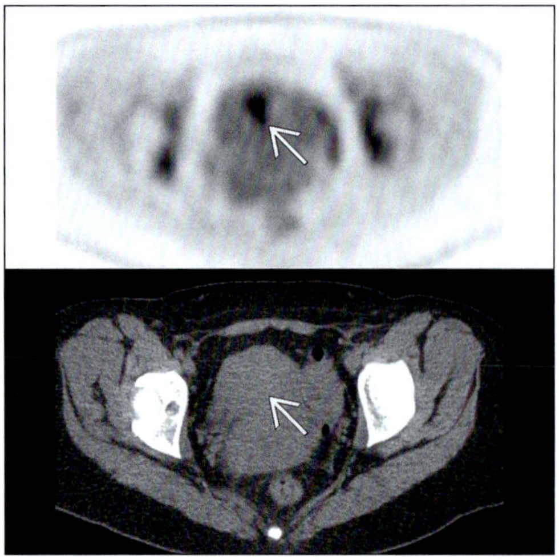

Axial PET (top) and CT (bottom) demonstrate increased FDG avidity in the endometrium ➔ secondary to menstruation.

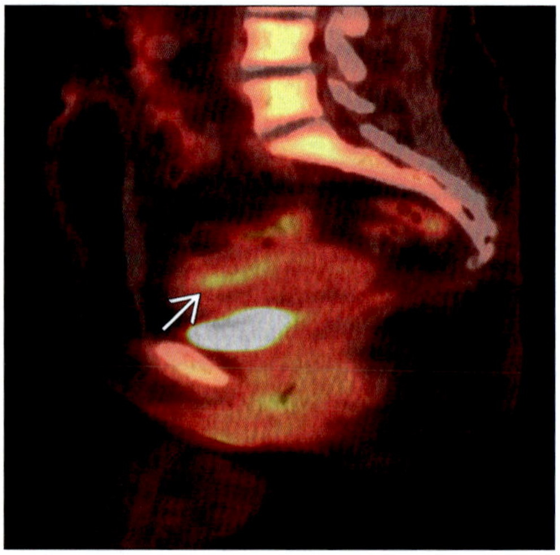

Sagittal fused PET/CT demonstrates increased FDG avidity in the endometrium ➔ secondary to menstruation.

CLINICAL SCENARIO

History

- 30-year-old woman with Hodgkin lymphoma status post chemotherapy

IMAGE INTERPRETATION

Pitfalls

- Misinterpretation of endometrial or ovarian uptake as malignancy (including in setting of known cervical cancer)

Actual Diagnosis

- Physiologic activity in uterine cavity premenopausal females

Clues to Correct Diagnosis

- Know phase of patient's menstrual cycle
- Compare with other available examinations to correlate for benign versus malignant anatomic lesions
- SUV alone cannot assess for primary malignancy

BACKGROUND

General

- Active menstruation is most common cause of uptake in endometrium without known malignancy
  - 2 peaks of ↑ uptake: Mid cycle and menstrual flow
- In premenopausal, FDG uptake in ovaries may be malignant or functional with high SUV (> 7.9) found to be highly specific for malignancy

Relevant Physiology

- Postmenopausal hormonal therapy is usually not associated with ↑ FDG uptake; therefore, uptake in this population may raise suspicion for malignancy

Relevant Pathology

- Benign lesions (e.g., serous & mucinous cystadenoma, dermoid cyst, endometriosis, inflammation & teratoma) can demonstrate FDG uptake

IMAGING FEATURES

CT

- Patterns of physiologic uptake in endometrium & ovaries can be correlated with hypoattenuating, linear/triangular appearance of endometrium and with presence of ovarian follicles
- Particularly useful with respect to evaluating for lymph node staging and detection of distant metastasis when used in conjunction with PET

PET/CT

- Patterns of physiologic activity
  - Endometrial activity tends to be linear or triangular with variable intensity, and can be most prominent during menstrual phase (also seen during ovulation)
  - Ovarian activity is also variable, but should only be seen during ovulatory phase of cycle
    - Seen in both, one, or neither adnexal regions
- Malignant & nonmalignant functional ovarian lesions have overlapping SUVs, therefore PET is limited in differentiating borderline malignant & benign tumors
  - Correlate with menstrual phase and imaging features
- Cervical, endometrial, vulvar, and ovarian carcinomas demonstrate ↑ FDG uptake with PET/CT playing role in lymph node staging and distant metastasis

RELATED REFERENCES

1. Kitajima K et al: Spectrum of FDG PET/CT findings of uterine tumors. AJR Am J Roentgenol. 195(3):737-43, 2010
2. Nishizawa S et al: Incidence and characteristics of uterine leiomyomas with FDG uptake. Ann Nucl Med. 22(9):803-10, 2008
3. Nishizawa S et al: Physiological 18F-FDG uptake in the ovaries and uterus of healthy female volunteers. Eur J Nucl Med Mol Imaging. 32(5):549-56, 2005
4. Lerman H et al: Normal and abnormal 18F-FDG endometrial and ovarian uptake in pre- and postmenopausal patients: assessment by PET/CT. J Nucl Med. 45(2):266-71, 2004

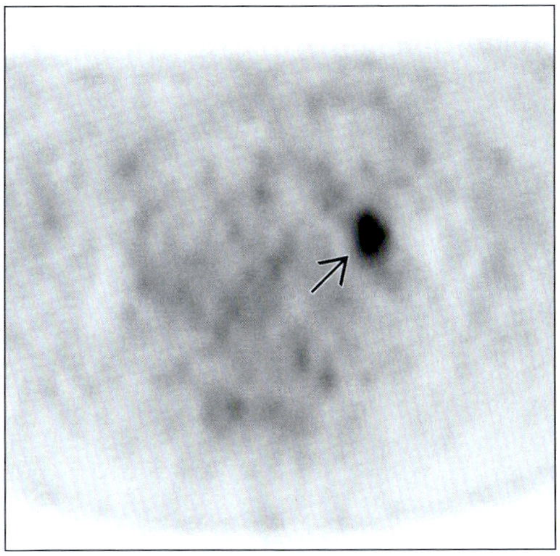

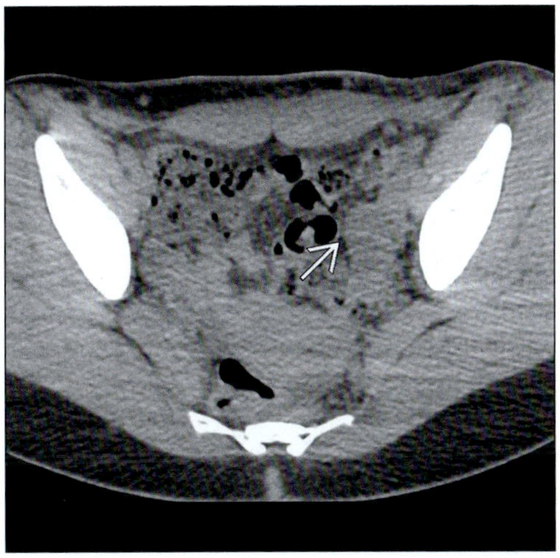

(Left) *Axial PET in a 22-year-old woman with mycosis fungoides undergoing restaging demonstrates increased radiotracer activity in the left ovary ⇨. While this was nonspecific on imaging, it ended up representing physiologic activity.* ***(Right)*** *Axial NECT in the same patient shows the left ovary ➡, which appears to be of normal size and morphology.*

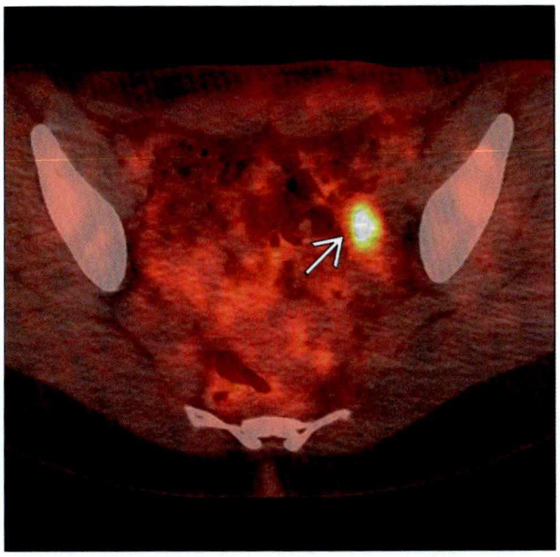

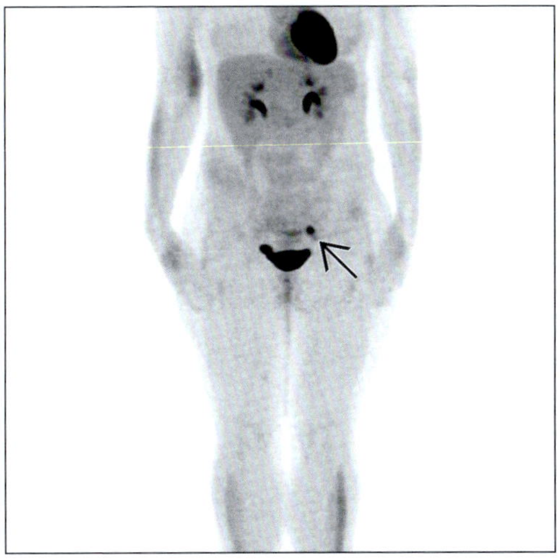

(Left) *Axial fused FDG PET/CT in the same patient demonstrates increased radiotracer activity in the left ovary ➡.* ***(Right)*** *Coronal MIP PET in the same patient demonstrates increased radiotracer activity in the left ovary ⇨.*

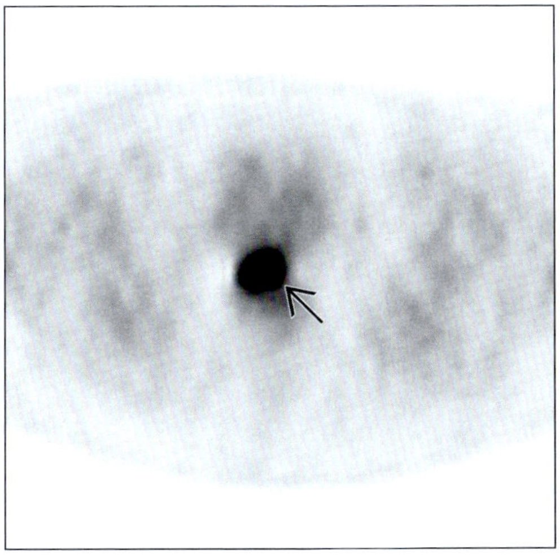

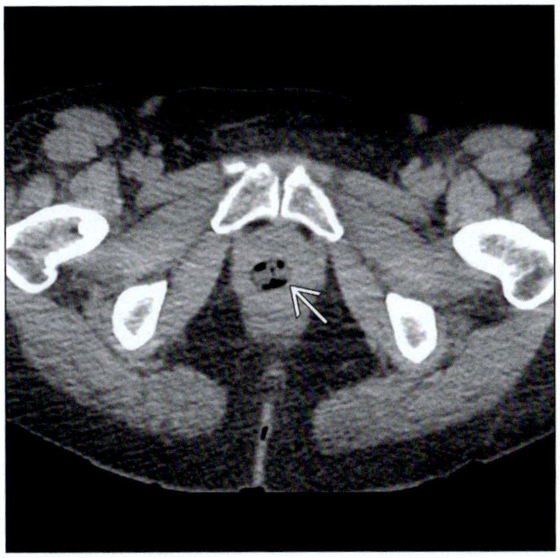

(Left) *Axial FDG PET in a 40-year-old woman with metastatic melanoma demonstrates increased radiotracer activity ⇨ (SUVmax: 34.1) in the region of vagina.* ***(Right)*** *Axial NECT in the same patient demonstrates that increased radiotracer activity on PET image correlates with a vaginal tampon ➡.*

PHYSIOLOGIC ACTIVITY IN FEMALE REPRODUCTIVE ORGANS

(Left) *Axial fused FDG PET/CT in the same patient demonstrates increased radiotracer activity on FDG PET image localizing to a tampon ➡ (SUVmax: 34.1).* *(Right)* *Sagittal fused FDG PET/CT in the same patient demonstrates increased radiotracer activity on FDG PET image localizing to a tampon ➡ (SUVmax: 34.1).*

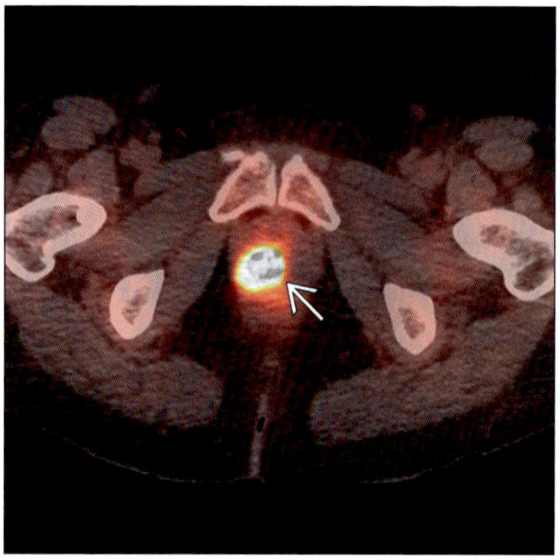

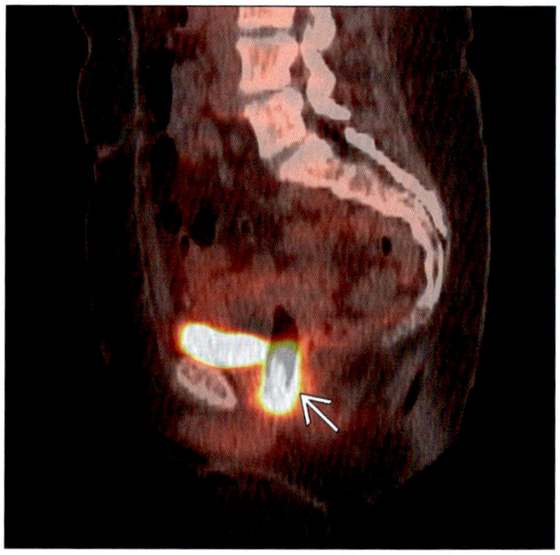

(Left) *Axial PET image in a 28-year-old woman with recurrent cervical cancer demonstrates focus of increased FDG activity ➡ (SUVmax: 4.6) in the left mid abdomen.* *(Right)* *Axial CECT in the same patient demonstrates transposed ovary ➡ in the left mid abdomen adjacent to a surgical clip and loops of bowel.*

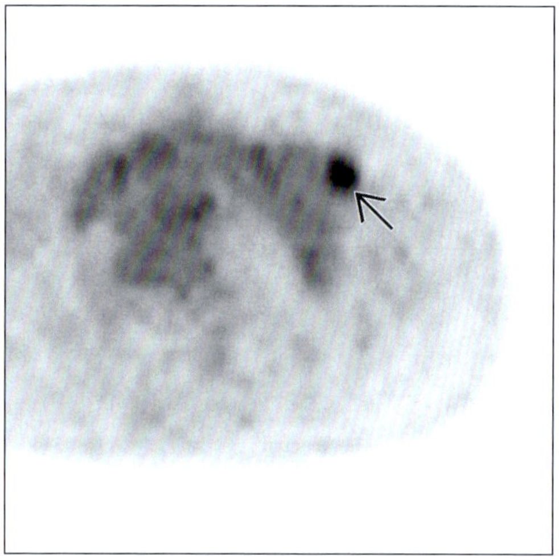

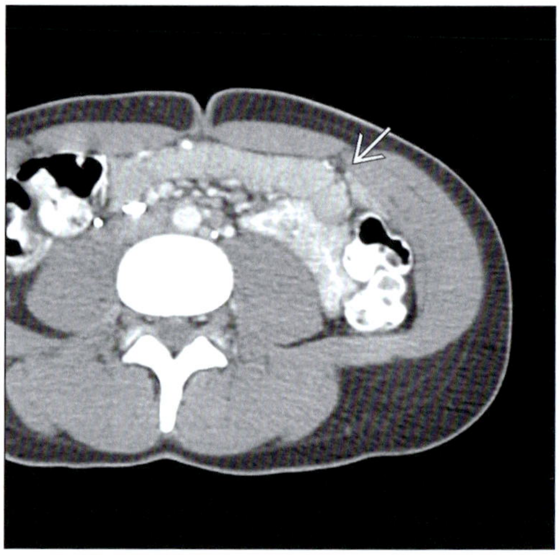

(Left) *Axial fused FDG PET/CT in the same patient demonstrates focus of increased FDG activity ➡ in the left mid abdomen.* *(Right)* *MIP image in the same patient demonstrates foci of increased FDG activity (SUVmax: 4.6) ➡ in the left mid abdomen, most compatible with physiologic activity within transposed ovaries.*

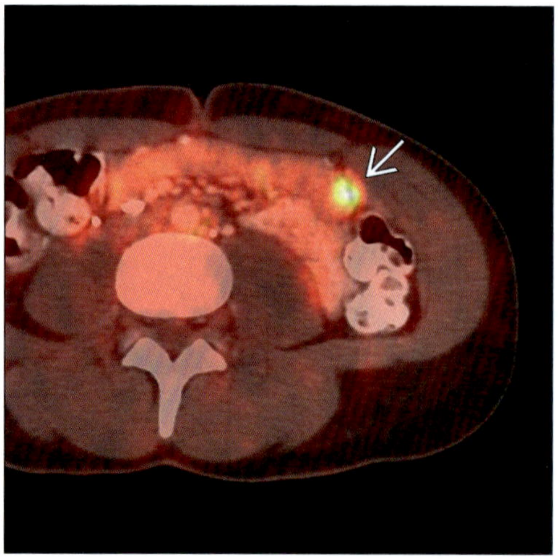

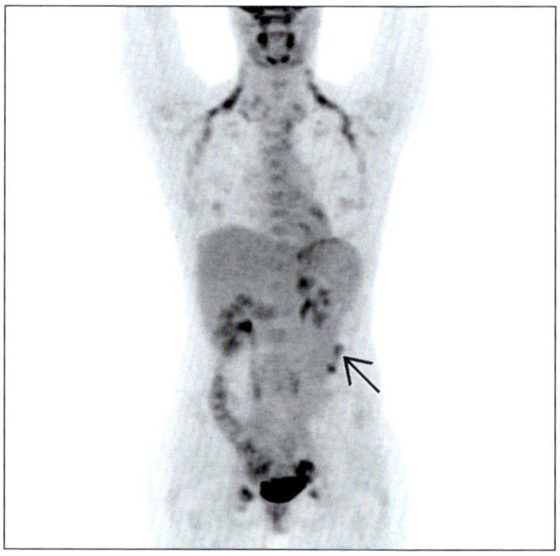

PHYSIOLOGIC ACTIVITY IN FEMALE REPRODUCTIVE ORGANS

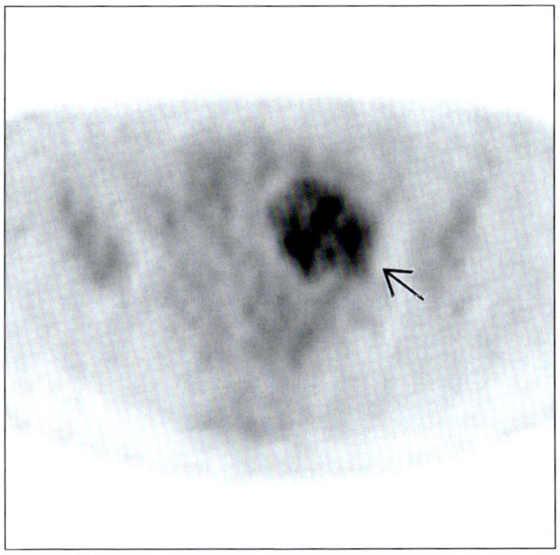

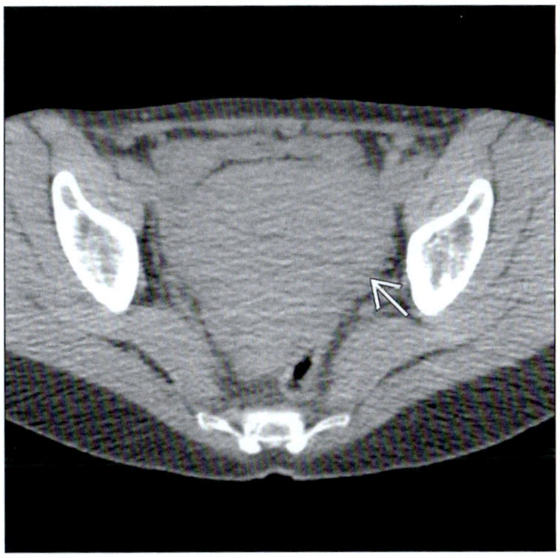

(Left) *Axial PET in a 34-year-old woman with Hodgkin lymphoma demonstrates increased radiotracer activity* → *(SUVmax: 6.4) at the left aspect of an enlarged uterus.* ***(Right)*** *Axial NECT in the same patient demonstrates the enlarged uterus with subtle evidence of a round isoattenuating mass* → *in the left uterine wall.*

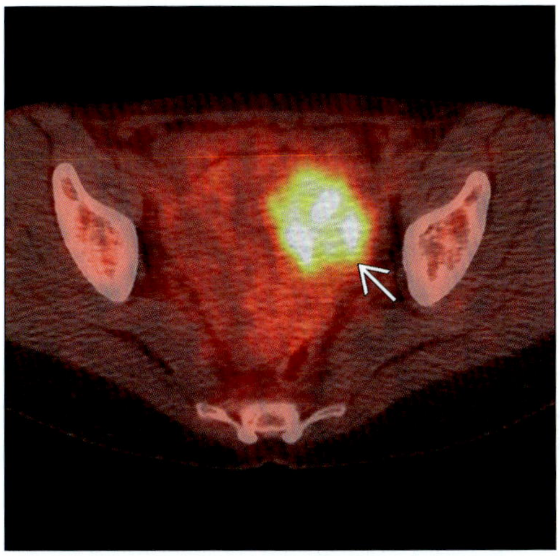

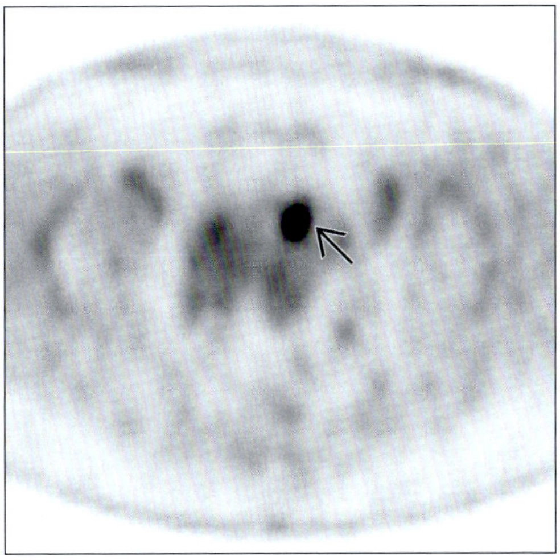

(Left) *Axial fused FDG PET/CT in the same patient demonstrates increased radiotracer activity* → *at the left aspect of the enlarged uterus.* ***(Right)*** *Axial PET in a 53-year-old postmenopausal female with newly diagnosed endometrial cancer demonstrates increased radiotracer activity* →.

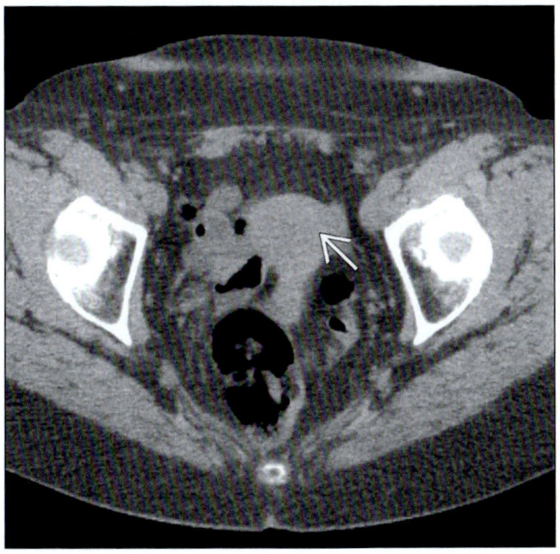

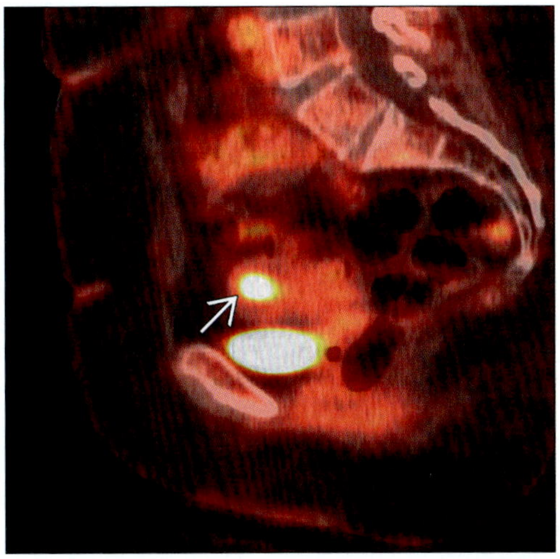

(Left) *Axial NECT in the same patient demonstrates no definite abnormality* →. ***(Right)*** *Sagittal fused FDG PET/CT in the same patient demonstrates increased radiotracer activity* → *in the endometrial canal, which was found to represent endometrial cancer. Increased FDG in the uterus and adnexa of postmenopausal females is always abnormal and should be further investigated.*

BOWEL UPTAKE SECONDARY TO METFORMIN

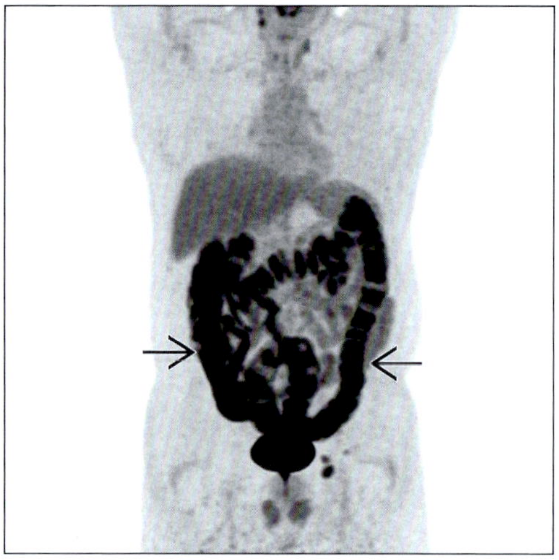

MIP demonstrates diffuse increased FDG-18 activity throughout the colon and loops of small bowel ➔, compatible with use of metformin.

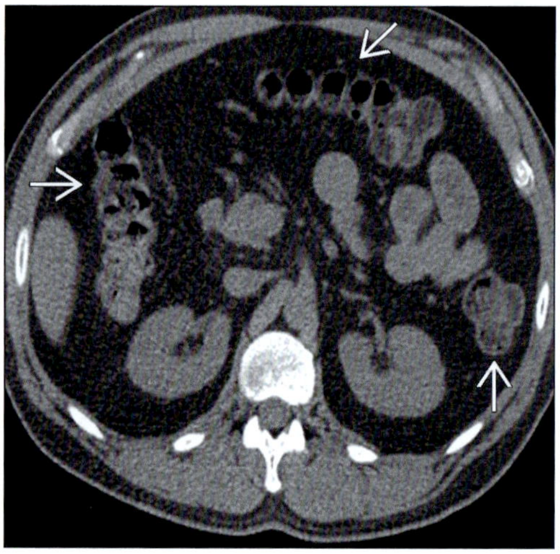

Axial CT demonstrates normal-appearing colon and loops of the small bowel ➔.

CLINICAL SCENARIO

History
- 42-year-old man with recurrent Hodgkin lymphoma and diabetes mellitus type II

IMAGE INTERPRETATION

Pitfalls
- Increased radiotracer activity within bowel may be mistakenly interpreted as malignancy or inflammation/infection
- On the other hand, increased uptake secondary to malignancy may be mistakenly attributed to metformin

Actual Diagnosis
- Bowel uptake secondary to metformin

Clues to Correct Diagnosis
- Primary clue is patient's medication history
- Attention should also be paid to start and duration of metformin therapy in comparing PET/CT exams
- If underlying concern for bowel malignancy or metastasis, stopping metformin 2 days prior to examination can decrease uptake within bowel

BACKGROUND

General
- Metformin is considered first-line oral therapy in treatment of type II diabetes mellitus

Relevant Anatomy
- Attention to distribution of bowel uptake and background level of uptake in surrounding bowel should be paid

Relevant Physiology
- Metformin causes increased FDG uptake in intestine through reduced glucose absorption and increased glucose utilization in small intestine

IMAGING FEATURES

CT
- Comparison of bowel wall morphology helps differentiate normal uptake due to metformin vs. uptake secondary to inflammation or malignancy

PET/CT
- Bowel uptake related to metformin will generally follow pattern
  - Large bowel > small bowel > duodenum (with little uptake in duodenum attributed to metformin)
    - Generally, uptake in cecum and right colon is higher because of abundant lymphocytes, which have increased glucose uptake regardless of metformin use
- Additional distribution of uptake can be beneficial in identifying etiology: Diffuse, segmental, or focal
  - Diffuse uptake is more suggestive of metformin-related uptake vs. underlying diffuse inflammation
  - Segmental uptake can be seen with underlying inflammation
  - Focal FDG uptake in bowel can be due to benign, cancerous or precancerous lesions including hyperplastic polyps or hemorrhoids, which may not be well evaluated on corresponding noncontrast images

RELATED REFERENCES

1. Yılmaz S et al: Metformin-Induced Intense Bowel Uptake Observed on Restaging FDG PET/CT Study in a Patient with Gastric Lymphoma. Mol Imaging Radionucl Ther. 20(3):114-6, 2011
2. Oh JR et al: Impact of medication discontinuation on increased intestinal FDG accumulation in diabetic patients treated with metformin. AJR Am J Roentgenol. 195(6):1404-10, 2010
3. Gontier E et al: High and typical 18F-FDG bowel uptake in patients treated with metformin. Eur J Nucl Med Mol Imaging. 35(1):95-9, 2008

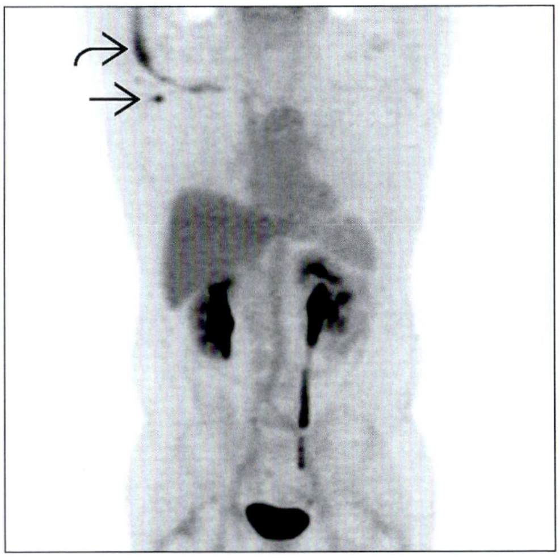

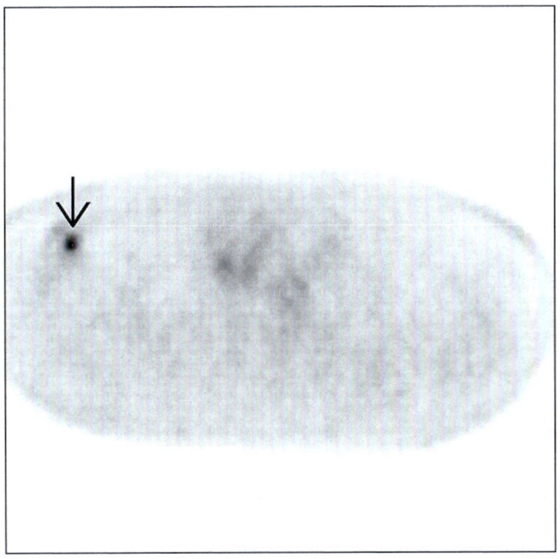

(Left) *MIP image in a 51-year-old man with squamous cell carcinoma of the tongue base demonstrates linear radiotracer activity along the right upper extremity and subclavian veins ↪. A focus of increased radiotracer uptake in the right axilla corresponds to a subcentimeter lymph node →. A portion of the dose infiltrated at the right antecubital fossa injection site.* ***(Right)*** *Axial PET in the same patient demonstrates a focus → of increased radiotracer uptake in the right axilla.*

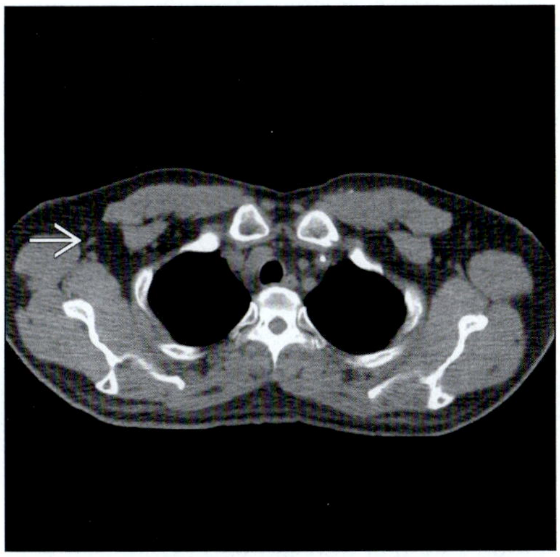

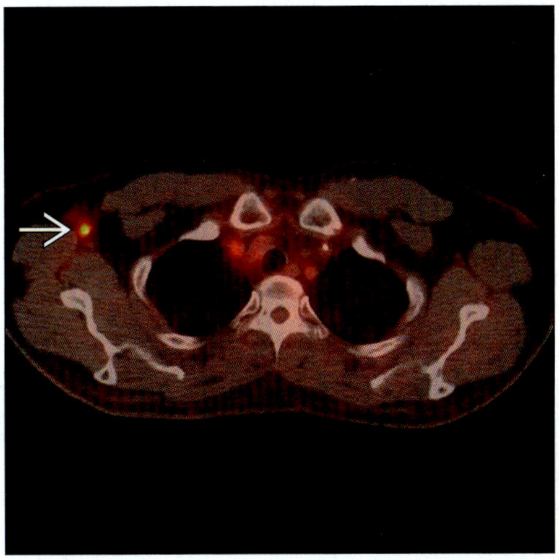

(Left) *The focus of increased radiotracer uptake in the right axilla corresponds to a subcentimeter lymph node →. This is a benign finding due to lymphatic drainage from the dose infiltration.* ***(Right)*** *Axial fused PET/CT in the same patient demonstrates a focus of increased radiotracer uptake in the right axilla corresponding to a subcentimeter lymph node →. This is a benign finding due to lymphatic drainage from the dose infiltration.*

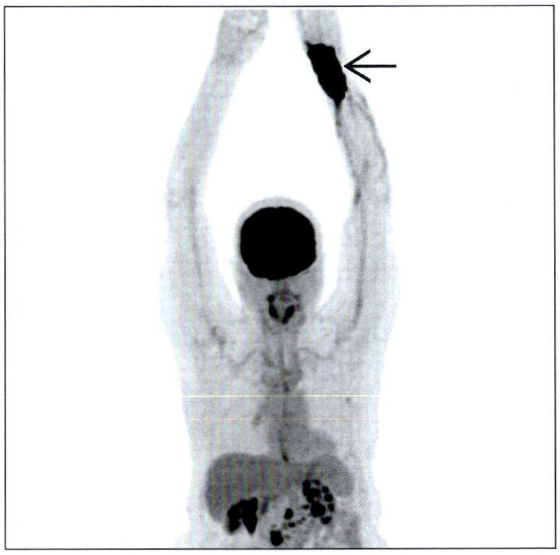

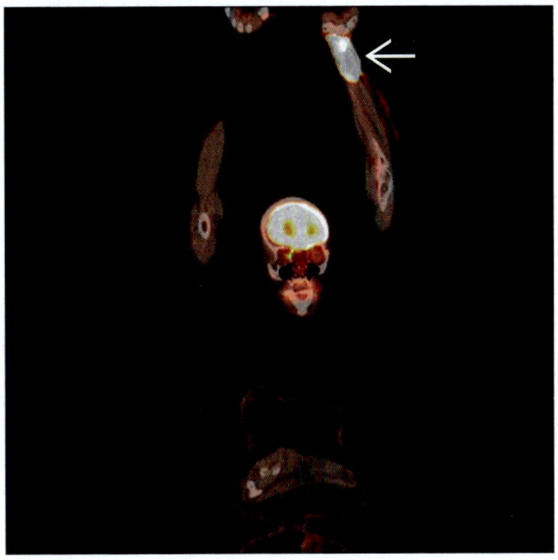

(Left) *MIP image in a 69-year-old woman with metastatic ovarian cancer demonstrates intense radiotracer activity at a radiotracer infiltration site in the left wrist →.* ***(Right)*** *Coronal fused PET/CT in the same patient demonstrates intense radiotracer activity at a radiotracer infiltration site in the left wrist →.*

POSTOPERATIVE UPTAKE AFTER TRANSURETHRAL PROSTATE RESECTION

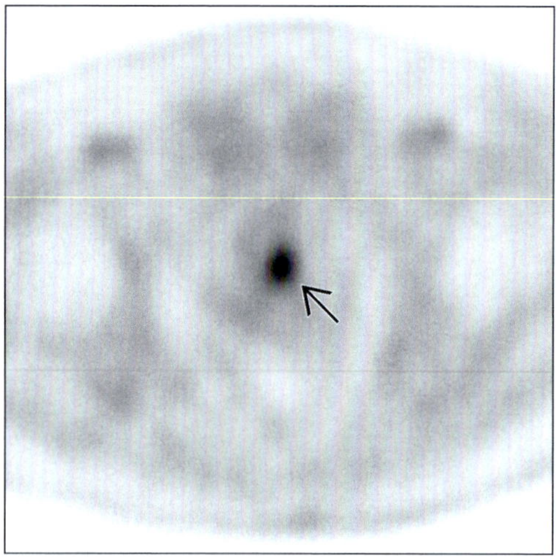

Axial PET demonstrates increased radiotracer activity ➔ in the pelvis.

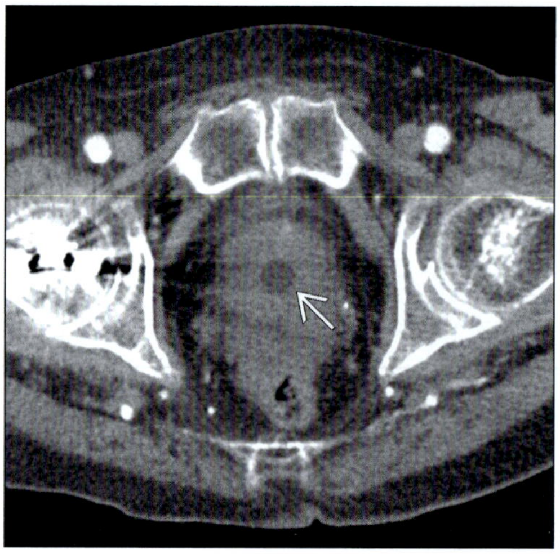

Axial CECT demonstrates a surgical defect ➔ from prior transurethral resection of prostate (TURP).

CLINICAL SCENARIO

History

- 44-year-old man with enlarged prostate gland due to benign prostatic hyperplasia

IMAGE INTERPRETATION

Pitfalls

- Uptake in prostatic defect after transurethral resection of prostate (TURP) can be mistaken for malignancy or inflammation

Actual Diagnosis

- Postoperative uptake after transurethral robotic-assisted prostatectomy

Clues to Correct Diagnosis

- Surgical and recent prostatic biopsy history
- Cylindrical focus of uptake surrounding prostatic urethra corresponding to defect in this region on CT
  - Tumor is generally round (or spherical) in shape
- Correlation with prostatic specific antigen is imperative in evaluating for primary or recurrent prostatic cancer

BACKGROUND

Epidemiology

- Benign prostatic hyperplasia is most common cause of lower urinary tract symptoms in elderly men

Relevant Anatomy

- 3 prostate zones: Central, transitional, and peripheral
  - Proximal prostatic urethra is surrounded by transitional zone and distal prostatic urethra is surrounded by peripheral zone
- TURP can be performed for persistent symptomatic benign prostatic hyperplasia
  - Typical procedure: Insert a resectoscope to remove urethral tissue surrounding prostatic urethra and bladder neck (including internal sphincter)
    - Once internal sphincter has been removed, continence is maintained by external sphincter within membranous urethra
    - Resulting defect is filled with urine on imaging

Relevant Physiology

- FDG-18 radiotracer demonstrates mild diffuse physiologic uptake in prostate and significant bladder uptake related to radiotracer excretion in genitourinary tract, limiting its evaluation in diagnosing and staging prostate cancer
- TURP defect will fill with contrast or any radiotracer excreted via genitourinary system

IMAGING FEATURES

CT

- Cylindrical, hypoattenuating defect in prostate gland, which will fill with contrast on delayed phase
- On single axial slice, defect may appear rounded
  - Persists on multiple axial slices and appears as a "U" shape extending from bladder on sagittal reconstruction image

PET/CT

- Cylindrical radiotracer uptake within prostate gland with additional visualization of U-shaped extension of adjacent bladder wall on sagittal images
- Usually TURP defect is central within prostate, whereas tumor is more peripheral in location
- SUV is unreliable in differentiating malignant and benign uptake

RELATED REFERENCES

1. Panebianco V et al: Advanced imaging for the early diagnosis of local recurrence prostate cancer after radical prostatectomy. Biomed Res Int. 2014:827265, 2014
2. Min DS et al: Effect of transurethral resection of the prostate based on the degree of obstruction seen in urodynamic study. Korean J Urol. 54(12):840-5, 2013

POSTOPERATIVE UPTAKE AFTER TRANSURETHRAL PROSTATE RESECTION

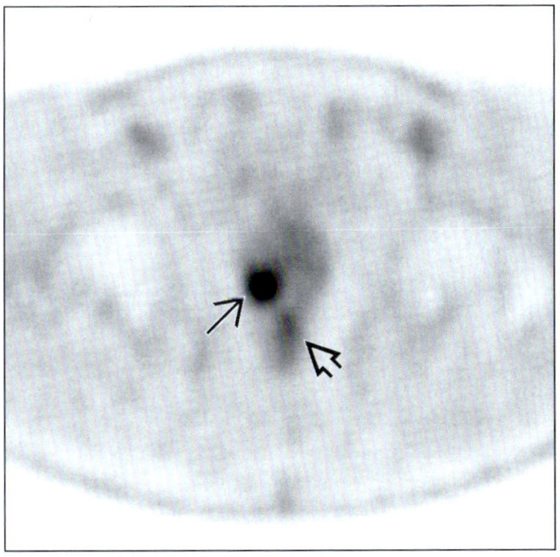

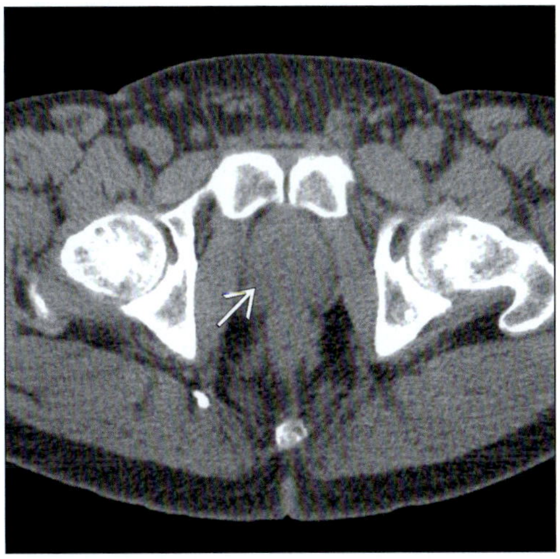

(Left) *Axial PET in a 68-year-old man with gastrointestinal stromal tumor demonstrates an incidental focus of increased FDG activity ➔ (SUVmax: 7.2) at the prostate gland on the right. Activity in the rectum ➔ is physiologic.* ***(Right)*** *Axial NECT demonstrates no definite CT abnormality in the peripheral zone of the prostate gland on the right ➔.*

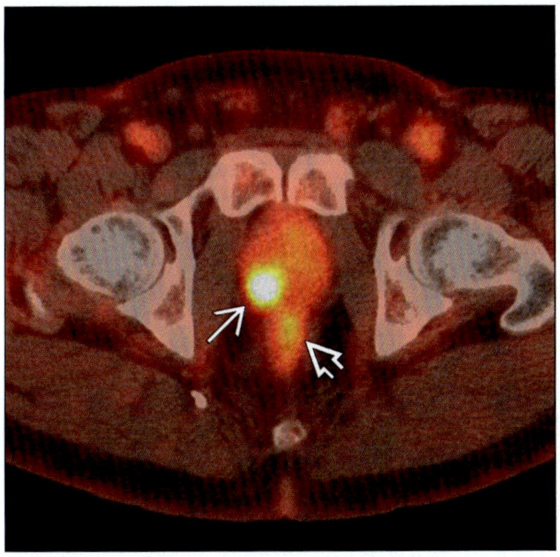

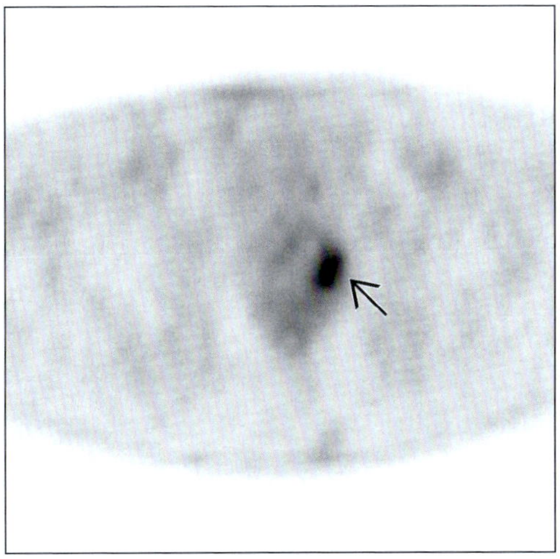

(Left) *Axial fused PET/CT in the same case demonstrates an incidental focus of increased FDG activity ➔ at the peripheral zone of the prostate gland on the right. Ultrasound-guided biopsy of the lesion was consistent with prostate adenocarcinoma. Activity in the rectum ➔ is physiologic.* ***(Right)*** *Axial PET in a 59-year-old man with a squamous cell carcinoma demonstrates a focus of increased radiotracer uptake ➔ at the periphery of the left prostate gland (SUVmax: 5.5).*

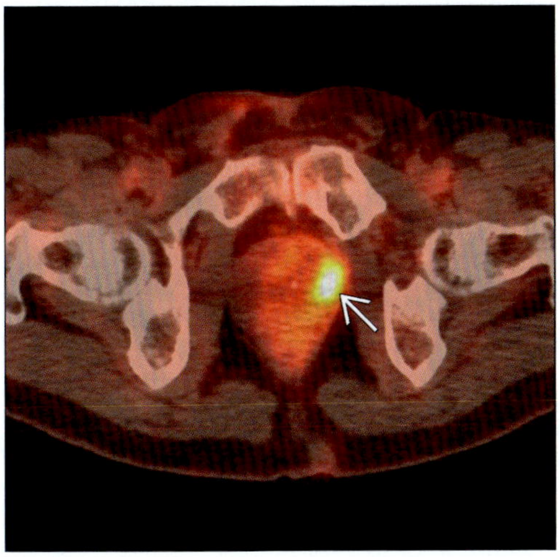

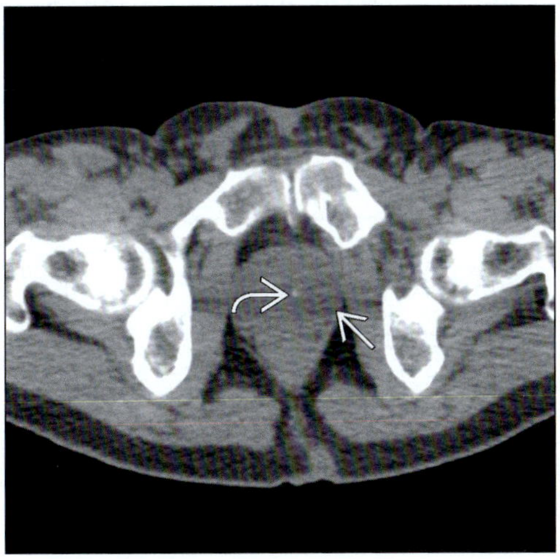

(Left) *Axial fused PET/CT in the same patient demonstrates a focus of increased radiotracer uptake at the periphery of the left aspect of the prostate gland ➔.* ***(Right)*** *Axial NECT in the same patient shows a vague area of low attenuation corresponding to the focus of increased radiotracer uptake at the periphery of the left aspect of the prostate gland ➔. Biopsy of this lesion revealed prostatitis. A tiny calcification ➔ is also noted.*

BOWEL UPTAKE SECONDARY TO DIVERTICULITIS

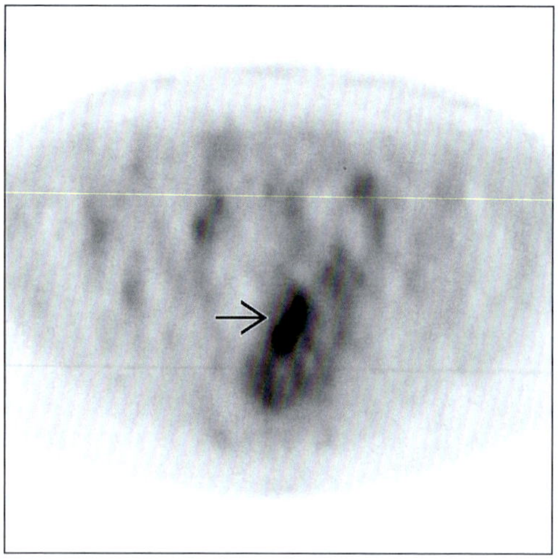

Axial PET demonstrates ↑ radiotracer activity (SUVmax: 12.8) ⇒ in sigmoid colon corresponding to an area of wall thickening, diverticulosis, and stranding of pericolonic fat on CT.

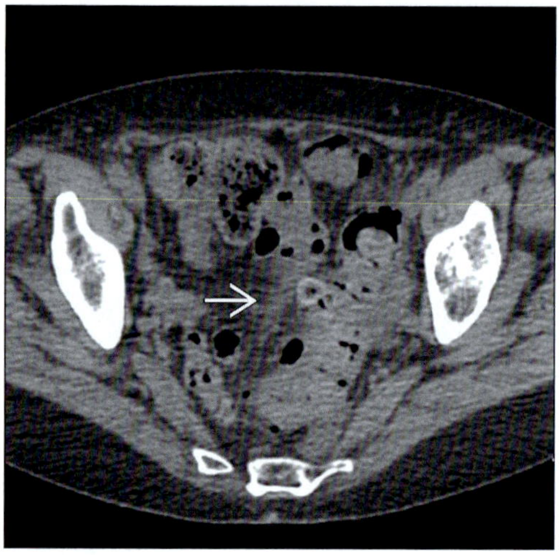

Axial CT demonstrates an area of bowel wall thickening, diverticulosis, and stranding of the pericolonic fat ⇒, compatible with diverticulitis.

CLINICAL SCENARIO

History

- 70-year-old woman with multiple myeloma

IMAGE INTERPRETATION

Pitfalls

- Focal uptake in or adjacent to bowel can be mistaken for malignancy, particularly in setting of known gastrointestinal tract malignancy
- Diverticulitis can lead to stenosis, which can be even more difficult to differentiate from malignancy

Actual Diagnosis

- Bowel uptake secondary to diverticulitis

Clues to Correct Diagnosis

- Underlying malignancy/indication for PET/CT and knowledge of where metastases generally occur
- Inflammatory change without underlying diverticular disease suggests unrelated inflammation in proper clinical setting, but may be difficult to distinguish from an incidental primary lesion based upon single study
- Correlation with sigmoidoscopy/colonoscopy and biopsy if performed
- Follow-up imaging may be necessary to monitor for resolution or interval growth in case of malignancy

BACKGROUND

Epidemiology

- 8.1-9.6% rate of diverticulitis in setting of underlying diverticulosis
- Patients with diverticulosis can develop colon cancer with propensity to involve same site

Relevant Anatomy

- Diverticula are "false diverticular" without muscular propria layer
- More commonly involve left hemicolon, specifically sigmoid colon
- Inflammation spreads into pericolonic fat

Relevant Physiology

- FDG uptake is present in any metabolically active process including inflammation or infection

IMAGING FEATURES

CT

- Wall thickening in setting of underlying colonic diverticula with adjacent mesenteric fat stranding and fluid
- Complications of diverticulitis include microperforation with abscess or stenosis

PET/CT

- Focal increased FDG uptake, particularly in left colon, and associated surrounding pericolonic inflammatory changes
- No definite SUV cutoff value for inflammation vs. malignancy
  - At times, further evaluation with colonoscopy and biopsy or follow-up imaging may be required to exclude synchronous malignancy

RELATED REFERENCES

1. Nishiyama N et al: Difficulty in differentiating two cases of sigmoid stenosis by diverticulitis from cancer. World J Gastroenterol. 18(27):3623-6, 2012
2. Metser U et al: Increased (18)F-fluorodeoxyglucose uptake in benign, nonphysiologic lesions found on whole-body positron emission tomography/computed tomography (PET/CT): accumulated data from four years of experience with PET/CT. Semin Nucl Med. 37(3):206-22, 2007
3. Kamel EM et al: Significance of incidental 18F-FDG accumulations in the gastrointestinal tract in PET/CT: correlation with endoscopic and histopathologic results. J Nucl Med. 45(11):1804-10, 2004

FDG UPTAKE IN SCLEROSING MESENTERITIS

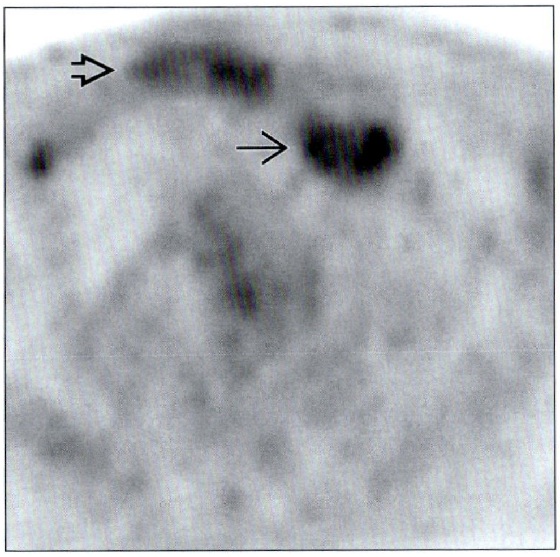

Axial PET shows ↑ radiotracer uptake (SUVmax: 4.2) ➙. Note the linear area of ↑ activity in the anterior abdominal wall ➯ at the site of a prior mesh repair.

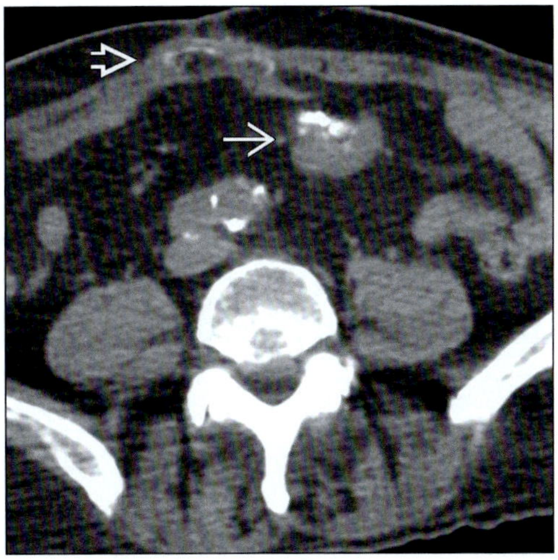

Axial NECT shows a soft tissue mass with coarse calcifications in mesentery ➙, representing biopsy-proven sclerosing mesenteritis. Prior anterior abdominal wall mesh repair ➯ is noted.

CLINICAL SCENARIO

History

- 80-year-old man with esophageal cancer

IMAGE INTERPRETATION

Pitfalls

- Increased uptake within soft tissue masses in mesentery may be mistaken for malignancy
- Even in PET/CT, variety of appearances with respect to degree of FDG uptake can be seen
- Malignancy or other inflammatory diseases can coexist with sclerosing mesenteritis

Actual Diagnosis

- FDG uptake in sclerosing mesenteritis

Clues to Correct Diagnosis

- Correlation with symptoms, laboratory markers, imaging findings over time, and degree of FDG uptake to differentiate benign sclerosing mesenteritis ± coexisting malignancy
- Patient's underlying primary malignancy history and related treatment, if known
- Definitive diagnosis may include laparotomy/biopsy

BACKGROUND

Epidemiology

- Prevalence based on CT scans: 0.6%
- Peak incidence: 6th-7th decades
- 69% linked to malignancy, particularly lymphoma
- Also associated with pancreatitis, infection, trauma, and surgery

Relevant Anatomy

- Generally involves small bowel mesentery, similar location to lymphoma

Relevant Physiology

- Fat necrosis and acute inflammation are predominant histological changes in sclerosing mesenteritis resulting in macrophage response
- Macrophages take up FDG-18 in inflammation, resulting in positive uptake on PET/CT

General

- Sclerosing mesenteritis is a benign process of unknown etiology affecting small bowel mesentery

IMAGING FEATURES

CT

- Increased soft tissue within mesenteric fat representing enlarged lymph nodes with similar appearances in underlying malignancies such as lymphoma or gastrointestinal stromal tumor
- Alternatively may present as thickening of small bowel mesentery
- Fat ring sign of hypoattenuating fatty halo surrounding soft tissue mass may distinguish mesenteritis from malignancy

PET/CT

- Varying degree of uptake within soft tissue masses in abdominal mesentery
- Lack of FDG uptake strongly suggests against tumor involvement

RELATED REFERENCES

1. Metser U et al: Increased (18)F-fluorodeoxyglucose uptake in benign, nonphysiologic lesions found on whole-body positron emission tomography/computed tomography (PET/CT): accumulated data from four years of experience with PET/CT. Semin Nucl Med. 37(3):206-22, 2007
2. Zissin R et al: Mesenteric panniculitis in oncologic patients: PET-CT findings. Br J Radiol. 79(937):37-43, 2006
3. Daskalogiannaki M et al: CT evaluation of mesenteric panniculitis: prevalence and associated diseases. AJR Am J Roentgenol. 174(2):427-31, 2000

HYPERATTENUATING CRESCENT SIGN

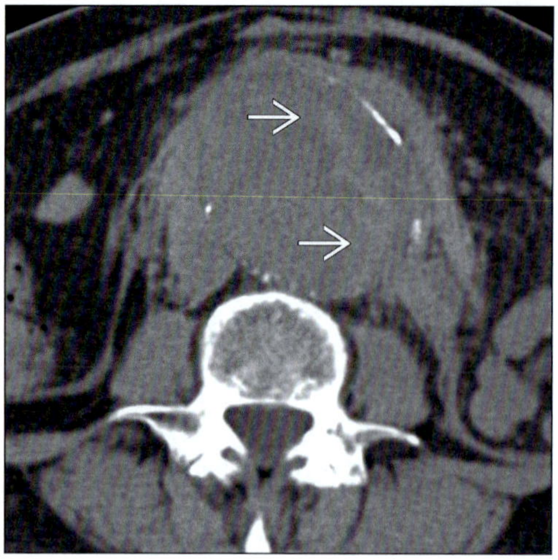

Axial NECT shows a crescent of high attenuation ➔ paralleling the left lateral wall of an abdominal aortic aneurysm.

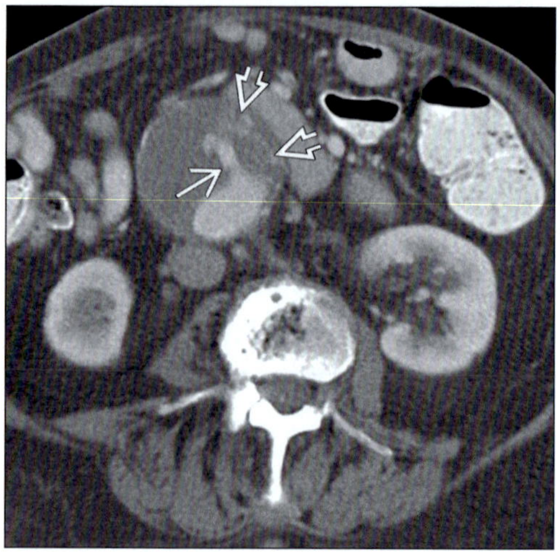

Axial CECT shows rupture of the mural thrombus with extension of contrast through a channel ➔ into the thrombus and contrast accumulation ➔ parallel to the aortic wall.

IMAGING FEATURES

Appearance

- Describes crescent-shaped area of increased attenuation within aortic wall or mural thrombus of abdominal aortic aneurysm (AAA)
  - Best demonstrated on nonenhanced CT images and is of higher attenuation than intraluminal aortic blood
  - On CECT, hyperattenuating crescent is of higher attenuation compared with adjacent psoas muscle

Clinical Significance

- One of the earliest and most specific imaging manifestations of acute or impending rupture of abdominal aortic aneurysm
  - Recognizing this sign can be lifesaving
- Sensitivity and specificity of hyperattenuating crescent sign to detect AAA rupture are 77% and 93%, respectively

Other Imaging Findings Predicting AAA Rupture

- Aneurysm rupture risk increases with size
  - 4 cm aneurysm: Risk of rupture is ~ 2% per year
  - 5-6 cm aneurysm: 3-15% per year
  - 6-7 cm aneurysms: 10-20% per year
  - 7-8 cm aneurysms: 20-40% per year
  - For those with diameter > 8 cm: 30-50% per year
- Increasing aneurysm size
  - Average expansion rate of 4 mm per year
  - With every 5 mm increase in diameter, there is doubling of rupture risk
  - Enlargement rate ≥ 10 mm per year is used as indication for surgical repair
- Focal discontinuity of aortic wall calcification
  - Most helpful when finding is new in comparison to previous studies
- Periaortic fat stranding
  - Frequently observed in impending rupture and may be earliest sign before complete AAA rupture
- Thrombus:lumen ratio
  - Decreases with increasing aneurysm size
  - ↓ volume of thrombus within aneurysm and enlargement of patent lumen is indicative of partial lysis of thrombus, which predisposes aneurysm to rupture

BACKGROUND

Explanation

- Hyperattenuating crescent sign represents blood penetrating through mural thrombus within AAA
- Then, blood extends around thrombus and is limited by aortic wall
- Finally, blood penetrates aortic wall and damages its muscle fibers → complete rupture

Epidemiology

- Rupture of AAA is a life-threatening complication
  - Mortality rates have been estimated to be 70–94%
  - Up to 62% of patients with a ruptured AAA will die before reaching emergency department
- Emergent surgical repair of a ruptured AAA has approximate mortality rate of 50%
- Elective repair of unruptured aneurysm has a mortality rate of 4%

RELATED REFERENCES

1. Vu KN et al: Rupture signs on computed tomography, treatment, and outcome of abdominal aortic aneurysms. Insights Imaging. 5(3):281-93, 2014
2. Rakita D et al: Spectrum of CT findings in rupture and impending rupture of abdominal aortic aneurysms. Radiographics. 27(2):497-507, 2007
3. Pillari GP: Crescent sign origin and the thrombus-to-lumen ratio in abdominal aortic aneurysm. Radiology. 214(2):604, 2000
4. Gonsalves CF: The hyperattenuating crescent sign. Radiology. 211(1):37-8, 1999

E

F

G

H

I

J

K

L

M

N

O

P

R

S

T

U

V

W

X